OXFORD MEDICAL PUBLICATIONS

Benzodiazepine Dependence

Benzodiazepine Dependence

Edited by

COSMO HALLSTRÖM

Department of Psychiatry
Charing Cross Hospital
London, UK

Oxford   New York   Tokyo
OXFORD UNIVERSITY PRESS
1993

Oxford University Press, Walton Street, Oxford OX2 6DP
Oxford   New York   Toronto
Delhi   Bombay   Calcutta   Madras   Karachi
Kuala Lumpur   Singapore   Hong Kong   Tokyo
Nairobi   Dar es Salaam   Cape Town
Melbourne   Auckland   Madrid
and associated companies in
Berlin   Ibadan

Oxford is a trade mark of Oxford University Press

Published in the United States
by Oxford University Press Inc., New York.

© Oxford University Press, 1993

A catalogue record for this book is available from the British Library

Library of Congress Cataloging in Publication Data
Benzodiazepine dependence / edited by Cosmo Hallström.
(Oxford medical publications)
Includes bibliographical references and index.
1. Benzodiazepine abuse.   2. Benzodiazepines—Physiological
effect   I. Hallström, Cosmo.   II. Series.
[DNLM: 1. Benzodiazepine Tranquillizers.   2. Substance Dependence.
QV 77.9 B4790158 1993]
RC568.B45B44   1993   616.86—dc20   93–20040
ISBN 0–19–262094–0 (H'bk)

Typeset by The Electronic Book Factory, Fife, Scotland
Printed in Great Britain by
Bookcraft Ltd, Midsomer Norton, Avon

Foreword

Professor Malcolm Lader

Tranquillity is a state of mind that has been sought by human beings for millennia. Starting with alcohol, cannabis, and opium, we have progressed to numerous synthetic products of the pharmaceutical industry, culminating in this century with the extensive use of, first, the barbiturates and, then, the benzodiazepines. Each new introduction was hailed as the panacea for all psychological ills; then later, as its drawbacks became increasingly evident, the pendulum swung just as far the other way and the tranquillizer was condemned as a poison. Finally, it became apparent that many of these compounds were useful in some types of patients but perhaps only in the short term.

The time has come to assess the latest in this apparently inexhaustible series of tranquillizers, namely, the benzodiazepines. Among the most successful drugs ever introduced, they still dominate the tranquillizer market. However, they are perceived to have major problems: they produce dose-related subjective sedation and psychomotor, cognitive, and memory impairment; paradoxical release of anxiety, anger, or hostility is not uncommon; rebound and withdrawal syndromes may attend discontinuation even after therapeutic dosage; abuse, either alone or in a polydrug context, is becoming increasingly common. The last two adverse effects have occasioned the greatest concern over the past decade.

This concern is not confined to the specialist pharmacologist or psychiatrist or even to the medical profession at large. The general public are acutely aware of the problems, which is not surprising in view of the fact that one in five women and one in 10 men have used these tranquillizers at some time. The media have been extensively involved and, more recently, the legal profession have mounted what may well be the largest personal injury case in legal history with thousands of claims launched by users of tranquillizers.

The concern also varies from country to country. In the UK, the drug regulatory authorities have issued warnings about long-term prescription. In the USA attempts to limit usage have been made, for example, in New York State. But in many other countries a *laissez-faire* attitude on the part of prescriber, patient, and public still prevails.

It is therefore most timely that a detailed account should be available of all these issues relating to the benzodiazepine tranquillizers. A most distinguished group of experts has been assembled by Dr Cosmo Hallström to provide chapters on each and every aspect of this topic. I am greatly honoured to have been invited to write this foreword to a book which is sure to become the standard reference source.

Contents

9 Oral and intravenous abuse of benzodiazepines   128

John Strang, Nicholas Seivewright, and Michael Farrell

**10 The assessment of anxiety and benzodiazepine
dependence**   143

John Pecknold

**11 The epidemiology of neurosis and benzodiazepine
use and abuse**   162

Hans-Ulrich Wittchen and Cecilia Ahmoi Essau

14 Pharmacological differences in the dependence
   potential of benzodiazepines   221
   Peter Tyrer

15 Benzodiazepine use and dependency in the elderly:
   striking a balance   238
   Raymond J. Ancill and William W. Carlyle

**19 Psychological treatments for benzodiazepine
dependence**   296

Susan Golombok and Anna Higgitt

**20 Pharmacological treatments for benzodiazepine
dependence**   310

Peter P. Roy-Byrne and James C. Ballenger

Contributors

Raymond J. Ancill, Division of Geriatric Psychiatry, 749 West 33rd Avenue, Vancouver, British Columbia V5Z 2K4, Canada.

James C. Ballenger, Department of Psychiatry, Institute of Psychiatry, Medical University of South Carolina, Charleston, South Carolina, USA.

Alyson Bond, Institute of Psychiatry, De Crespigny Park, London SE5 8AF, UK.

Stefan Borg, Karolinska Institute, Department of Psychiatry, Box 12500, S-11281 Stockholm, Sweden.

Sten Carlsson, Karolinska Institute, Department of Psychiatry, Box 12500, S-11281 Stockholm, Sweden.

William W. Carlyle, Division of Geriatric Psychiatry, 749 West 33rd Avenue, Vancouver, BC V5Z 2K4, Canada.

Anthony Clift, 133 Manchester Old Road, Middleton, Manchester M24 4DZ, UK.

Cecilia Ahmoi Essau, Max Planck Institute of Psychiatry, Clinical Institute (Clinical Psychology), Kraepelinstrasse 2–10, 8000 Munich 40, Germany.

Michael Farrell, Drug Unit, National Addiction Centre, The Maudsley, Denmark Hill, London SE5 8AZ, UK.

Sandra E. File, Psychopharmacology Research Unit, UMDS Division of Pharmacology, University of London, Guy's Hospital, London SE1 9RT, UK.

Peter Fonagy, Psychoanalysis Unit, c/o Department of Psychology, University College London, Gower Street, London WC1E 6BT, UK.

Jonathan Gabe, Sociology Division, Legal, Political, and Social Sciences, South Bank University, 103 Borough Road, London SE1 0AA, UK.

Paul Glue, Clinical Pharmacology, Schering Plough Research Unit, 2015 Galloping Hill Road, Kenilworth, NJ 07033, USA.

Susan Golombok, Clinical and Health Psychology Research Centre, City University, Northampton Square, London EC1V 0HB, UK.

Ann Hackmann, Department of Psychiatry, Warneford Hospital, Oxford OX3 7JX, UK.

Cosmo Hallström, Department of Psychiatry, Charing Cross Hospital, London W6 BRF, UK.

Moira Hamlin, Department of Psychology, UBHT NHS Trust, Bristol BS19 3SG, UK.

Anna Higgitt, St Charles's Hospital, Exmoor Street, London W10 6DZ, UK.

Malcolm Lader, Institute of Psychiatry, De Crespigny Park, London SE5 8AF, UK.

Pierre Lafolie, Department of Clinical Pharmacology, Karolinska Hospital, Box 60500, S-10401 Stockholm, Sweden.

David Nutt, Psychopharmacology Unit, University of Bristol School of Medical Sciences, University Walk, Bristol BS8 1TD, UK.

John Pecknold, Community Psychiatry Centre, Douglas Hospital, Verdun, Quebec H4H IR3, Canada.

Hannes Pétursson, Department of Psychiatry, Borgarspítalinn, IS108 Reykavík, Iceland.

Karl Rickels, Psychopharmacology Research and Treatment Unit, Science Center, 3600 Market Street, Philadelphia, Pennsylvania 19104, USA.

Peter P. Roy-Byrne, Harborview Medical Center ZA-15, 325 Ninth Avenue, Seattle, Washington 98104, USA.

Carl Salzman, Department of Psychiatry, Harvard Medical School and Massachusetts Mental Health Center, 74 Fenwood Road, Boston, Massachusetts 02115, USA.

Edward Schweizer, Psychopharmacology Research and Treatment Unit, Science Center, 3600 Market Street, Philadelphia, Pennsylvania 19104, USA.

Nicholas Seivewright, Department of Psychiatry, University of Manchester, Rawnsley Building, Manchester Royal Infirmary, Oxford Road, Manchester M13 9WL, UK.

Richard J. Simpson, Forth Valley GP Research Group, Department of Psychology, University of Stirling, Stirling FK9 4LA, Scotland.

John Strang, Addiction Research Unit, National Addiction Centre, The Maudsley/Institute of Psychiatry, Denmark Hill, London SE5 8AF, UK.

Mark Tattersall, The Gordon Hospital, Bloomburg Street, London SW1V 2RH, UK.

Peter Tyrer, Academic Unit of Psychiatry (St Mary's Hospital Medical School), St Charles's Hospital, Exmoor Street, London W10 6DZ, UK.

Eric Watsky, Department of Psychiatry, Harvard Medical School and Massachusetts Mental Health Center, 74 Fenwood Road, Boston, Massachusetts 02115, USA.

Frank Wells, Association of the British Pharmaceutical Industry, 12 Whitehall, London SW1A 2DY, UK.

Susan Wilson, Department of Medicine, Science and Technology, Psycho-pharmacology Unit, University of Bristol School of Medical Sciences, University Walk, Bristol BS8 1TD, UK.

Hans-Ulrich Wittchen, Department of Evaluation Research, Max Planck Institute of Psychiatry, Kraepelinstrasse 10, 8000 Munich 40, Germany.

1 Why people take benzodiazepines

Moira Hamlin

Benzodiazepines are one of the most controversial group of psychotropic drugs currently in use. Their introduction as a safe effective alternative to barbiturates in the 1960s was generally welcomed with a subsequent meteoric rise in prescriptions. In 1980 it was estimated that one billion doses per day were taken worldwide. As problems of dependence and withdrawal emerged considerable attention was focused on these important issues, but the fundamental question of *why* people take benzodiazepines is relatively unexplored.

Looking at reasons why people take benzodiazepines can be likened to peeling an onion. Simple starting points from the trite, 'because they were prescribed' or 'to relieve symptoms of anxiety', give way to more complex issues of the medicalization of personal problems and individual/organizational power and control within Western society. Benzodiazepine use must be viewed within a context—it is not something separate from the rest of a person's life. It should be acknowledged that we live within a culture which seeks 'instant cures' and 'a pill for every ill' and this forms a backdrop to drug-taking behaviour that is influenced by many interacting psychosocial and medical factors.

Presenting problems

Benzodiazepines have generally been prescribed for minor affective problems. As many as 30 per cent of patients seen in general practice present with problems that are primarily emotional in origin. A study carried out for the television programme '*That's life*' (Lacey and Woodward 1985) found that work stress, headaches, loneliness, postnatal depression, bereavement, and relationship difficulties were cited as reasons for initial prescriptions. A proportion of patients have also received benzodiazepine prescriptions for physical complaints, notably back pain, hypertension, cardiovascular disease, arthritis, and premenstrual symptoms. A substantial number of people, about one-fifth of long-term users, were first prescribed benzodiazepines following a bereavement.

Anxiety or sleep disorders have featured largely in medical diagnoses of presenting problems. A related difficulty with assigning such broad general categories has been to use benzodiazepines as a 'blunderbuss' remedy to encompass a wide range of psychological problems and life stresses. Partly this has arisen from confusion about the nature of 'anxiety' itself within a medical framework. It should also be remembered that benzodiazepines, in any case, are only a symptomatic treatment and any underlying psychological problems remain. Tyrer *et al*. (1985) described these drugs as 'a dam acting merely to stem the flow of anxiety'.

In many cases psychological problems exist prior to a benzodiazepine prescription and continue despite the use of such medication. A very high proportion of long-term users continue to regularly consult their general practitioner for psychological problems. In a study by Catalan *et al*. 1984, where patients received either a benzodiazepine prescription or brief counselling from the general practitioner, both methods achieved the same results. However, one-third of patients were not helped by either method suggesting that there is a group of people who present with more severe psychological problems.

Why do doctors prescribe benzodiazepines?

The relatively few studies that have attempted to answer the question of why doctors prescribe benzodiazepines have been unsuccessful in explaining more than a small proportion of variance between doctors. An interesting early study using a postal questionnaire to assess general practitioners' attitudes was carried out by Linn (1971). This revealed that doctors with a working-class background were more likely to be in favour of prescribing benzodiazepines. Doctors working in isolation or in single-handed practices also have the highest rates of benzodiazepine prescribing. It is easy to understand why a full waiting room and a large list lead to feelings of time pressure and benzodiazepine prescriptions as an 'easy option'.

There is no doubt that doctors came under pressure from extensive promotion of benzodiazepines by the drug industry, particularly in the 1960s and 1970s. Despite the fact that there were few differences between the benzodiazepines, compounds were marketed on the basis of differentiation. With so many similar products, the manufacturers felt they needed to promote them on a grand scale, so that doctors could tell them apart. Medawar (1992) cites the example of Roche in 1970, who spent 44 per cent of their promotion budget on sales representatives, who were making over 1000 visits a week to doctors; 16 per cent of the budget went on 500 whole-page advertisements in 25 different medical journals and 97 separate promotional mailings were carried out for Librium and Valium. In response to these differing claims for benzodiazepines, doctors were encouraged to look for clinical symptoms that fitted in with the marketing profile of the drugs. A former senior writer in a drug firm (Hemminki 1975) stated, 'As an advertising man I can assure you that advertising which does not work does not continue to run. If experience did not show beyond doubt that the great majority of doctors are splendidly responsive to current ethical advertising, new techniques would be devised in short order.'

The role of the doctor has also changed in line with general changes in society. He or she is increasingly turned to for counselling and advice on emotional and social problems as much as for physical disease. Although doctors increasingly receive more training in such areas, few would claim to be sufficiently equipped to cope with the volume and range of demands for psychosocial interventions. Yet they are continually faced with patients who are obviously distressed and asking for help. Pressure to prescribe benzo-diazepines also comes from patients themselves. It is therefore important to appreciate the external influences impinging on doctors to prescribe and their internal responses, which reflect their desire to alleviate distress. Benson (1988) makes a similar point, 'Undoubtedly irresistible compassion is behind most benzodiazepine dependence. The feeling that some help must be given, however imperfect, is deeply ingrained and hard to resist.'

Many studies have looked at the symbolic function of the prescribing pad and its use has been found to be a routine behaviour for general practitioners. More attention should be paid to these factors and the prescription pad should not be used as a means of opting out of a discussion of the patient's emotional and social problems. It is also true that, where doctors hold more negative attitudes towards the use of drugs for social problems and everyday stress, fewer benzodiazepines are prescribed. Sometimes, even with a will to reduce prescribing, it is difficult. The drugs may have been initially prescribed from another source, a different practice, or on hospital discharge. In general practice partners, trainees, and locums may also see the same patient.

Women are prescribed twice as many benzodiazepines as men, and women perceived by doctors as having two or more social problems are likely to receive longer treatment. As the length of treatment increases, the probability of stopping medication decreases. It has also been noted that benzodiazepines tend to be prescribed more frequently to older people and, on a long-term basis, to members of lower socio-economic groups.

Interestingly, it is evident that many doctors do now offer alternatives to benzodiazepines, such as counselling and support, or recommend relaxation techniques such as yoga. Concern about these drugs does feature in medical training, and younger general practitioners, in particular, have become more aware of the problems.

Prior to increased public awareness about benzodiazepines, a sizeable proportion of people were unaware that they were taking these drugs. In the BBC television *'That's Life'* survey, 50 per cent of people claimed they did not know they were taking benzodiazepines. Reasons for initial prescriptions were also not always known, but evidence from numerous studies indicates that benzodiazepines are prescribed for a wide variety of symptoms and disorders. In the early days of benzodiazepines their scope was apparently vast: 'whatever the diagnosis' claimed the advertisements for Librium on the assumption that anxiety was present in any disorder. Up to one-third of long-term users were initially prescribed benzodiazepines following a bereavement and repeat prescriptions were continued, often for many years. It is now acknowledged that benzodiazepines can interfere with the normal process of mourning. Adjustment may be severely inhibited and denial reinforced. Since 1988 the UK Committee on Safety of Medicines (CSM) has cautioned its use for bereavement.

To alleviate anxiety is the main reason given for benzodiazepine prescriptions, at least in the young and middle-aged. Subsumed within that large category lie more specific problems related to occupational stress, conflict within relationships, disruptive family life, phobias, and life transitions. Benzodiazepines are also prescribed for social problems such as poor living conditions. A high proportion of people receive benzodiazepines for physical symptoms such as headaches and premenstrual and menopausal symptoms as well as for relief of chronic physical ailments such as arthritis and cardiovascular disease.

Benzodiazepines are also prescribed for depression, although this should not be a primary indication for benzodiazepines. Their use in cases of depression may have serious consequences and can precipitate suicide. Since 1988 the Royal College of Psychiatrists and the CSM have drawn attention to this problem.

Sleep disorders form another category of use, particularly in the elderly. About two-thirds of the population report an average duration of sleep of between 7 and 8 hours per night, but, as age advances, an increasing proportion sleep for 5 hours or less. Estimates suggest an annual incidence of around 4 per cent insomnia in an adult general-practice population.

There is no doubt that lack of sleep has a debilitating effect on daytime functioning and a feeling of well-being. Yet have we been too ready to prescribe benzodiazepines for the elderly? About 10–15 per cent of the elderly population take a hypnotic drug each night. The elderly are particularly vulnerable to the effects of drug accumulation as with age, the body becomes less efficient at clearing drugs from the body. Major adverse effects can include respiratory depression and physical injury caused by 'sudden falls' resulting from unsteadiness or drowsiness. Oversedation, on the other hand, leads to confusion and impaired memory. As hypnotic use has continued to rise in recent years it seems as if many elderly users are unnecessarily exposed to these risks. Non-pharmacological methods that have been developed for sleep disorders should be used more as the first line of defence.

It is clear from the wide range of presenting symptoms discussed so far that benzodiazepines seem to have been used as a blunderbuss remedy to encompass a wide range of psychological and medical problems. Estimates from the USA suggest that one-third of patients prescribed a benzodiazepine may be wrongly diagnosed and therefore treated inappropriately. In addition, concern has been expressed in the UK that a significant proportion of drugs are incorrectly prescribed on pharmacological grounds. There are repeat prescriptions that are unnecessarily prolonged, incorrect dosages, and combinations of drugs with similar actions.

Why do people take benzodiazepines?

So far we have considered the more objective reasons why benzodiazepines are prescribed, but people are not merely passive recipients of medication: their perceptions of the drugs are important to consider. In two studies (Helman 1981*a,b*) suggested that patients' subjective beliefs about benzodiazepines play a major role in determining whether they will become chronic users of benzodiazepines. He further hypothesized, on the basis of patients' beliefs and expectations of benzodiazepines, that there were three main patient groups. He categorized these as 'tonic', 'food', and 'fuel', which were conceptualized as a continuum of perceived control over the drug. Patients in the 'tonic' group had maximal control over the drug, which they could use in a flexible way as needed. In the 'fuel' group benzodiazepines played an important and constant part in the patients' daily lives. However, in the 'food' group only minimal control was exerted over the drug. Patients in this group gave the impression they would disintegrate without it. They took benzodiazepines at fixed times and at inflexible dosages.

From a sociological perspective, Gabe and Thorogood (1986) argue that it is insufficient to focus on the meaning of benzodiazepines *per se*; rather meaning must be seen in the context of people's everyday lives. They take the position that benzodiazepines can be viewed as a resource to help people manage their everyday lives. Access to three resources—paid work, children, and partners—had an important influence on the use of benzodiazepines for long-term users. What is not clear, however, is whether long-term users have less access to resources because the effects of benzodiazepines limit a person's ability to use available resources, or whether reduced access to resources leads to benzodiazepine use. The authors also found that the meaning of benzodiazepine use varied across the sample. For some, benzodiazepines seemed to be perceived solely as a *life-line*, something they depended upon in order to keep going in daily life. Others appeared to see the drug as a *stand-by* to be kept in reserve and used occasionally as problems arose. Some even seemed to draw on both sets of meanings.

Cooperstock and Lennard (1979) were interested in the function the drug played in an individual's life and their investigations focused on the social roles their subjects fulfilled. They considered that women took benzodiazepines because of role conflicts inherent in their expected gender role. Conversely, men's benzodiazepine use enabled them to feel in control of situations they found stressful.

When patients are asked directly why they have continued to take benzodiazepines, many clearly have complex feelings about their drug use. In a survey of the general population in 1989 almost 10 per cent of people did not know why they had taken them. However, large numbers continue benzodiazepine use, not because they feel benefit, but because they think they are dependent and wish to avoid withdrawal. Some feel that the drugs are positively harming them while others feel they give peace of mind. Ambivalence about continued drug use is a striking feature of long-term users. In one research study conducted by the author self-concept was investigated using repertory grid techniques. It was found that people had an idealized and unrealistic picture of what kind of person they would be *without* taking benzodiazepines. There was a large discrepancy between this picture and how they saw themselves currently taking benzodiazepines. They often had high expectations and hopes that the drugs would help them, yet this seemed to wax and wane when confronted with the reality of actual benefit received.

Research on patients' subjective experience illustrates the need to consider benzodiazepine users as a heterogeneous group, not a homogeneous one as is often implied. Benzodiazepines can be perceived and used in different ways, irrespective of the patient's diagnosis or the particular drug prescribed. Analyses based on the patients' subjective experience of the drug offer an alternative way to predict those most at risk of being long-term users.

Psychologists have looked for underlying psychological mechanisms in an attempt to explain long-term benzodiazepine use. A social learning perspective attempts to go beyond limited pharmacological explanations, which concentrate on the characteristics of the drug, and instead emphasizes the many interacting factors that need to be taken into consideration. Benzodiazepine use is determined by many influences, which include biological, social, and psychological factors.

Initially, benzodiazepines have a pleasant anxiolytic effect. The benzodiazepines therefore act as powerful reinforcers. Once physical dependence is established the drugs may act as negative reinforcement; they are then taken to avoid unpleasant withdrawal symptoms. The phenomenon of gradient of reinforcement helps to explain that behaviour can have both rewarding and punishing consequences because it is the immediate consequences that are the most important in shaping habitual behaviour. Benzodiazepine users frequently state that they worry about the long-term damage to their health and they would like to withdraw, but this appears to take second place to their immediate short-term goal of reducing anxiety or avoiding withdrawal symptoms.

An important aspect in the process is the role of cognitions. Expectations of anxiety reduction and appraisal of what might happen when the medication is stopped contribute to the drug use. Secondary reinforcement is also important. If the benzodiazepine reduces anxiety in a stressful situation then a powerful association is built up so that the next time a similar situation occurs the individual is more likely to take a benzodiazepine.

How effective are benzodiazepines?

Despite early claims of efficacy and lack of dependence problems with benzodiazepines, evidence has continued to accumulate regarding the disadvantages of these drugs. First, we need to remind ourselves what the drugs were meant to accomplish. Having been established as the treatment of choice for anxiety it seems as if the fact that they were only ever a *symptomatic* treatment was overlooked. Although the benzodiazepines can relieve the symptoms of anxiety in the short term and can have a significant placebo effect, they do not necessarily affect the anxiety state itself.

Rickels *et al.* (1990) found that, despite receiving daily medication, 84 per cent of patients still met the DSM-IIIR (*Diagnostic and statistical manual of mental disorders*; APA 1987) criteria for current psychiatric illness. In general practice Catalan *et al.* (1988) found that, of the 43 per cent of patients who could be classified as psychiatrically unwell, long-term psychotropic drug treatment was wholly or partly ineffective in alleviating their symptoms. In addition, relapse rates following withdrawal of medication are high. Rickels *et al.* (1980) found a relapse rate of 81 per cent for anxious patients after short-term benzodiazepine treatment. The same research group later estimated the frequency of relapse after stopping benzodiazepines to be between 63 and 81 per cent.

Even their efficacy for treating symptoms has been questioned. The Committee on the Review of Medicines (1980) stated that 'there was little convincing evidence that benzodiazepines were efficacious in the treatment of anxiety after four months continuous treatment'. The guidelines issued by the Committee on Safety of Medicines (CSM) in 1988 gave stronger voice to concerns about the drugs' effects and emphasized the need for short-term treatment only. In the Nottingham study comparing drug and psychological treatments, Tyrer *et al.* (1988) found that diazepam became progressively less effective after 4 weeks of treatment.

Users themselves frequently report that they think benzodiazepines are of benefit to them. In a survey for the *Women's Own* magazine in 1979 about three-quarters of the respondents considered the drug helpful. This confirmed the finding of an earlier survey by Parry *et al.* (1973) that looked at national patterns of psychotropic drug use. It is interesting to see how this view began to change in later years as public awareness of the drugs developed. By 1983 when the BBC Television programme 'That's life' conducted their survey fewer than one-third of respondents claimed the benzodiazepines helped them 'a lot' in the first few months. The placebo effect of benzodiazepines and the effect of cognitive attributions about benzodiazepine use are likely to have significant impact on the effectiveness of the drugs. People need to attribute meaning to what they do and it is probably difficult to take medication for long periods of time without perceiving it as helpful to some extent. Research on personality variables and benzodiazepines is inconclusive; however, a consistent theme over a number of studies indicates the presence of a high degree of passivity. It could therefore be predicted that this fits in with an emphasis on external control factors being important to such people. A benzodiazepine, as an external agent, would be seen as more powerful than the individual's internal coping mechanisms and ability to affect the external environment.

The effect of benzodiazepines on psychological functioning, both cognitive and emotional, has clear disadvantages. Numbing of the emotions or 'emotional anaesthesia' is described repeatedly in subjective reports by users. It is not uncommon for women particularly to comment, once they have withdrawn, that they have missed a considerable part of their lives. Typical descriptions include phrases such as 'I felt like a zombie', 'it was like being wrapped in cotton wool', 'I missed my children growing up'. Although they were present in the home, the quality of their relationships and interactions was seriously impaired. The sense individuals give is of not being fully in touch with what they feel—they are aware of what is happening in their environment, they often respond, but they are not fully engaged in what is happening to them: the edge of the feeling has been blunted.

Emotional distress is not an adequate indication for the prescription of benzodiazepines—yet this appears to be a common reason for their use. What is often not sufficiently recognized is that they may actually interfere with the individual's normal coping skills. Their willingness and ability to confront the issues causing distress can be severely reduced, e.g. they do not resist the development of avoidance behaviour.

Since the 1960s a large number of studies have provided clear evidence that single doses of these drugs impair cognitive functioning. Short-term use has been shown to impair memory, reasoning, and physical coordination. In one of the few studies with chronic users Golombok *et al.* (1988) found that long-term use adversely affected tasks involving visual–spatial ability and sustained attention. The drugs have only recently entered the time period when long-term effects become clear. The important question of whether they cause structural brain changes remains unresolved. Initial research with computerized tomography (CT) scans, which indicated that long-term users had enlarged cerebral ventricles, has not been replicated conclusively.

Are there alternatives to benzodiazepines?

Undoubtedly, benzodiazepines offer benefit in short-term relief of disabling anxiety in a crisis. However, their role over the last three decades has gradually become narrower and more focused. We started in the 1960s from a position where benzodiazepines were seen to have almost universal benefit. Now, current guidelines emphasize their disadvantages and urge 2–4 week use only where anxiety is severe. In practice, benzodiazepines have been prescribed mainly to deal with minor affective problems, particularly in general practice, where such problems make up to 30 per cent of the case load. If benzodiazepines are of limited use in dealing with such emotional and social problems, are there any effective alternatives?

Psychological treatments offer the potential to develop more effective coping strategies that enhance the individual's skills and abilities, rather than relying on a drug, an external agent. Historically, the earliest psychological interventions have their roots in behavioural methods based on principles of learning and conditioning. Sustained and rigorous attempts were made to evaluate their effectiveness and clear benefits were found, particularly for specific, circumscribed fears.

More recently, most attention has been given to cognitive–behavioural treatments for emotional disorders. Worry, apprehension, negative think-ing, and misperception all play a major role in such problems. This has led to a greater emphasis on methods of self-control, such as relaxation training, anxiety-management training, and cognitive therapy. In a review of behavioural and cognitive treatments of panic disorder and agoraphobia, Michelson and Marchione (1991) concluded that cognitive–behaviour therapy (CBT) studies show consistently positive findings with substantive therapeutic gains. In another review of two decades of CBT and pharmacological panic disorder research, Clum (1989) found that overall CBT was found to be more effective (74 per cent success) and had significantly lower relapse rates than pharmacotherapy. However, further studies are now needed to compare CBT and alternative psychological and pharmacological treatments over long-term follow-ups.

A similar picture emerges with psychological treatment for depression. Cognitive therapy has been a promising innovation, with many studies showing that it has an effect, although the size of the effect is still under debate. In a large-scale study by the National Institute of Mental Health (Elkin *et al.* 1989) two brief psychotherapies were investigated: cognitive–behaviour therapy and interpersonal psychotherapy. Overall there were little differences found between the psychotherapies and the standard ref-erence treatment, imipramine plus clinical management. However, the study looked only at the short-term effectiveness of the treatment. Follow-up data that demonstrated the effectiveness of the therapies but provided only limited support for *specific* effects of CBT was provided by Imber *et al.* (1990).

Clearly, psychological methods offer a valuable alternative to benzo-diazepines. However, more research is needed to determine the size of therapeutic effect and to match patient characteristics to specific interven-tions. It should also be recognized that applying sophisticated psychological methods requires skill and there are only a limited number of psychologists available to carry out such methods. In any case the methods are not always suitable for everyone. One way forward is to develop a model that considers the different levels of intervention required for different types of benzodiazepine users (Fig.1.1).

A parallel can be drawn with smoking research where two-thirds of individuals can give up on their own or with minimal support. A good example in the benzodiazepine field is the study by Catalan *et al.* (1984), where brief counselling by the general practitioner was as effective as benzodiazepines. There is scope for further development of minimal interventions including brief counselling methods, self-help literature, and short-term professional input followed by self-help. Research is needed to look at the effectiveness of these and other minimum interventions and to determine for which patients they are most suited. Catalan *et al.*'s study also revealed that one-third of patients were not helped by either benzodiazepines or brief counselling. This suggests the need for a different level of intervention, which requires more skilled and intensive input. The author has found that this group can be further subdivided into two levels. Level 2 also includes information about benzodiazepines and their effects but adds a short-term psychological intervention of 8–15 sessions. This might be for individuals or groups. Level 3 is reserved for a smaller proportion of people who have severe psychological problems in addition to benzodiazepine dependence. They may require a range of psychological treatments and longer-term therapy of up to 30 sessions.

Understanding about the long-term effects of benzodiazepines is still poor. As the data sheets still say, 'little is known about the efficacy or safety of benzodiazepines in long-term use'. The enthusiasm that once welcomed the 'new wonder drugs' has given way over the years to a more realistic appraisal of the drugs and their limitations. Clearly, caution rather than complacency is needed in the next decade.

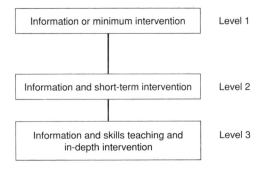

Fig. 1.1. Different levels of intervention required for different types of benzodiazepine users.

References

APA (American Psychiatric Association) (1987). *Diagnostic and statistical manual of mental disorders* (3rd edn, revised), American Psychiatric Press, Washington, DC.

Benson, P. (1988). Too much or too little compassion. *British Medical Journal*, **297**, 801.

Catalan, J., Gath, D., Edmonds, G., Ennis, J., Bond, A., and Martin, P. (1984). The effects of non-prescribing of anxiolytics in general practice. *British Journal of Psychiatry*, **144**, 593–610.

Catalan, J., Gath, D.H., Bond, A., Edmonds, G., Martin, P., and Ennis, J. (1988). General practice patients on long-term psychotropic drugs. *British Journal of Psychiatry*, **152**, 399–405.

Clum, G.A. (1989). Psychological interventions versus drugs in the treatment of panic. *Behaviour Therapy*, **20**, 429–57.

Committee on the Review of Medicines (1980). Systematic review of the benzodiazepines. *British Medical Journal*, **280**, 910–12.

Cooperstock, R. and Lennard, H.L. (1979). Some social meanings of tranquillizer use. *Sociology of Health and Illness*, **1**, 331–47.

Elkin, I., Shea, M.T., Watkins, J.T., Imber, S.D., Sotsky, S.M., Collins, J.F., Glass, D.R., Pilkonis, P.A., Leber, W.R., Docherty, J.P., Fiester, S.J., and Parloff, M.B. (1989). National Institute of Mental Health Treatment of depression collaborative research program. *Archives of General Psychiatry*, **46**, 971–82.

Gabe, J. and Thorogood, N. (1986). Prescribed drugs and the management of everyday life: the experiences of black and white working class women. *The Sociological Review*, **34**, 737–72.

Golombok, S., Moodley, P., and Lader, M. (1988). Cognitive impairment in long-term benzodiazepine users. *Psychological Medicine*, **18**, 365–74.

Helman, C.G. (1981*a*) Patients' perceptions of psychotropic drugs. *Journal of the Royal College of General Practitioners*, **31**, 107–12.

Helman, C.G. (1981*b*) 'Tonic', 'Fuel' and 'Food'. Social and symbolic aspects of the long-term use of psychotropic drugs. *Social Science and Medicine*, **15B**, 521–33.

Hemminki, E. (1975). The role of prescriptions in therapy. *Medical Care*, **13**, 150–9.

Imber, S.P., Pilkonis, P.A., Sotsky, S.M., Elkin, I., Watkins, J.T., Collins, J.F., Shea, M.T., Leber, W.R., and Glass, D.R. (1990). Mode specific effects among three treatments for depression. *Journal of Consulting and Clinical Psychology*, **58**, 352–9.

Lacey, R. and Woodward, S. (1985). *That's life: survey on tranquillisers*. BBC in association with MIND, London.

Linn, L. S. (1971). Physician characteristics and attitudes toward legitimate use of psychotherapeutic drugs. *Journal of Health and Social Behaviour*, **12**, 331–40.

Medawar, C. (1992). *Power and dependence: social audit on the safety of medicines*. Social Audit Ltd, London.

Michelson, L.K. and Marchione, K. (1991). Behavioural cognitive and pharmacological treatments of panic disorder with agoraphobia: critique and synthesis. *Journal of Consulting and Clinical Psychology*, **59**, 100–14.

Parry, H., Balter, I., Mellinger, G., Gisin, I., and Manheimer, D. (1973). National patterns of psychotropic drug use. *Archives of General Psychiatry*, **28**, 769–83.

Rickels, K., Case, W.G., and Diamond, L. (1980). Relapse after short-term drug therapy in neurotic outpatients. *International Pharmacopsychiatry*, **15**, 186–92.

Rickels, K., Schweizer, E., Case, G., and Greenblath, D.J. (1990). Withdrawal reactions from chlordiazepoxide (Librium). *Psychopharmacologia*, **2**, 63–8.

Tyrer, P. J., Murphy, S., Oates, G., and Kingdon, D. (1985). Psychological treatment for benzodiazepine treatment. *Lancet*, **i**, 1042–3.

Tyrer, P., Murphy, S., Kingdon, D., Brothwell, J., Gregory, S., Seivewright, N., Ferguson, B., Barczak, P., Darling, C., and Johnson, A.L. (1988). The Nottingham study of neurotic disorder: a comparison of drug and psychological treatments. *Lancet*, **ii**, 235–40.

2 Rational prescribing of benzodiazepines

Carl Salzman and Eric Watsky

Benzodiazepines are among the most widely prescribed psychotropic drugs in the world. Although prescribed primarily for acute anxiety and stress conditions, benzodiazepines are now also used regularly for the treatment of panic and agoraphobic conditions, sleep, and behavioural control of psychotic patients.

One-year usage rates of benzodiazepines around the world suggest that the availability and use by adults is high, ranging from 6 to over 25 per cent (Mellinger and Balter 1981, 1983; Balter *et al.* 1984; Mellinger *et al.* 1984*a,b*; APA Task Force 1990). In the USA two-thirds of this use is for 60 days or under. Nevertheless, such widespread availability and use have raised questions regarding possible overuse and misuse of benzodiazepines. In turn, such reappraisal of the prescription of this class of compounds argues for a discussion of rational versus irrational prescription.

Rational prescription of benzodiazepines requires simultaneous consideration of the therapeutic indications and efficacy of these drugs balanced against their potential for toxicity and dependence. Most clinicians would argue that rational prescription occurs when the therapeutic efficacy clearly outweighs toxicity and/or dependence. Most would also agree that, when the opposite condition obtains, drug treatment should not continue. However, there are many clinical situations in which the initial rational use of benzodiazepines may become irrational as treatment continues. In certain cases non-pharmacological treatment is preferred even if drug treatment has little risk of toxicity or dependence. Lastly, there may be differences among patients so that rational treatment for one patient may be irrational for another with similar symptoms. Rational prescription, therefore, must also consider appropriate duration of treatment and limitations of such treatment.

This chapter will review the common uses of benzodiazepines for typical clinical indications, focusing first on their acute use and then on their chronic use. Within each category the risks versus benefits of their use will be examined.

Treatment of acute anxiety and stress situations

Throughout human history, compounds with sedative/hypnotic properties have been used to ameliorate acute stress and anxiety conditions. Until the development of benzodiazepines virtually all such agents (e.g. alcohol, barbiturates, bromides, propanediols) carried risks of substantial toxicity, including overdose lethality, as well as dependence and severe withdrawal states (Salzman 1984). The development of benzodiazepine anti-anxiety agents heralded a new era in the pharmacological treatment of acute anxiety. These compounds were more potent (on a per milligram basis) than previous drugs. Initially, their toxicity was believed to be low, and dependence and withdrawal were not considered to be clinically significant problems. Over the 3 decades of their clinical availability, however, it has become apparent that benzodiazepines have a toxic profile similar to other sedative/hypnotics, although considerably less severe and life-threatening. It has also become apparent that benzodiazepines, in a dose- and time-related fashion, can induce a state of physiological dependence with a clinically predictable and identifiable abstinence syndrome upon abrupt withdrawal (Lader and Pétursson 1981; Pétursson and Lader 1984; APA Task Force 1990). In most cases, however, toxicity, dependence, and withdrawal are related to dose and duration of treatment so that brief therapeutic treatment with benzodiazepines may lead to reduction of stress and anxiety without serious negative reactions. As a consequence, this class of compounds has become the most widely used pharmacological agent for the treatment of acute stress and anxiety.

At present benzodiazepines are usually considered for use when stress situations or the development of acute anxiety compromise the individual's ability to function normally. This is commonly seen during acute crisis and acute illness. Typically, low-to-moderate therapeutic doses are prescribed for these conditions over a period of days or weeks; most prescription is for under 60 days. For most patients, the therapeutic gains achieved by low-dose short-term treatment greatly outweigh toxicity and dependence potential so that this constitutes their rational use (Rickels 1983; Woods *et al.* 1988).

The effect of benzodiazepines in reducing acute stress and anxiety is well known and has been documented numerous times. This has been well discussed elsewhere (e.g. Greenblatt and Shader 1974; Greenblatt *et al.* 1983*a,b*; Trimble 1983; Tyrer 1983; Woods *et al.* 1987; APA Task Force 1990). In general, benzodiazepines seem to be indicated in patients needing immediate symptom relief from stress or anxiety (Cowley and Dunner 1991). Reduction in anxiety and stress may help the individual to function better, avoiding the use of other more dangerous sedative/hypnotic drugs (such as alcohol) (Forster and Marmer 1991). The following vignette illustrates the successful prescription of a benzodiazepine for the management of acute stress and anxiety. (*NB*. Mention of a specific benzodiazepine compound in these vignettes does not constitute an endorsement of any particular compound;

similarly, no criticism is implied if a particular drug is not mentioned in a vignette.)

Dr A, a 33-year-old physician, provided emergency medical care on an urban street corner to the victim of a gunshot wound. After the patient was safely delivered to an emergency room, the doctor began to worry about possible exposure to Aids. Over the next several weeks the doctor became progressively convinced of exposure and became acutely anxious, although the shooting victim tested negatively for the HIV virus. Symptoms included tension, agitation, disruption of sleep, decreased ability to concentrate, and a forgetfulness at work. He became increasingly preoccupied and found that his ability to provide care to his patients diminished. Diazepam 5 mg was prescribed on a four times daily and at night basis.

Because Dr A's symptoms interfered with his daily activities, reduction of anxiety restored him to normal functioning, which in turn further helped reduce anxiety. Similar use of short-term benzodiazepines occurs very frequently in stress situations associated with acute medical illness or treatment. Thus, it is very common for physicians to prescribe benzodiazepines daily (as well as for sleep) to patients who are undergoing medical or surgical treatment, or who are recuperating from medical or surgical illness. Such short-term benzodiazepine use may also be successfully used after acute traumatic experiences, e.g. earthquake, rape, war-time trauma (Feldman 1987).

Clinical experience and research data (APA Task Force 1990) suggest that the toxic risk of such short-term treatment is minimal. In cases of severe anxiety and stress, *not* treating a patient with a benzodiazepine might be considerably more hazardous than acute treatment. For younger adults low-to-moderate therapeutic doses of benzodiazepines prescribed for periods of less than 4 months are unlikely to produce toxic consequences that outweigh the therapeutic effect (APA Task Force 1990). Some patients, however, may become disinhibited by benzodiazepines with a resulting increase in anger and aggression (Gardos *et al.* 1968; Salzman *et al.* 1974, 1975; Lion *et al.* 1975; Kochansky *et al.* 1978; Rosenbaum *et al.* 1984; Gardner and Cowdry 1985; Dietch and Jennings 1988). For other patients, depressive symptoms may emerge following benzodiazepine administration (Lydiard *et al.* 1987). Moreover, dependence, as defined by clinically significant withdrawal symptoms, is unlikely to develop in response to therapeutic doses when treatment is for under 4 months for long-half-life benzodiazepines and for under 2–3 months for short-half-life compounds (APA Task Force 1990). Elderly patients, however, are more likely to become sedated, to have more difficulty with co-ordinated motor movement, and to fall and sustain fractures when taking a benzodiazepine than younger adults. Furthermore, they are more likely to be taking a medication that may adversely interact with a benzodiazepine. There are no data to suggest that short-term use of benzodiazepines for acute stress or anxiety leads to prolonged use, dependence, or abuse of benzodiazepines.

The following vignette illustrates the use of benzodiazepines to manage acute anxiety in an elderly person in whom the toxic effects of the drug were greater than its therapeutic effect.

Mrs B, an 82-year-old widow, decided after many months to sell her home and move to a retirement community. When the her house was put up for sale, Mrs B began to experience difficulty falling asleep, as well as awakening frequently at night. During the day she found herself tense, preoccupied, and jittery. She could not sit still and could not concentrate while reading or watching television. Because of her obvious symptoms of anxiety and associated sleep disturbance, her internist prescribed lorazepam 0.5 mg thrice daily and at bedtime. Over the weeks that followed, Mrs B became progressively more forgetful, lost all ability to concentrate, and began to talk about feeling hopeless. She became preoccupied and anxious about her rapidly failing memory. At first it was assumed that these symptoms were the result of the change in her life status as well as her advanced age. However, as they did not improve with supportive and psychotherapeutic measures, it was decided to discontinue the lorazepam. Within a week of discontinuance, Mrs B's dysphoric symptoms began to subside, and her concentration and attention span improved. She reported to her children that she felt that her thinking was 'clearer', and remarked that her anxiety had actually increased when she experienced failing cognitive function while on medication.

This vignette illustrates potential toxic consequences of short-term benzodiazepine prescription, which are more likely in an older patient. The emergence of depressive symptoms as well as memory impairment may cause further upset to a patient, and even confuse the clinical picture (Salzman *et al.* 1990). Similar concern could be expressed about the influence of short-term benzodiazepines on driving skills in the elderly, about excessive daytime sedation, and about the possible interaction between the sedative effects of benzodiazepines and other sedating medically overprescribed or over-the-counter compounds. For younger adults, interaction of acutely prescribed benzodiazepines with alcohol is a primary concern, especially since the patient may already have increased alcohol consumption in an effort to deal with the acute stress or anxiety.

It is important to note that the clinical usefulness of benzodiazepines under conditions of acute stress and anxiety does not suggest that all such conditions should be treated by benzodiazepines. The decision not to use these drugs for treatment of acute anxiety partly depends on the aetiology of the anxiety and the availability of alternative treatments. For psychologically induced stress or for anxiety that results from environmental stress, psychological treatment or environmental intervention, respectively, may be more efficacious. Some studies have suggested that brief counselling or psychotherapy may be as efficacious as benzodiazepine treatment (Shapiro *et al.* 1983; Catalan *et al.* 1984; Cohen 1987). Relaxation training, cognitive behavioural therapy, or simple supportive measures may also be effective. For some patients, the classical psychodynamic formulation of anxiety as a signal of underlying psychic conflict may be applicable and indicate the need for psychotherapeutic intervention rather than simple symptom reduction.

Treatment of chronic anxiety

Most patients who receive benzodiazepines as part of treatment for chronic stress or anxiety fall into one of two categories. The first and larger group is comprised of older people who tend to have medical illness (Rickels *et al.* 1984; APA Task Force 1990). In many cases they are taking prescribed medications for their medical condition, are in pain, and suffer from depressive symptoms as well as anxiety. As a group, these patients experience considerable therapeutic benefit from benzodiazepines. Reduction of daytime tension and anxiety and improvement of nighttime sleep typically provides a sense of improved well-being and, in some cases, may actually assist the healing process (Fernandez and Levy 1991). For some patients, such as those with orthopaedic disorder or hypertension, the relaxant properties of benzodiazepines may prevent the worsening of symptoms, if not actually assisting in symptom reduction. Studies indicate that patients not only find these benzodiazepines helpful, but tend to treat them somewhat reverentially: they never increase the dose or self-medicate, nor do they abuse the benzodiazepines in any manner. They are typically scrupulous about not mixing the drugs with alcohol, and tend to be very high compliers with doctors' prescription regimens. Their physicians similarly believe the benzodiazepines to be a therapeutic part of the overall treatment programme. Consequently, for these chronic, medically ill patients, ongoing therapeutic doses of benzodiazepines represent rational prescribing. The following vignette illustrates such a case.

Mrs C, a 55-year-old woman, had sustained a serious hip fracture in an automobile accident. She had undergone several surgical procedures, but was left with residual pain. Her orthopaedic treatment included ongoing administration of non-narcotic analgesics, non-steroidal anti-inflammatories, and a low dose of a benzodiazepine. The patient remained on this regimen for more than 20 years until her death due to an unassociated cancer of the lymphatic system. She remarked, over the course of her chronic disability, that the benzodiazepine that she took was an essential part of her treatment programme providing emotional as well as muscle relaxation; without the benzodiazepine she required higher analgesic doses. She ridiculed statements in the media that these drugs were destructive to people's health.

The second group of patients with chronic anxiety are patients with chronic psychiatric or emotional disorder. Commonly they have mixed anxiety and depressive states and have personality disorders (patients with panic disorder will be considered separately in the next section). These patients represent a large proportion of out-patient psychiatric and psychotherapeutic practice and are also seen for treatment by general practitioners and family physicians. Many have lifelong symptoms of anxiety, dysthymia, and a fluctuating mood disturbance. Some are hypochondriacal and have somatic concern or preoccupation; others have 'free-floating' anxiety, a non-specific worry that seems to attach itself to various aspects of the patient's life. Because of the severity of their anxiety symptoms, some of these patients are started on benzodiazepines for acute symptoms and then become chronic users when the symptoms persist or recur.

Thus, for some patients, chronic benzodiazepine use is therapeutic, and represents rational prescribing. Reduction of chronic or recurrent anxiety improves daily functioning and enhances the individual's sense of well-being and self-control. Such long-term use is not necessarily associated with toxicity, dose escalation, or abuse, as illustrated in the following vignette.

Mr D, a 48-year-old school teacher, was a 'worrier' his whole life. He functioned well, however, although he was constantly tense, apprehensive, vigilant, and had difficulty falling and staying asleep. Past age 40, he began to notice episodes of increased anxiety, usually associated with somatic symptoms, that began to interfere with his daily functioning. Recognizing that these symptoms could be relieved by increasing his modest daily alcohol intake, he sought medical assistance and was prescribed oxazepam, 15 mg, four times daily. Typically, Mr. D would take the oxazepam as prescribed for approximately 4–6 months, finding the drug helpful. He would then gradually discontinue the treatment, restarting only when anxious again. He never increased his dose beyond the prescribed amount and did not experience toxic or withdrawal symptoms.

Mr D illustrates a common pattern of long-term intermittent benzodiazepine use. The therapeutic effect outweighs either the toxicity, which is minimal, or the development of dependence, which is not inevitable; there is no dose escalation nor progression towards drug misuse or abuse. Another vignette illustrates a similar pattern of chronic use that is continual, rather than intermittent, but without hazards.

Dr E, a 63-year-old psychiatrist, suffered from anxiety and labile hypertension for more than 20 years. He was maintained on prazepam 7.5 mg twice daily in conjunction with a β-blocking cardiovascular drug; taken together, his blood pressure was well controlled. Mindful of the potential hazards of chronic benzodiazepine use, Dr E also underwent psychotherapy and had his medication closely monitored by a psychopharmacologist. He never varied his prescribed dose and experienced no toxicity.

For some patients, however, the indications for chronic benzodiazepine prescription are less clear, and long-term prescribing may not always be so rational. Among patients with chronic anxiety disorder there is a group with personality disorder whose anxiety is persistent and disabling. These patients typically are dependent on other people, drugs, or alcohol (or even psychotherapy) for reassurance and for reduction of worry. It is this group of patients for whom chronic benzodiazepine use may not be therapeutic and may even lead to dependence, overuse, and, possibly, abuse. Some patients, for example, will self-medicate and adjust their own benzodiazepine dose without medical supervision, gradually increasing their dose beyond recommended levels. Others may obtain benzodiazepines from several sources and gradually escalate the dose; still others may use benzodiazepines as part of a pattern of alcohol or substance abuse.

Mr F, a 24-year-old self-employed musician, appeared in an out-patient psychiatric clinic. Saying that he had just moved to Boston from another city and that his benzodiazepine prescription had expired, he was becoming acutely anxious without his medication. He gave a history of chronic, recurrent anxiety that had been well controlled with alprazolam. He asked for a prescription for his drug by name, dose, and prescribing directions. Suspicion about possible benzodiazepine misuse or abuse arose when the patient himself told the doctor that he might have a withdrawal seizure if his prescription were not renewed.

Mr F represents a small group of chronically anxious patients who may potentially abuse benzodiazepines. Miss G in the following vignette is a more typical, difficult patient who is not likely to be considered a true drug abuser, but whose use of benzodiazepines raises questions of rational prescription.

Miss G, a 26-year-old store manager, frequently sought medical and psychiatric attention in emergency rooms and clinics. She always appeared on the verge of a serious crisis—jobs ending, lovers leaving, parents misunderstanding. Invariably, psychotherapy or counselling would be recommended to her, along with benzo-diazepine treatment for her chronic, crippling anxiety. However, she would often miss follow-up appointments (or come late) and seemed unable to sustain any therapeutic relationship. As she became well known in the medical and psychiatric clinics of Boston, it became apparent that she sometimes obtained benzodiazepines from several medical sources simultaneously. She denied doing this deliberately, but seemed to genuinely lose her prescriptions or misplace the medications. She claimed that the benzodiazepines were essential to her ability to function, yet she rarely reported significant anxiolytic relief, despite taking high doses over a period of many years.

Mr F and Miss G illustrate two patterns of chronic benzodiazepine use that may not be rational. Although neither experienced toxicity, there was little evidence of any meaningful sustained therapeutic effect. Because both patients took high doses for long periods of time, they were subject to the development of dependence and withdrawal symptoms; it is possible that some of their motivation for continuing high-dose benzodiazepine treatment was to avoid the development of discontinuance symptoms.

The abuse of benzodiazepines alone is unusual, although common among polysubstance abusers. More typical is the patient with a personality disorder who starts taking benzodiazepines for the resolution of acute symptoms, but then continues to take the medication beyond clear clinical indications. Serious consequences of high-dose chronic benzodiazepine use may result.

Mrs H, a 42-year-old professional woman, was initially prescribed benzodiazepines for anxiety that developed after serious complications with home renovation. Although she initially found chlordiazepoxide, 10 mg four times daily, to be helpful, her anxiety persisted beyond realistic reasons for feeling anxious. Reassurances from her family were not helpful, and she requested an increased benzodiazepine dose. Her physician, empathizing with her plight, and not thinking of her as a 'drug-abusing type' concurred with the dose increase. But symptom relief was short-lived and she soon requested another dose increase. Over the course of several months, her initial dose doubled, then trebled, and finally quadrupled. When she finally presented for psychotherapeutic consultation, she was taking more than five times the suggested daily anti-anxiety dose. Her thinking was confused, her memory impaired, and she staggered and frequently fell while walking; extended hospitalization was required to taper and discontinue the medication.

Chronic benzodiazepine treatment can also be hazardous to older patients. Although initially responding to treatment without toxicity, most people often become progressively more sensitive to the sedating and psychomotoric toxic effects of benzodiazepines as they age (Salzman 1992). However, since the toxic effects only begin to appear years after the initial benzodiazepine prescription they may be mistaken for the natural consequences of ageing or for a developing neuropsychiatric disorder.

Mrs I was a 75-year-old woman with symptoms of Alzheimer's disease. She was sometimes disoriented, often forgetful, and had poor attention and concentration. Her symptoms seemed somewhat worse in the evening when she became agitated, restless, and irritable. Initially it was believed that Mrs I was suffering from age-associated memory impairment, which was to be expected in a woman of her age. As her symptoms progressed and interfered with her function, however, a provisional clinical diagnosis of Alzheimer's dementia was made, and it was suggested to her family that institutionalization might be necessary. A consulting psychiatrist noted that the patient had been taking diazepam 20 mg/day for more than 20 years and suggested that it be gradually tapered and discontinued. Within 3 weeks of discontinuance the patient's mental status had markedly improved. She was no longer confused, forgetful, or disoriented. Her memory function was consistent with that of a woman her age, and there was no evidence of a progressive dementing disorder.

The use of benzodiazepines for treatment of chronic anxiety, therefore, must be made with a careful appraisal of the clinical needs of the patient and with a regard to the possible consequences many years after prescribing has been initiated. For some psychiatric patients, and elderly patients in particular, the toxic or dependence-inducing consequences of chronic prescription may ultimately outweigh the therapeutic benefit. For patients with ongoing serious medical illness, however, the use of benzodiazepines as an adjunctive treatment may be helpful and rational.

Treatment of panic disorder

High-potency benzodiazepines, alprazolam (Alexander and Alexander 1986; Charney *et al.* 1986; Dunner *et al.* 1986; Liebowitz *et al.* 1986; Rickels *et al.* 1987; Sheehan 1987; Ballenger *et al.* 1988; Noyes *et al.* 1988*a*; Pecknold *et al.* 1988; Charney and Woods 1989; Uhlenhuth *et al.* 1989) and clonazepam (Pollack *et al.* 1986; Spier *et al.* 1986; Tesar and Rosenbaum 1986; Cohen and Rosenbaum 1987; Tesar *et al.* 1987; Schweizer *et al.* 1988*a*; Tesar 1990; Cowley and Dunner 1991) in particular, are among the treatments that are used regularly for panic anxiety and agoraphobic disorder. Recently, three other high-potency short-half-life benzodiazepines, lorazepam, bromazepam, and adinazolam, have been shown to have antipanic efficacy (Charney *et al*. 1987; Howell *et al*. 1987; Fogelson 1988; Schweizer *et al*. 1988*a*; Charney and Woods 1989; Tesar 1990; Cowley and Dunner 1991). Studies suggest that alprazolam demonstrates at least moderate efficacy in 82 per cent of panic disorder patients, with at least half becoming free of panic attacks. Case studies have indicated that clonazepam, like alprazolam, also has antipanic efficacy when used on a chronic basis. These benzodiazepines are sometimes recommended for patients with panic disorder who require immediate symptom relief, or who are sensitive to antidepressant side-effects (Cowley and Dunner 1991). They may also be added to antidepressants as an adjunct medication. Since panic disorder is a chronic illness, the use of benzodiazepines is usually limited to an adjunctive role or early symptom relief until the effects of antidepressants are experienced. Benzodiazepines are also helpful for the treatment of sleep disturbance associated with panic and agoraphobic disorders.

The use of a benzodiazepine for the primary treatment of chronic panic and agoraphobic disorders as opposed to the use of other psychotropic drugs such as antidepressants, requires an appraisal of efficacy versus toxicity of these two different classes of therapeutic agents. Although there are no clear data demonstrating the superior efficacy of one versus the other drug class, some clinicians believe that the benzodiazepines may be superior for the chronic treatment of mild-to-moderate panic anxiety, whereas antidepressants are superior for moderate-to-severe symptoms (Salzman and Green 1987). The side-effect profiles of these two classes of compounds, are however, quite different. Benzodiazepines are preferred for patients who are likely to be sensitive to the α-blocking, or anticholinergic properties of antidepressants. The antidepressants, on the other hand, may be preferred for patients who are sensitive to the sedating or psychomotor toxic properties of these compounds, who have been dependent on alcohol or other sedative–hypnotics, or who may be at risk for drug abuse. Furthermore, as noted, some patients who take benzodiazepines chronically may experience an increase in aggressive behaviour. The following vignettes illustrate a patient who was successfully treated for a panic disorder with a benzodiazepine, and a patient for whom a benzodiazepine produced unacceptable toxic effects.

Mr J was a 32-year-old advertising executive with a long history of panic disorder. He finally sought treatment when his symptoms interfered with travel necessitated by his work. Because his symptoms were only of moderate severity, alprazolam was elected as the initial treatment. He experienced almost immediate relief from 0.5 mg thrice daily, but after 2 or 3 weeks complained that he was still having breakthrough panic attacks. Doses of alprazolam were gradually increased by 0.5 mg increments to a total daily dose of 3 mg. At this dose, he was completely free from panic anxiety and was functioning normally at his job. He did not experience daytime sedation, psychomotor impairment, depression, or memory dysfunction, and was delighted with the course of his treatment. At two-year follow-up, he had been maintained on the same dose without further breakthrough of panic anxiety.

Mr J also illustrates an observation reported in research studies of alprazolam treatment of panic disorder: patients who are successfully treated do not escalate their dose, do not abuse their medication, and find it helpful. Some patients, however, do not have this positive outcome.

Mrs K presented for treatment because of progressively increasing panic attacks. She had been anxious all her life, and had experienced undiagnosed panic attacks. At age 36, however, following a serious illness of one of her children, she reported a marked increase in both the frequency and severity of these panic attacks which eventually began to interfere with her ability to work, and to care for her children at home. Because of concern over antidepressant side-effects, Mrs K was begun on clonazepam, 0.5 mg twice daily, with gradual dose increases up to 2 mg/day. At this dose her panic anxiety was significantly diminished. However, Mrs K was troubled by significant daytime sedation which did not pass over the course of time; she was also frequently unsteady. It was decided to discontinue the clonazepam and to begin treatment with an antidepressant. The dose of clonazepam was decreased by 0.25 mg/week, but the patient experienced severe rebound panic disorder necessitating an even more gradual discontinuance schedule. It took the patient $2^{1/2}$ months of gradual discontinuance before she was off clonazepam.

Benzodiazepine discontinuance can be difficult for some patients. Rebound symptoms, particularly rebound anxiety and panic symptoms, may be so disabling that some patients are unwilling or unable to discontinue their benzodiazepine treatment despite an equivocal therapeutic effect (APA Task Force 1990). Because treatment of panic anxiety and agoraphobic symptoms requires chronic use of high benzodiazepine doses (3–5 times higher than usual anti-anxiety doses), these patients are at increased risk for toxicity and the development of physiological dependence. Significant discontinuance symptoms have been reported when panic-disorder patients attempt to discontinue their benzodiazepine treatment (Noyes *et al.* 1984, 1988*a,b*; Smith and Wesson 1985; Pecknold *et al.* 1988), even with gradual dose reduction (Fyer *et al.* 1987). Thus, although benzodiazepines may be a rational treatment for panic anxiety and agoraphobic symptoms, clinicians must carefully weigh the potential risks of these drugs against the risks of antidepressants, which are also therapeutically useful. Benzodiazepines, if successful, are likely to be used at high doses with consequent increased risk of dependence and clinically significant discontinuance symptoms.

Treatment of sleep

Benzodiazepines are commonly used to treat sleep that has been acutely disturbed by illness and stress. Because the safety margin of benzodiazepines is considerably greater than that of other sedative hypnotics such as barbiturates and non-barbiturate hypnotics, they are used with confidence by clinicians to help patients whose sleep is acutely disturbed (Pascualy 1991). It is not unusual, therefore, to observe a majority of patients in a general hospital who are taking a benzodiazepine for sleep. Out-patients suffering from medical illness or acute psychiatric disturbance may also be helped over a period of temporary sleep disruption as illustrated in the following vignettes.

Mrs L, a 48-year-old psychologist, fell in the bathtub, sustaining a fracture of her clavicle. Since analgesics alone were unable to help her sleep, alprazolam, 0.125 mg, was prescribed nightly. On this dose Mrs L was able to sleep without interruption. She maintained this dose for 5 weeks of recuperation and then discontinued without difficulty.

Mrs M, a 76-year-old woman, was grieving because of the death of her husband. She found that she was unable to sleep, and a benzodiazepine was prescribed. Estazolam 1 mg (the recommended geriatric dose) was prescribed for nightly use over a 3-week period. Mrs M was able to sleep through the acute grieving process and not suffer any loss of her own health.

Benzodiazepines are sometimes used to treat chronic sleep disturbance. Studies have suggested, however, that, after 30 consecutive nights of use, this class of drugs loses its hypnotic efficacy due to the development of tolerance to the sedative effects. Nevertheless, some patients insist that they sleep better every night with a benzodiazepine. For some patients, a gradual increase in dose of benzodiazepines is necessary to maintain sleep, and this may lead to overuse of these compounds and serious consequences as illustrated in the following vignette.

Mrs O, a 55-year-old poet, began to have trouble sleeping and was prescribed diazepam 5 mg at night. Initially, this prescription was helpful, but over the course of 6 weeks she found it necessary to increase the dose to 10 mg. A diagnosis of depression was made and the patient was offered antidepressant treatment. She refused, however, stating that she was only depressed because she could not sleep, rather than not sleeping because she was depressed. She insisted that benzodiazepines had been helpful and that she needed to continue the medication.

Over the next 6 months the patient gradually convinced her psychiatrist to continue prescribing diazepam, and the dose gradually escalated to 75 mg nightly. Although Mrs O could sleep using these gradually increasing doses, she became so sedated and unsteady during the day that she was essentially non-functional. Attempts to lower the dose resulted in a night without sleep and the patient being frantic. Ultimately, hospitalization was necessary to gradually discontinue Mrs O from benzodiazepines and begin antidepressant treatment.

It is also not uncommon to observe elderly patients who take benzodiazepines chronically for sleep. Surveys of nursing-home drug prescribing reveal that the use of benzodiazepines for sleep is a common practice (Beers *et al.* 1988; Avorn *et al.* 1989). Although some older patients may insist that these drugs are necessary for sleep, benzodiazepines cause cognitive impairment in older patients when prescribed acutely, and recent data suggest that their chronic use in elderly nursing-home residents produces a cognitive impairment that resembles mild-to-moderate Alzheimer's dementia. When the benzodiazepine hypnotics are discontinued, cognitive function dramatically improves (Salzman *et al.* 1990). This is illustrated in the following vignette.

Mr P, an 83-year-old retired lawyer, was placed on temazepam, 15 mg nightly, when he entered a nursing home. He continued to take this drug nightly for the next 3 years. It was noticed that Mr P was progressively more forgetful, disoriented, and confused during the day. His activities declined and he spent most of his time sitting alone in the day room. Temazepam was gradually decreased and, 3 weeks after the last dose, the nursing home staff noticed an improvement in Mr P's mood and willingness to interact with other nursing home residents. Psychological tests administered before and after temazepam discontinuance revealed a statistically significant improvement in delayed recall.

Treatment of psychosis

Studies of the treatment of schizophrenia with benzodiazepines have yielded inconsistent results (Beckmann and Haas 1980; Jimerson *et al.* 1982; Nostoros *et al.* 1982, 1983), and most clinicians do not use benzodiazepines as the sole treatment for this disorder (Schatzberg and Cole 1981; Karson *et al.* 1982; Csernansky *et al.* 1984, 1988; Wolkowitz *et al.* 1986, 1988). Benzodiazepines are commonly used, however, as an adjunct to neuroleptic treatment of schizophrenia, especially for the control of acute disruptive behaviour (Arana *et al.* 1986; Bacher *et al.* 1986; Campbell and Simpson 1986; Cohen 1991). The technique for behavioural control involves the intramuscular administration of a high-potency, short-half-life benzodiazepine such as lorazepam in conjunction with a neuroleptic, usually also administered intramuscularly (Guz *et al.* 1972; Bick and Hannah 1986; Modell 1986; Ward *et al.* 1986; Mendoza *et al.* 1987; Garza-Trevino and Hollister 1988). Studies have suggested that most behaviour can be brought under control with only one or two such injections (Salzman *et al.* 1986, 1991).

Mr R, a 21-year-old college student, became acutely delusional over the course of several weeks prior to examinations. On admission to the hospital he was fearful, suspicious, and menacing. Within the first 2 days he began threatening the staff and other patients despite treatment with haloperidol. When he assaulted another patient on the third hospital day, lorazepam 0.5 mg was given intramuscularly in conjunction with 5 mg of haloperidol. A second injection of each drug was given 1 hour later; Mr R was now calmed and exhibiting controlled behaviour. He was continued on oral haloperidol without further need of lorazepam.

Although there are a few acute hazards to the use of adjunct benzo-diazepines for behavioural control, many clinicians maintain these patients on benzodiazepines in the belief that this class of compounds will *prevent* future violence or disruptive behaviour. There are no data to support this supposition, however, and, consequently, some patients with schizophrenia are maintained on benzodiazepines without clear-cut therapeutic indication. A recent report has suggested that chronic use of benzodiazepines may result in lower overall neuroleptic dosage for these patients, but this work needs to be further confirmed (Baldessarini *et al.* 1988).

Mr S, a 30-year-old unemployed auto mechanic, was also assaultive during a hospitalization for schizophrenic decompensation. His behaviour was controlled with clonazepam 0.5 mg given orally three or four times a day. Because of his past history of violence this treatment regimen was continued with gradually increasing doses to a total of 4 mg of clonazepam each day. Over the next 2 years, Mr S continued to be intermittently psychotic and assaultive without any evidence that the clonazepam was attenuating his violent behaviour. Nevertheless, the hospital staff was reluctant to discontinue the clonazepam for fear that his violence and psychosis might further escalate.

In recent years, high-potency benzodiazepines such as clonazepam or lorazepam have been used either alone or as an adjunct for the treatment of acute manic states (Dever and Schweizer 1988; Chouinard *et al.* 1983; Victor *et al.* 1984; Freinhar and Alvarez 1985; Greenspan and Levin 1985; Modell *et al.* 1985; Adler 1986; Santos and Morton 1987, 1989; Cohen *et al.* 1987; Lenox 1988). This technique seems to be effective for some patients with little hazard. Whether or not benzodiazepines are more therapeutic or as therapeutic as other pharmacological means of controlling manic excitement has not yet been determined. High doses, however, are sometimes necessary, which may result in progressive daytime toxicity, especially of the long-half-life benzodiazepine, clonazepam. If manic patients are maintained on benzodiazepines, then, like schizophrenic patients, they will become dependent on the drugs. Since there are no data to support the ongoing maintenance treatment of mania with benzodiazepines, this dependence may not be counterbalanced by therapeutic effect.

Discussion

Given the available clinical and research information, it is probably safe to say that the pharmacological class of benzodiazepine compounds is effective and safe; when used in appropriate clinical conditions, their efficacy exceeds their potential for liability from toxicity or dependence. Rational prescribing of benzodiazepines, therefore, depends as much on a careful and accurate appraisal of the needs of an individual patient, as on knowledge of the pharmacology of the drug. Rational use of these drugs occurs when the following three conditions are met: (1) the patient's clinical condition warrants treatment; (2) pharmacotherapy is warranted; (3) benzodiazepines are the best choice among the available psychotropic drugs. In consideration of these three factors, the following principles of rational benzodiazepine prescription may be developed.

1. Acute anxiety, stress, and disrupted sleep constitute the most common and reasonable indications for benzodiazepine treatment. Benzodiazepines

should be considered when anxiety, stress, or insomnia threaten the patient's usual physical or emotional equilibrium and interfere with usual functioning. However, the presence of anxiety, stress, or insomnia is not an automatic indication for the use of a benzodiazepine (or any psychotropic drug).

2. Rational chronic treatment with benzodiazepines is most appropriate for *some* patients with chronic anxiety that is associated with ongoing medical illness and for *some* patients with panic attack and agoraphobic symptoms. The presence of anxiety in medical illness, however, does not constitute an automatic indication for long-term treatment with benzodiazepines, nor does a diagnosis of panic/agoraphobia.

3. Long-term use of benzodiazepines for symptomatic relief of patients with personality disorder or recurrent intrapsychic conflict may not always be appropriate treatment. Clinicians should always carefully evaluate such patients with the knowledge that the efficacy of benzodiazepines in such patients may be questionable and that a possible development of toxicity and dependence may outweigh any modest therapeutic benefit.

4. The use of benzodiazepines to treat chronic sleep disturbance is the least rational use of these drugs. Although a few patients may require chronic benzodiazepines for sleep on a nightly basis for many years, it is likely that most chronic benzodiazepine hypnotic use is preventing rebound insomnia rather than promoting genuine sleep. Since chronic benzodiazepine hypnotic use may produce daytime toxicity, especially in the elderly, clinicians should endeavour to limit chronic benzodiazepine hypnotic prescription whenever possible.

Since anxiety, panic, and insomnia, are subjective experiences, it may be difficult for some clinicians to make appropriate clinical judgements about the rational use of benzodiazepines. Prescribing these drugs depends partly on the clinician's own treatment philosophy. Some clinicians believe that immediate symptom relief is their primary treatment strategy; others are more likely to seek the cause of the symptoms rather than immediately treat. Still other factors unrelated to the patient's clinical state may also impinge upon the clinical decision to use or not use benzodiazepines. For example, it is possible that patients who seek treatment in a very busy clinic setting or who do not speak the language of the clinician with facility may not always receive benzodiazepine treatment on a rational basis. It is also possible that some patients with serious symptoms may be undermedicated because the clinician either subscribes to an exclusive psychodynamic role of the aetiology of the symptoms, or the patients minimize or are unable to describe their subjective experiences. Lastly, because benzodiazepines have been discussed at length in the media for more than a decade, some patients may have misinformation about the appropriate use of these drugs and either not wish to take them when indicated or wish to take them when not indicated. Clinicians must take into consideration all of these non-pharmacological factors when weighing the decision to use benzodiazepines. Benzodiazepine use and other treatment modalities are not mutually exclusive, and rational prescribing should be the rule regardless of circumstances.

Benzodiazepines are neither panaceas nor poisons. When used appropriately, they are effective and safe compounds. Their inappropriate use stems not from their own pharmacological properties, however, but from the misapplication of the usual standards of good clinical practice. Like any other medication they should be used when indicated, at the lowest effective doses, and for the briefest period of time. For those patients whose symptoms or illness require treatment outside the usual acute–treatment parameters, a constant reappraisal of risk versus benefit must be made. It is hoped that clinicians will not abandon the use of benzodiazepines from fear of overuse or misuse, but will continue to evaluate the appropriate use of these medications for each individual patient. It is similarly hoped that patients can be educated about the safe clinical use of benzodiazepines so that they can assist the physician in rational decision-making processes. Lastly, it should be emphasized that for many patients treatment is not simply a matter of drug versus no drug; benzodiazepines, like other psychotropic drugs, are most typically part of an overall treatment programme. Patients are not well served when clinicians, researchers, consumer advocates, or the media attempt to promote conflict between two treatment strategies that are not in opposition to each other but that work best together.

References

Adler, L.W. (1986). Mixed bipolar disorder responsive to lithium and clonazepam. *Journal of Clinical Psychiatry*, **47**, 49–50.

Alexander, P.E. and Alexander, D.D. (1986). Alprazolam treatment for panic disorders. *Journal of Clinical Psychiatry*, **47**, 301–4.

APA Task Force (American Psychiatric Association Task Force) (1990). *Benzodiazepine dependence, toxicity, and abuse*. American Psychiatric Press Inc, Washington, DC.

Arana, G.W., Ornsteen, M.L., Kanter, F., Friedman, H.L., Greenblatt, D.J., and Shader, R.I. (1986). The use of benzodiazepines for psychotic disorders: a literature review and preliminary clinical findings. *Psychopharmacology Bulletin*, **22**, 77–87.

Ashton, H. (1984). Benzodiazepine withdrawal: an unfinished story. *British Medical Journal*, **88**, 1135–40.

Avorn, J., Dreyer, P., Connelly, K., and Soumerai, S.B. (1989). Use of psychoactive medications and the quality of care in rest homes. Findings and policy implications of a statewide study. *New England Journal of Medicine*, **320**, 227–33.

Bacher, N.M., Lewis, H.A., and Field, P.B. (1986). Combined alprazolam and neuroleptic drug in treating schizophrenia. *American Journal of Psychiatry*, **143**, 1311–12.

Baldessarini, R.J., Cohen, B.M., and Teicher, M.H. (1988). Significance of neuroleptic dose and plasma level in the pharmacological treatment of psychoses. *Archives of General Psychiatry*, **45**, 79–91.

Ballenger, J.C., Burrows, G.D., DuPont, R.L., Lesser, I.M., Noyes, R., Pecknold, J.C., Rifkin, A., and Swinson, R.P. (1988). Alprazolam in panic disorder and agoraphobia: results from a multicenter trial. *Archives of General Psychiatry*, **45**, 413–22.

Balter, M.B., Manheimer, D.I., Mellinger, G.D., and Uhlenhuth, E.H. (1984). A cross-national comparison of anti-anxiety sedative drug use. *Current Medical Research and Opinion*, **8** (suppl.), 5–20.

Beckmann, H. and Haas, S. (1980). High dose diazepam in schizophrenia. *Psychopharmacology, Berlin*, **71**, 171–9.

Beers, M., Avorn, J., Soumerai, S.B., Everitt, D.E., Sherman, D.S., and Salem, S. (1988). *Journal of the American Medical Association*, **260**, 3016–20.

Bick, P.A. and Hannah, A.L. (1986). Letter: Intramuscular lorazepam to restrain violent patients. *Lancet*, **i**, 206.

Campbell, R. and Simpson, G.M. (1986). Alternative approaches in the treatment of psychotic agitation. *Psychosomatics*, **27** (suppl.), 23–6.

Catalan, J., Gath, D., Edmonds, G., Ennis, J., Bond, A., and Martin, P. (1984). The effects of non-prescribing of anxiolytics in general practice. I. Controlled evaluation of psychiatric and social outcome. *British Journal of Psychiatry*, **144**, 593–602.

Charney, D.S. and Woods, S.W. (1989). Benzodiazepine treatment of panic disorder: a comparison of alprazolam and lorazepam. *Journal of Clinical Psychiatry*, **50**, 418–23.

Charney, D.S., Woods, S.W., Goodman, W.K., Rifkin, B., Kinch, M., Aiken, B., Quadrino, L.M., and Heninger, G.R. (1986). Drug treatment of panic disorder: the comparative efficacy of imipramine, alprazolam, and trazodone. *Journal of Clinical Psychiatry*, **44**, 580–6.

Charney, D.S., Woods, S.W., Goodman, W.K., Heninger, G.R. (1987). The efficacy of lorazepam in panic disorders. A paper read before the 140th Annual Meeting of the American Psychiatric Association, Chicago, 11 May 1987.

Chouinard, G., Young, S.N., and Annable, L. (1983). Antimanic effect of clonazepam. *Biological Psychiatry*, **18**, 451–66.

Cohen, L.S. and Rosenbaum, J.F. (1987). Clonazepam: new uses and potential problems. *Journal of Clinical Psychiatry*, **48** (suppl.), 50–5.

Cohen, S. (1991). Benzodiazepines in psychotic and related conditions. In *Benzodiazepines in clinical practice: risks and benefits* (ed. P.P. Roy-Byrne and D.S. Cowley), pp.57–72. American Psychiatric Press, Washington, DC.

Cohen, S., Khan, A., and Johnson, S. (1987). Pharmacological management of manic psychosis in an unlocked setting. *Journal of Clinical Psychopharmacology*, **7**, 261–4.

Cohen, S.I. (1987). Letter: Are benzodiazepines useful in anxiety? *Lancet*, **ii**, 1080.

Cohen, J.B. and Wilcox, C.S. (1984). Long-term comparison of alprazolam, lorazepam and placebo in patients with an anxiety disorder. *Pharmacotherapy*, **4**, 93–8.

Cowley, D.S. and Dunner, D.L. (1991). Benzodiazepines in anxiety and depression. In *Benzodiazepines in clinical practice: risks and benefits* (ed. P.P. Roy-Byrne and D.S. Cowley), pp.35–56. American Psychiatric Press, Washington, DC.

Csernansky, J.G., Lombrozo, L., Gulevich, G.D., Hollister, L.E. (1984). Treatment of negative schizophrenic symptoms with alprazolam: a preliminary open-label study. *Journal of Clinical Psychopharmacology*, **4**, 349–52.

Csernansky, J.G., Riney, S.J., Lombrozo, L., Overall, J.E., Hollister, L.E. (1988).

Double-blind comparison of alprazolam, diazepam, and placebo for the treatment of negative schizophrenic symptoms. *Archives of General Psychiatry*, **45**, 655–9.

Dever, A. and Schweizer, E. (1988). Letter: Rapid remission of organic mania after treatment with lorazepam. *Journal of Clinical Psychopharmacology*, **8**, 227–8.

Dietch, J.T. and Jennings, R.K. (1988). Aggressive dyscontrol in patients treated with benzodiazepines. *Journal of Clinical Psychiatry*, **49**, 184–8.

Dunner, D.L., Ishiki, D., Avery, D.H., Wilson, L.G., and Hyde, T.S. (1986). Effect of alprazolam and diazepam on anxiety and panic attacks in panic disorder: a controlled study. *Journal of Clinical Psychiatry*, **47**, 458–60.

Feldman, T.B. (1987). Letter: Alprazolam in the treatment of posttraumatic stress disorder. *Journal of Clinical Psychiatry*, **48**, 216–17.

Fernandez, F. and Levy, J.K. (1991). Use of benzodiazepines in the medically ill. In *Benzodiazepines in clinical practice: risks and benefits* (ed. P.P. Roy-Byrne and D.S. Cowley), pp.177–200. American Psychiatric Press, Washington, DC.

Fogelson, D.L. (1988). Letter: Lorazepam and oxazepam in the treatment of panic disorder. *Journal of Clinical Psychopharmacology*, **8**, 150.

Fontaine, R. (1989). Clonazepam for panic disorders and agitation. *Psychosomatics*, **26**, 13.

Forster, P. and Marmar, C.R. (1991). Benzodiazepines in acute stress reactions: benefits, risks, and controversies. In *Benzodiazepines in clinical practice: risks and benefits* (ed. P.P. Roy-Byrne and D.S. Cowley), pp.73–90. American Psychiatric Press, Washington, DC.

Freinhar, J.P. and Alvarez, W.H. (1985). Use of clonazepam in two cases of acute mania. *Journal of Clinical Psychiatry*, **46**, 29–30.

Fyer, A.J., Liebowitz, M.R., Gorman, J.M., Campeas, R., Levin, A., Davies, S.O., Goetz, D., and Klein, D.F. (1987). Discontinuation of alprazolam treatment in panic patients. *American Journal of Psychiatry*, **144**, 303–8.

Gardner, D.L. and Cowdry, R.W. (1985). Alprazolam-induced dyscontrol in border-line personality disorder. *American Journal of Psychiatry*, **142**, 98–100.

Gardos, G., Dimascio, A., Salzman, C., and Shader, R.I. (1968). Differential actions of chlordiazepoxide and oxazepam on hostility. *Archives of General Psychiatry*, **18**, 757–60.

Garza-Trevino, E.S. and Hollister, L. (1988). Haloperidol combined with lorazepam for agitation. In *Continuing medical education syllabus and scientific proceedings*, p. 75. American Psychiatric Press, Washington, DC.

Greenblatt, D.J. and Shader, R.I. (1974). *Benzodiazepines in clinical practice*. Raven Press, New York.

Greenblatt, D.J., Shader, R.I., and Abernethy, D.R. (1983*a*). Current status of benzodiazepines, Part I. *New England Journal of Medicine*, **309**, 354–8.

Greenblatt, D.J., Shader, R.I., and Abernethy, D.R. (1983*b*). Current status of benzodiazepines, Part II. *New England Journal of Medicine*, **309**, 410–16.

Greenspan, D. and Levin, D. (1985). Use of clonazepam in a patient with schizoaffective disorder. *American Journal of Psychiatry*, **142**, 774–5.

Guz, I., Moraes, R., and Sartoretto, J.N. (1972). The therapeutic effects of lorazepam in psychotic patients treated with haloperidol: a double-blind study. *Current Therapy Research*, **14**, 767–74.

Howell, E.F., Laraia, M., Ballenger, J.C., *et al.* (1987). Lorazepam treatment of panic disorder. A paper read before the 140th Annual Meeting of the American Psychiatric Association, Chicago, 13 May 1987.

Jimerson, D.C., van Kammen, D.P., Post, R.M., Docherty, J.P., Bunney, W.E.

(1982). Diazepam in schizophrenia: a preliminary double-blind trial. *American Journal of Psychiatry*, **139**, 489–91.

Karson, C.N., Weinberger, D.R., Bigelow, L., Wyatt, R.J. (1982). Clonazepam treatment of chronic schizophrenia: negative results in a double-blind, placebo-controlled trial. *American Journal of Psychiatry*, **139** (12), 1627–8.

Kochansky, G.E., Salzman, C., Shader, R.I., Harmatz, J.S., and Ogletree, A.M. (1978). The differential effects of chlordiazepoxide and oxazepam on hostility in a small group setting. *American Journal of Psychiatry*, **132**, 861–3.

Lader, M. and Petursson, H. (1981). Benzodiazepine derivatives—side effects and dangers. *Biological Psychiatry*, **16**, 1195–201.

Lenox, R. (1988). Clinical management of manic agitation: double-blind comparison of lorazepam vs. haloperidol. In Proceedings of the American College of Psychopharmacology, San Juan, Puerto Rico, December 1988.

Liebowitz, M.R., Fyer, A.J., and Gorman, J.M. (1986). Alprazolam in the treatment of panic disorders. *Journal of Clinical Psychopharmacology*, **6**, 13–20.

Lion, J.R., Azcarate, C., and Koepke, H.H. (1975). 'Paradoxical rage reactions' during psychotropic medication. *Diseases of the Nervous System*, **36**, 557–8.

Lydiard, R.B., Laraia, M.T., and Ballenger, J.C. (1987). Emergence of depressive symptoms in patients receiving alprazolam for panic disorder. *American Journal of Psychiatry*, **144**, 664–5.

Mellinger, G.D. and Balter, M.B. (1981). Prevalence and patterns of use of psychotherapeutic drugs: results from a 1979 national survey of American adults. In *Epidemiological impact of psychotropic drugs* (ed. G. Tognoni, C. Bellantuono, and M. Lader), pp.117–35. Elsevier North Holland Inc, New York.

Mellinger, G.D. and Balter, M.B. (1983). Psychotherapeutic drugs: a current assessment of prevalence and patterns of use. In *Society and medication: conflicting signals of prescribers and patients* (ed. J.P. Morgan and D.V. Kagan), pp.137–44. DC Heath and Co, Lexington, Kentucky.

Mellinger, G.D., Balter, M.B., and Uhlenhuth, E.H. (1984a). Anti-anxiety agents: duration of use and characteristics of users in the USA. *Current Medical Research and Opinion*, **8** (suppl.), 21–36.

Mellinger, G.D., Balter, M.B., and Uhlenhuth, E.H. (1984b). Prevalence and correlates of the long-term regular use of anxiolytics. *Journal of the American Medical Association*, **251**, 375–9.

Mendoza, R., Djenderedjian, A.H., Adams, J., Ananth, J. (1987). Midazolam in acute psychotic patients with hyperarousal. *Journal of Clinical Psychiatry*, **48**, 291–2.

Modell, J.G. (1986). Letter: Further experience and observations with lorazepam in the management of behavioral agitation. *Journal of Clinical Psychopharmacology*, **6**, 385–7.

Modell, J.G., Lenox, R.H., and Weiner, S. (1985). Inpatient clinical trial of lorazepam for the management of manic agitation. *Journal of Clinical Psychopharmacology*, **5**, 109–13.

Nostoros, J.N., Suranyi-Cadotte, B.E., Speers, R.C., Schwartz, G., Nair, N.P.V. (1982). Diazepam in high doses is effective in schizophrenia. *Progress in Neuropsychopharmacology and Biological Psychiatry*, **6**, 513–16.

Nostoros, J.N., Nair, N.P.V., Pulman, J.R., Schwartz, G., Bloom, D. (1983). High doses of diazepam improve neuroleptic-resistant chronic schizophrenic patients. *Psychopharmacology*, **81**, 42–7.

Noyes, R., Anderson, D.J., Clancy, J., Crowe, R.R., Slymen, D.J., Ghoneim,

M.M., *et al.* (1984). Diazepam and propranolol in panic disorder and agoraphobia. *Archives of General Psychiatry*, **41**, 287–92.

Noyes, R.J. Jr, DuPont, R.L., Pecknold, J.C., Rifkin, A., Rubin, R.T., Swinson, R.P., Ballenger, J.C., and Burrows, G.D. (1988*a*). Alprazolam in panic disorder and agoraphobia: results from a multicenter trial. *Archives of General Psychiatry*, **45**, 423–8.

Noyes, R. Garvey, M.J., Cook, B.L., Perry, P.J. (1988*b*). Benzodiazepine withdrawal: a review of the evidence. *Journal of Clinical Psychiatry*, **49**, 382–9.

Pascualy, R. (1991). Benzodiazepines and sleep. In *Benzodiazepines in clinical practice: risks and benefits* (ed. P.P. Roy-Byrne and D.S. Cowley), pp.91–110. American Psychiatric Press, Washington, DC.

Pecknold, J.C., Swinson, R.P., Kuch, K., and Lewis, C.P. (1988). Alprazolam in panic disorder and agoraphobia: results from a multicenter trial. *Archives of General Psychiatry*, **45**, 429–35.

Pétursson, H. and Lader, M. (1984). *Dependence on tranquillizers*. Oxford University Press, New York.

Pollack, M.H. (1990). Long-term management of panic disorder. *Journal of Clinical Psychiatry*, **51** (suppl.), 11–13.

Pollack, M.H., Tesar, G.E., and Rosenbaum, J.F. (1986). Clonazepam in the treatment of panic disorder and agoraphobia: a one year follow-up. *Journal of Clinical Psychopharmacology*, **6**, 302–4.

Rickels, K. (1983). Benzodiazepines in the treatment of anxiety: North American experiences. In *The benzodiazepines: from molecular biology to clinical practice* (ed. E. Costa), pp.295–310. Raven Press, New York.

Rickels, K., Case, G.W., Winokur, A., Swenson, C. (1984). Long-term benzodiazepine therapy: benefits and risks. *Psychopharmacology Bulletin*, **20**, 608–15.

Rickels, K., Feighner, J.P., and Smith, W.T. (1985). Alprazolam, diazepam, imipramine, and placebo in outpatients with major depression. *Archives of General Psychiatry*, **42**, 134–41.

Rickels, K., Schweizer, E. (1987). Current pharmacotherapy of anxiety and panic. In *Psychopharmacology: The third generation of progress* (ed. H. Meltzer) pp.1193–203. Raven Press, New York.

Rosenbaum, J.F. (1990). A psychopharmacologist's perspective on panic disorder. *Bulletin of the Menninger Clinic*, **54**, 184–98.

Rosenbaum, J.F., Woods, S.W., Groves, J.E., and Klerman, G.L. (1984). Emergence of hostility during alprazolam treatment. *American Journal of Psychiatry*, **141**, 792–3.

Salzman, C. (1984). Benzodiazepine habituation and withdrawal. *Family Practice Recertification*, **6** (suppl.), 39–47.

Salzman, C. (1989). Treatment with antianxiety agents. In *American Psychiatric Association Task Force. Treatments of psychiatric disorders*, pp.2036–52. American Psychiatric Association, Washington, DC.

Salzman, C. (1991). Pharmacological treatment of anxiety. In *Anxiety in the elderly* (ed. C. Salzman and B. Lebowitz). Springer Verlag, New York.

Salzman, C. (1992). *Clinical geriatric psychopharmacolgy* (2nd edn). Williams & Wilkins, Baltimore, Maryland.

Salzman, C. and Green, A.I. (1987). Differential therapeutics: psychopharmacology. In *American Psychiatric Association Annual Review*, Vol. 6 (ed. R.E. Hales and A.J. Frances), pp.415–27. American Psychiatric Association, Washington, DC.

Salzman, C., Kochansky, G.E., Shader, R.I., Porrino, L.J., Harmatz, J.S., and Swett,

C.P. Jr (1974). Chlordiazepoxide-induced hostility in a small group setting. *Archives of General Psychiatry*, **31**, 401–5.

Salzman, C., Kochansky, G.E., Shader, R.I., Hermatz, J.S., Ogletree, A.M. (1975). Is oxazepam associated with hostility? *Diseases of the Nervous System*, **36**, 30–2.

Salzman, C., Green, A.I., Rodriguez Villa, F., Jaskiw, G.E. (1986). Benzodiazepines in combination with neuroleptics for the management of severe disruptive behavior. *Psychosomatics*, **27**, 17–21.

Salzman, C., Fisher, J., Nobel, K., and Wolfson, A. (1990). Abstract: Reversibility of benzodiazepine-induced memory impairment. In *Proceedings of the American College of Neuropsychopharmacology*. San Juan, Puerto Rico, December 1990.

Salzman, C., Solomon, D., Miyawaki, E., Glassman, R., Rood, L., Flowers, E., and Thayer, S. (1991). Parenteral lorazepam versus parenteral haloperidol for the control of psychotic disruptive behavior. *Journal of Clinical Psychiatry*, **52**, 177–80.

Santos, A.B. and Morton, W.A. (1987). More on clonazepam in manic agitation. *Journal of Clinical Psychopharmacology*, **7**, 439–40.

Santos, A.B. and Morton, W.A. (1989). Use of benzodiazepines to improve management of manic agitation. *Hospital and Community Psychiatry*, **40**, 1069–71.

Schatzberg, A.F. and Cole, J.O. (1981). Benzodiazepines in the treatment of depressive, borderline personality and schizophrenic disorders. *British Journal of Clinical Pharmacology*, **11**, (suppl.), 17–22.

Schweizer, E., Fox, I., Case, G., Rickels, K. (1988*a*). Lorazepam vs. alprazolam in the treatment of panic disorder. *Psychopharmacology Bulletin*, **24**, 224–7.

Schweizer, E., Rickels, K., Zavodnick, S., *et al.* (1988*b*). Clinical and medication status at 1 year follow-up after maintenance treatment of panic disorder. Presented at the CINP Congress, Munich, August 1988.

Shapiro, A.K., Struening, E.L., Shapiro, E., Milcarek, B.I. (1983). Diazepam: how much better than placebo? *Journal of Psychiatric Research*, **17**, 51–73.

Sheehan, D.V. (1987). Benzodiazepines in panic disorder and agoraphobia. *Journal of Affective Disorders*, **13**, 169–81.

Smith, D.E. and Wesson, D.R. (1985). Benzodiazepine dependency syndromes. In *The benzodiazepines. Current standards for medical practice* (ed. D.E. Smith and D.R. Wesson), pp.235–48. MTP Press Ltd, Lancaster, England.

Spier, S.A., Tesar, G.E., Rosenbaum, J.F., Woods, S.W. (1986). Treatment of panic disorder and agoraphobia with clonazepam. *Journal of Clinical Psychiatry*, **47**, 238–42.

Tesar, G.E. (1990). High-potency benzodiazepines for short-term management of panic disorder: the U.S. experience. *Journal of Clinical Psychiatry*, **51** (suppl.), 4–10.

Tesar, G.E. and Rosenbaum, J.F. (1986). Successful use of clonazepam in patients with treatment-resistant panic disorder. *Journal of Nervous and Mental Disorders*, **174**, 477–82.

Tesar, G.E., Rosenbaum, J.F., and Pollack, M.H. (1987). Clonazepam versus alprazolam in the treatment of panic disorder: interim analysis of data from a prospective, double-blind, placebo-controlled trial. *Journal of Clinical Psychiatry*, **48** (suppl.), 16–19.

Trimble, M.R. (1983). *Benzodiazepines divided*. John Wiley & Sons, New York.

Tyrer, P. (1983). The place of tranquilizers in the management of stress. *Journal of Psychosomatic Research*, **27**, 385–90.

Uhlenhuth, E.H., Matuzas, W., Glass, R.M., Easton, C. (1989). Response of panic disorder to fixed doses of alprazolam or imipramine. *Journal of Affective Disorders*, **17**, 261–70.

Victor, B.S., Link, N.A., Binder, R.L., Bell, I.R. (1984). Use of clonazepam in mania and schizoaffective disorders. *American Journal of Psychiatry*, **141**, 1111–12.

Ward, M.E., Saklad, S.R., and Ereshefsky, L. (1986). Letter: Lorazepam for the treatment of psychotic agitation. *American Journal of Psychiatry*, **143**, 1195–6.

Wolkowitz, O.M., Pickar, D., Doran, A., Breier, A., Tarell, J., Paul, S.M. (1986). Combination alprazolam–neuroleptic treatment of the positive and negative symptoms of schizophrenia. *American Journal of Psychiatry*, **143**, 85–7.

Wolkowitz, O.M., Breiz, A., Doran, A., Kelsoe, J., Lucas, P., Paul, S.M., Pickar, D. (1988). Alprazolam augmentation of the antipsychotic effects of fluphenazine in schizophrenic patients. *Archives of General Psychiatry*, **45**, 664–72.

Woods, J.H., Katz, J.L., and Winger, G.(1987). Abuse liability of benzodiazepines. *Pharmacological Reviews*, **39**, 251–419.

Woods, J.H., Katz, J.L., and Winger, G.(1988). Use and abuse of benzodiazepines. *Journal of the American Medical Association*, **260**, 3476–80.

3 The risks of taking benzodiazepines

Alyson Bond

It is easy to forget when writing about the risks of benzodiazepines that this group of drugs is one of the safest psychotropics to be synthesized so far and that, prior to their introduction, the risks of taking the alternatives were far greater. However, it is this very quality, safety, that led to their overprescribing in the 1960s and 1970s when they were variously and imaginatively named 'a bonanza' (Tyrer 1974) and 'the opium of the masses' (Lader 1978). The growth and extent of their prescription outside psychiatry for minor symptomatology has perhaps changed the definition of the risks. The risks of taking a benzodiazepine have then become not the province of the individual prescriber or recipient but those of society itself.

All drugs have risks. There is no such thing as an entirely safe drug but risks must be carefully balanced against benefits. In the case of severe chronic pervasive anxiety, benzodiazepine use, even chronic treatment, may be justified but even then the patient should be seen and assessed regularly. In the case of moderate, intermittent periods of anxiety and worry, benzodiazepine use should be limited and, in cases of reality-based worries, stress reactions, and bereavement, benzodiazepines should not be used. The greatest risk of benzodiazepine treatment is now thought to be dependence but that will be dealt with in other chapters. I shall discuss the other risks under three broad headings: biological; psychological; and social.

Biological risks

Although benzodiazepines are comparatively safe drugs they do carry certain biological risks. They may affect the central control of endocrine function and some benzodiazepines have been shown to increase plasma cortisol, prolactin concentrations, and growth hormone secretion (Ashton 1986). Because they are prescribed to twice as many women as men, their risks in pregnancy and breastfeeding are particularly important. All the benzodiazepine derivatives are lipophilic and exhibit rapid placental transfer with significant fetal uptake of the drug (Kanto 1982). Various deformaties in children exposed to benzodiazepines *in utero* have been described (Barry and St Clair 1987; Laegreid *et al.* 1987) but, in the absence of any controlled studies, a true estimate of the fetal risks apart from 'floppy infant syndrome' or neonatal depression is impossible. Meanwhile their use in pregnant women is contraindicated, especially in the first trimester. Benzodiazepines also pass into breast milk but the amount of drug transferred seems to be small unless maternal doses are very high (Buist *et al.* 1990). A short-acting benzodiazepine with less accumulation in plasma is recommended.

The elderly are another group to whom benzodiazepines are more commonly prescribed. They are also at greater risk because elimination half-lives are longer and accumulation of both the parent compound and the active metabolites is more likely to occur in this group. This leads to excessive sedation shown in ataxia, dysarthria, and toxic confusional states, which may be difficult to distinguish from dementia (Larson *et al.* 1987) and which are certainly worse in those with pre-existing cognitive impairment. The elderly who are prescribed benzodiazepines are also more likely to be suffering from general ill health and to be taking other prescribed drugs (Nolan and O'Malley 1988; Morgan 1990) and there is a risk of potentiation and central nervous system depression. The most common interaction, however, is with alcohol. This is a major cause for concern.

Psychological risks

Mental health

The use of benzodiazepines to treat stress and bereavement reactions has suppressed traumatic memories, including those of childhood sexual abuse and previous acts of violence, that can be vividly evoked upon withdrawal many years later (Risse *et al.* 1990). It seems that benzodiazepines may delay the normal posttraumatic stress reaction, which might have been dealt with in counselling. Although our techniques of counselling and dealing with posttraumatic stress disorder have become much more specific and skilful since the introduction of benzodiazepines, many people might have been able to mourn or cope with various types of abuse with the help of friends and relatives. The enlightened, perhaps only seeking some reassurance or guidance from their general practitioner, realized this and never took the prescribed tranquillizer. Others desisted after a few days because they disliked the feeling of being out of control. Yet many others persisted despite side-effects because, like smoking, they thought 'it was the thing to do' and, unlike smoking, it had been recommended by their doctor. It is not known if this group has special characteristics that separate them from other groups and lead to long-term dependence.

Just as benzodiazepines suppress these emotions, they can mask more serious psychiatric illness. Used correctly for a short period of time with concomitant advice, it has been suggested that they may be prophylactic and protect against the development of depression. However, they have also been implicated in an increased risk of impulsive suicide (Zisook and DeVaul 1977) and recently they have been shown to impede the full therapeutic effect of unilateral electroconvulsive therapy in depressed in-patients (Pettinati *et al.*

1990). If their use is continued for several years, more severe psychiatric illness may emerge on withdrawal (Olajide and Lader 1984). This illness is not a direct consequence of withdrawal but may not have been evident previously because of treatment with benzodiazepines.

Subjective sedation

Sedation is a known side-effect of benzodiazepines as it is of several other major groups of psychotropics. Despite improved specificity of action in comparison to the barbiturates, drowsiness or tiredness is still the most common side-effect even of the newer benzodiazepines (Dawson *et al.* 1984). Sedation is also the most common subjective side-effect in healthy volunteers and it can be detected on visual analogue scales after each dose even after a week's treatment (Bond *et al.* 1983). Although tolerance is said to occur in chronic use, this may in fact be an adjustment of expectation of normal alertness as patients on long-term treatment often exhibit a certain lack of spontaneity and a general dulling, which remits on withdrawal. Several prisoners who were compulsorily withdrawn from benzodiazepines admitted feeling better than they had felt for many years (Brown 1978). It must be stressed, however, that the withdrawal period was long and hard and that these prisoners were generally not being treated for chronic anxiety states. On the contrary, benzodiazepines were being used to sedate and control disruptive behaviour without any proven efficacy.

Objective effects in volunteers

Sedation can also be measured objectively in the laboratory. As the benzo-diazepines have been the most widely prescribed group of psychotropic drugs, they have also been the most widely investigated and so this section must of necessity be only a brief summary of such work. An excellent review appears in Woods *et al.* (1987). Most of the work has been conducted in healthy volunteers and this will be discussed first. Early work showed that psychological impairment could be measured on a variety of tasks several hours after consumption. A review of 27 studies (Wittenborn *et al.* 1979) indicated a positive relationship between magnitude of effect and dosage level but was unable to discriminate between benzodiazepines because of the few studies comparing different compounds and the diversity of the psychomotor tests used. However, it was possible to conclude that the functions showing consistent impairment were) : (1) speed of repetitive movements; and (2) acquisition of new material. There was little evidence that benzodiazepines affected faculties of visual–spatial, perceptual, verbal, and arithmetical ability, and the authors therefore concluded that there was relatively little indication at that time that well established higher mental faculties were adversely affected.

As well as acute effects, benzodiazepines have been shown to produce impairment for up to a day after use as hypnotics, even when several hours of sleep have intervened. A review of 52 studies (Johnson and Chernik 1982) concluded that all hypnotics produce decrements in performance the next day, the extent of this impairment being dependent on dose but not consistently on half-life. Most of the tasks used were psychomotor although some (digit symbol substitution test (DSST), sorting, cancellation) also had a cognitive element. The functions that showed consistent impairment were: (1) speed of performance, which the authors related to sedation and central nervous system depression, but also (2) anterograde memory, i.e. memory for information learned after drug administration. The latter effect, although well known and indeed very useful in the case of benzodiazepines used intravenously as pre-operative sedatives (Milligan *et al.* 1987), was not expected to accompany oral nighttime administration. These two factors did not differ between healthy volunteers and insomniac patients.

Putting the results of these two reviews together there is some considerable agreement. Both reviews found that tasks involving speed and learning were most affected and those involving co-ordination and spatial abilities were least affected. The difference between them was in the sensitivity of the critical flicker fusion threshold (CFFT) but an earlier review of CFFT and psychotropic drugs (Smith and Misiak 1976) found that the threshold was altered in 65 per cent of studies and the threshold was decreased by sedative drugs. This lends support to the findings of Wittenborn *et al.* (1979) and has been confirmed in several studies since (Hindmarch 1988).

The results of studies on higher functions, showing that learning and anterograde memory are the most sensitive and retrograde memory the least sensitive to benzodiazepine effects, have been further clarified by a specialized review on memory and benzodiazepines (Curran 1986). This review confirmed that memory for information acquired pre-drug (retrograde memory) was not impaired by benzodiazepines and may even be improved acutely (retrograde facilitation) because of reduced retroactive interference from other information acquired post drug intake. Anterograde amnesia was again shown to be common with all benzodiazepines. The most sensitive tasks were those of increased complexity and involving a delay in recall because more demands were made on memory.

If we summarize the functions most affected by benzodiazepines, also taking into account later work, we are able to draw three major conclusions as shown in Table 3.1. These effects were mainly found in healthy volunteer subjects. This is important because these studies offer precise, controlled measurement of performance changes pre- and post-drug and allow us to determine which functions are potentially impaired by the substance rather than by the illness or therapeutic response. It is also important to remember that benzodiazepines have often been prescribed to normal healthy people with a transient problem whose functioning pre-drug would be closer to that of normal volunteers than to that of psychiatric patients with more serious or chronic problems.

Table 3.1. Major effects of benzodiazepines on performance

Speed of repetitive movements

In simple motor tests, e.g. tapping or sorting
As a component of more complex tests, e.g. cancellation or scanning
In the time domain of tasks of old learning, e.g. arithmetic

Acquisition of new material

In coding tests, e.g. DSST
In learning tests, e.g. paired associates

Anterograde amnesia

In recall tasks
In delayed retrieval

There is some evidence that tolerance develops to the sedative effects of benzodiazepines after 1 or 2 weeks of continuous administration. However, because of the few studies completed with more than 1 or 2 weeks of treatment using therapeutic doses, in which clear tolerance has been shown, this widely held belief is difficult to substantiate with more complex or cognitive tasks. In fact, such patient work as has been done tends to negate it.

Objective effects in patients

Anxiety itself can be a potent impairer of performance. Benzodiazepines are often assumed to counteract these debilitating effects of anxiety but we found some years ago that, although patients' performance was indeed impaired pretreatment, it was not improved by several weeks of benzodiazepine medication (Bond *et al.* 1974*a,b*). There are, in fact, too few studies in patient populations to determine if their responses differ greatly from those of controls. It is evident from the review on hypnotics that insomniacs do not differ from controls in their experience of effects on performance and there is some evidence that similar functions are affected in anxious patients too (Linnoila *et al.* 1983; Woods *et al.* 1987). Similar functions to those in normal controls were also affected in patients with panic disorder (Roy-Byrne *et al.* 1990), although in this small study it was found that the patients were less sensitive to the effects of diazepam and required three times as much drug to obtain the same effects. A study of an acute dose in 22 long-term users revealed impairment on a delayed recall task (Lucki *et al.* 1986) and a more recent study in long-term users (Golombok *et al.* 1988) showed that performance was still impaired after at least 1 year's treatment as compared to that of two control groups. The tasks affected were again those requiring the ability to perform simple repetitive tasks and the acquisition of new material. In addition, tasks measuring visual–spatial ability showed impairment but, surprisingly, memory tasks did not. The authors explain the discrepancy with previous work on visual–spatial ability as being due to their tasks requiring more elaborate processing of information, but there is no convincing explanation for their lack of memory effects. In a recent, as yet unpublished study we have found both psychomotor and memory effects to be still measurable after 8 weeks of treatment in agoraphobic patients taking a relatively high dose of alprazolam (mean dose, 5.25 mg) compared to those taking placebo (Bruce, Bond, Curran, and O'Sullivan, personal communication).

Risk of accidents

It has been suggested that the use of benzodiazepines contributes to an increased risk of accidents both on the road and elsewhere. Formal studies of the risk of road accidents have approached the problem from two different angles. On the one hand, numerous laboratory tasks of simulated driving and even real driving tasks, both under controlled conditions named 'closed course' and in real traffic in a specially monitored car (O'Hanlon and de Gier 1986), have been developed. On the other hand, epidemiological investigations have concentrated on implying drug intake from self-report or prescription monitoring or more scientifically from measuring benzo- diazepine levels in the body fluids of people involved in accidents. Generally, benzodiazepines have been shown to adversely affect both simulated driving performance and actual driving ability. These methods have been criticized as not analogous to 'real' driving (Woods et al. 1987) but some agreement has been shown between the different methods, at least for alcohol effects (Gawron and Ranney 1988). One prospective epidemiological study carried out in the UK (Skegg et al. 1979) estimated the relative risk of an accident in which injury or death occurred to be 4.9 times greater when 'tranquillizers' were deemed (by prescription) to be present. However, epidemiological studies also suffer from many uncontrolled variables. First, psychiatric or medical patients may be at increased risk for accidents regardless of whether or not they are taking medication. Second, the fact that drugs were pre- scribed does not mean they were being taken at the time of the accident. Third, even if drugs can be detected this does not mean that they were behaviourally active at the time of the accident. Fourth, the presence of other drugs as well as alcohol is frequently a complicating factor. This means that a causal relationship can seldom be assumed. Epidemiological studies have found a frequency of benzodiazepine use ranging from 0.8 to 20 per cent but those studies that have attempted most control and have used a reference group, who were driving at similar locations and times to those at which accidents occurred, have not consistently demonstrated that benzodiazepine users are overrepresented either in the population of arrested drivers or of those involved in road traffic accidents whether fatal or not.

Far fewer studies have attempted to examine the incidence of benzo-diazepine use in other types of accident. One study of accident- and injury-related health-care utilization in the USA (Oster *et al*. 1987) did find that benzodiazepine users were significantly more likely to experience an accident, estimated from their use of accident-related health care, than non-users, but they were also more likely to use non-accident-related health care, which means that this group may just be more likely to use any sort of health care facilities more, presumably including benzodiazepines. There is thus little evidence to implicate the use of benzodiazepines as causal in industrial accidents. However, there is some evidence that the elderly may be more prone to fall while receiving such medication although this may not result in increased bone fractures (Hale *et al*. 1985). Hale *et al*.'s study was based on interview data, but another study of hospitalized patients found no difference in falls among younger patients but confirmed that patients over 70 years old who fell were more likely to have received a prescription for flurazepam (Kramer and Schoen 1984). Benzodiazepines have also been implicated in drug-associated hospital admissions (Kruse 1990).

Social risks

Benzodiazepine use has been found to affect a wide range of social behaviours with the type and severity of effects probably depending on the individual compound, route of administration, dose, and chronicity of usage as well as on the social circumstances themselves. Chronic use has often been said to cause an apathetic state with dulling of emotions. This observation has not been confirmed in a widespread study of social behaviours. Caplan *et al*. (1985) found no difference between diazepam users and non-users with respect to the relationship between social stresses and emotions. This difference may be explained by different populations of users. The apathetic state has usually been noted in or complained of by those wishing to come off long-term treatment and may also be more prevalent with benzodiazepines other than diazepam, whereas the study groups were chosen because they had recently filed a prescription for diazepam. In fact patients switched from lorazepam to diazepam prior to withdrawal in our department often report a dramatic temporary improvement in mood and social functioning (Morton, personal communication). Another study, again looking at diazepam, also found no difference in supervisor's ratings of work performance (Proctor 1981). Absenteeism, although less in users of no medication, did not differ between those reporting use of diazepam and those reporting use of some other medication.

Benzodiazepines have also been implicated in the risk of child abuse and reports have emerged of patients committing uncharacteristic antisocial acts such as shoplifting or sexual offences. However, some patient reports of sexual assault when, for example, benzodiazepines have been used for minor surgery have been shown to be due to fantasies (Brahams 1990). There is, in fact, little hard evidence for any of these reports, but they may be linked to disinhibition and other paradoxical effects that will be discussed under aggression.

Risk of abuse

Benzodiazepines can lead to euphoria (Griffiths *et al.* 1984) and therefore do have some abuse liability especially when used in high doses or intravenously. It has been shown that both abstinent alcoholics and the sons of alcoholics experience drug-induced changes in euphoria in response to benzodiazepines (Ciraulo *et al.* 1988, 1989) and may therefore be at high risk for abuse. Benzo-diazepines are also used by multiple drug users to potentiate opioid effects and temper the effects of stopping stimulants. It is rare for benzodiazepines to be abused on their own but this is partly due to their insolubility in water. Thus, when temazepam was marketed in the UK in liquid-filled capsules to speed absorption, drug-abusers were quick to employ syringes to inject the contents and this led eventually to the withdrawal of this formulation. As the recreational use of benzodiazepines is largely confined to people who already abuse other drugs it seems likely that they do not have a great inherent potential for abuse but are chosen when other supplies are not available. It should be noted here that patients generally do not escalate their doses of benzodiazepines but often remain on the same dose for years.

Enhancement of aggression

In their early development, benzodiazepines were claimed not only to be anxiolytic and calming but also to have anti-aggressive properties. This was despite the facts that the animal literature had always been equivocal on this point (Rodgers and Waters 1985) and that the first reports of rage attacks had come soon after release (Boyle and Tobin 1961). Such attacks have been labelled as paradoxical reactions as they tend to occur in isolated cases and frequently at high doses (Bond and Lader 1979). Nevertheless, they have continued to be reported at a fairly constant rate and with newer benzodiazepines (Rosenbaum *et al.* 1984). Problems of disinhibition and increased hostility have also been noted following the general use of benzodiazepines (Zisook and DeVaul 1977; Pyke and Kraus 1988) and their use as anticonvulsants particularly in children (Browne 1978). These clinical observations have led to more precise laboratory investigations. A variety of techniques has been used (Bond 1990) and, in all the studies that have been done, increased aggressive responding has consistently been found after benzodiazepines. However, differential effects have also been shown depending on the compound used. In particular, oxazepam, which is very similar to its chlorinated derivative lorazepam, has not been shown to affect aggression and is therefore the recommended benzodiazepine when there is any evidence of poor impulse control or personality disorder (Salzman *et al.* 1975; Lion 1979). In contrast to this evidence, benzodiazepines have been used successfully in the management of aggressive behaviour (Bond and Lader 1979), and it has been suggested from animal work that benzodiazepines enhance aggression only when basal levels are low to moderate (Mos and Olivier 1987). Although early case reports often cited patients who had experienced previous episodes of disturbed behaviour, later reports cite patients with no previous history of aggressive dyscontrol (Dietch and Jennings 1988), and high doses are frequently used in the control of severe disruptive behaviour in psychiatric hospitals. In particular, intramuscular lorazepam is an effective means of sedating assaultive patients when administered in conjunction with intramuscular haloperidol. However, this is only effective as an acute measure for 'rapid tranquillization', and there is no support for the routine or maintenance use of benzodiazepines in conjunction with neuroleptic treatment for the prevention of disruptive behaviour (Salzman 1988).

Interaction with alcohol

All the aforementioned effects of benzodiazepines are increased by their combination with alcohol. Effects on performance are generally additive (Sellers and Busto 1982), and there is some evidence for potentiation after acute doses although cross-tolerance may occur in chronic use. Behavioural effects such as disinhibition or aggression are enhanced by the addition of alcohol, and severe confusion and aggressive and violent outbursts, including acts culminating in murder, often with ensuing memory loss have been reported. It is likely that alcohol is the dominant partner in this combination but patients should be warned of the risks of taking alcohol or indeed any other central nervous system depressant while being prescribed a benzodiazepine.

Summary

The major risks of benzodiazepines come from their widespread use. Their biological risks are not severe compared to those of other psychotropic medication, but they should be used cautiously in pregnant women and the elderly. They may suppress traumatic memories and mask serious psychiatric disorder. They have replicable effects on behaviour, in particular on sedation, speed of repetitive movements, new learning, and anterograde memory, which have been shown in both volunteers and patients. They may increase accidents, particularly in the elderly. They are abused by alcoholics and multiple drug users. They have been implicated in both a general disinhibition of social behaviour and, in particular, in an increase in irritability and hostility leading to aggression in certain circumstances. While this chapter is not concerned with differences between benzodiazepines, it should be noted that oxazepam seems to differ from other benzodiazepines in terms of dependence and abuse potential, withdrawal problems, and effects on memory and aggression, and, therefore, in its 'risk potential'.

References

Ashton, H. (1986). Adverse effects of prolonged benzodiazepine use. *Adverse Drug Reaction Bulletin*, **118**, 440–3.

Barry, W.S. and St Clair, S.M. (1987). Exposure to benzodiazepines in utero. *Lancet*, i, 1436–7.

Bond, A.J. (1990). Pharmacological manipulation of aggressiveness and impulsiveness in healthy volunteers. *Clinical Neuropharmacology*, **13** (Suppl. 2), 251–2.

Bond, A.J. and Lader, M.H. (1979). Benzodiazepines and aggression. In *Psychopharmacology of aggression* (ed. M. Sandler), pp. 173–82. Raven Press, New York.

Bond, A.J., James, D.C., and Lader, M.H. (1974*a*). Physiological and psychological measures in anxious patients. *Psychological Medicine*, **4**, 364–73.

Bond, A.J., James, D.C., and Lader, M.H. (1974*b*). Sedative effects on physiological and psychological measures in anxious patients. *Psychological Medicine*, **4**, 374–80.

Bond, A., Lader, M., and Shotriya, R. (1983). Comparative effects of a repeated dose regime of diazepam and buspirone on subjective ratings, psychological tests and the EEG. *European Journal of Clinical Pharmacology*, **24**, 463–7.

Boyle, D. And Tobin, J.M. (1961). Pharmaceutical management of behaviour disorders: chlordiazepoxide in covert and overt expressions of aggression. *Journal of the Medical Society of New Jersey*, **58**, 427–9.

Brahams, D. (1990). Medicine and the law; benzodiazepines and sexual fantasies. *Lancet*, **335**, 157.

Brown, C.R. (1978). The use of benzodiazepines in prison populations. *Journal of Clinical Psychiatry*, **39**, 219–22.

Browne, T.R. (1978). Clonazepam. *New England Journal of Medicine*, **299**, 812–16.

Buist, A., Norman, T.R., and Dennerstein, L. (1990). Breastfeeding and the use of psychotropic medication: a review. *Journal of Affective Disorders*, **19**, 197–206.

Caplan, R.D., Andrews, F.M., Conway, T.L., Abbey, A., Abramis, D.J., and French, J.R.P. (1985). Social effects of diazepam use: a longitudinal field study. *Social Science and Medicine*, **21**, 887–98.

Ciraulo, D.A., Barnhill, J.G., Greenblatt, D.J., Shader, R.I., Ciraulo, A.M., Tarmey, M.F., Molloy, M.A., and Foti, M.E. (1988). Abuse liability and clinical pharmacokinetics of alprazolam in alcoholic men. *Journal of Clinical Psychiatry*, **49**, 333–7.

Ciraulo, D.A., Barnhill, J.G., Ciraulo, A.M., Greenblatt, D.J., and Shader, R.I. (1989). Parental alcoholism as a risk factor in benzodiazepine abuse: a pilot study. *American Journal of Psychiatry*, **146**, 1333–5.

Curran, H.V. (1986). Tranquillising memories: a review of the effects of benzodiazepines on human memory. *Biological Psychology*, **23**, 179–213.

Dawson, G.W., Jue, S.G., and Brogden, R.N. (1984). Alprazolam. A review of its pharmacodynamic properties and efficacy in the treatment of anxiety and depression. *Drug Evaluation*, **27**, 132–47.

Dietch, J.T. and Jennings, R.K. (1988). Aggressive dyscontrol in patients treated with benzodiazepines. *Journal of Clinical Psychiatry*, **49**, 184–8.

Gawron, V.J. and Ranney, T.A. (1988). The effect of alcohol dosing on driving performance on a closed course and in a driving simulator. *Ergonomics*, **31**, 1219–44.

Golombok, S., Moodley, P., and Lader, M. (1988). Cognitive impairment in long-term benzodiazepine users. *Psychological Medicine*, **18**, 365–74.

Griffiths, R.R., McLeod, D.R., Bigelow, G.E., Liebson, I.A., and Roache, J.D. (1984). Relative abuse liability of diazepam and oxazepam: behavioural and subjective dose effects. *Psychopharmacology*, **84**, 141–54.

Hale, W.E., Marks, R., and Stewart, R.B. (1985). Antianxiety drugs and central nervous system symptoms in an ambulatory elderly population. *Drug Intelligence and Clinical Pharmacy*, **19**, 37–40.

Hindmarch, I. (1988). Information processing, critical flicker fusion threshold and benzodiazepines: results and speculations. In *Benzodiazepine receptor ligands, memory and information processing. Psychometric, psychopharmacological and clinical issues, Psychopharmacology Series no.6* (ed. I. Hindmarch and H. Ott), pp.78–89. Springer-Verlag, Heidelberg.

Johnson, L.C. and Chernik, D.A. (1982). Sedative–hypnotics and human performance. *Psychopharmacology*, **76**, 101–13.

Kanto, J.H. (1982). Use of benzodiazepines during pregnancy, labour and lactation, with particular reference to pharmacokinetic considerations. *Drugs*, **23**, 354–80.

Kramer, M. and Schoen, L.S. (1984). Problems in the use of long-acting hypnotics in older patients. *Journal of Clinical Psychiatry*, **45**, 176–7.

Kruse, W.H.H. (1990). Problems and pitfalls in the use of benzodiazepines in the elderly. *Drug Experience*, **5**, 328–44.

Lader, M. (1978). Benzodiazepines—The opium of the masses. *Neuroscience*, **3**, 159–65.

Laegreid, L., Olegard, R., and Wahlstroms, C.N. (1987). Abnormalities in children exposed to benzodiazepines in utero. *Lancet*, **i**, 108–9.

Larson, E.B., Kukull, W.A., Buchner, D., and Reifler, B.V. (1987). Adverse drug reactions associated with global cognitive impairment in elderly persons. *Annals of Internal Medicine*, **107**, 169–73.

Linnoila, M., Erwin, C.W., Brendle, A., and Simpson, D. (1983). Psychomotor effects of diazepam in anxious patients and healthy volunteers. *Journal of Clinical Psychopharmacology*, **3**, 88–96.

Lion, J.R. (1979). Benzodiazepines in the treatment of aggressive patients. *Journal of Clinical Psychiatry*, **40**, 70–1.

Lucki, I., Rickels, K., and Geller, A.M. (1986). Chronic use of benzodiazepines and psychomotor and cognitive test performance. *Psychopharmacology*, **88**, 426–33.

Milligan, D.W., Howard, M.R., and Judd, A. (1987). Premedication with lorazepam before bone marrow biopsy. *Journal of Clinical Pathology*, **40**, 696–8.

Morgan, K. (1990). Hypnotics in the elderly. What cause for concern? *Drugs*, **40**, 688–96.

Mos, J. and Olivier, B. (1987). Pro-aggressive actions of benzodiazepines. In *Ethopharmacology of agonistic behaviour in animals and humans* (ed. B. Olivier, J. Mos, and P.F. Brain), pp. 187–206. Martinus Nijhoff, Dordrecht.

Nolan, L. and O'Malley, K. (1988). Patients, prescribing, and benzodiazepines. *European Journal of Clinical Pharmacology*, **35**, 225–9.

Olajide, D. and Lader, M.H. (1984). Depression following withdrawal from long-term benzodiazepine use: a report of four cases. *Psychological Medicine*, **14**, 937–40.

O'Hanlon, J.F. and de Gier, J.J. (1986). *Drugs and driving*. Taylor and Francis, London.

Oster, G., Russell, M.W., Huse, D.M., Adams, S.F., and Imbimbo, J. (1987). Accident- and injury-related health-care utilization among benzodiazepine users and nonusers. *Journal of Clinical Psychiatry*, **48** (suppl.) 17–21.

Pettinati, H.M., Stephens, S.M., Willis, K.M., and Robin, S.E. (1990). Evidence for less improvement in depression in patients taking benzodiazepines during unilateral ECT. *American Journal of Psychiatry*, **147**, 1029–35.

Proctor, R.C. (1981). Prescription medication in the workplace:occupational absenteeism, accidents, and performance when using non-psychoactive and psychoactive medication. *North Carolina Medical Journal*, **42**, 545–7.

Pyke, R.E. and Kraus, M. (1988). Alprazolam in the treatment of panic attack patients with and without major depression. *Journal of Clinical Psychiatry*, **49**, 66–8.

Risse, S.C., Whitters, A., Burke, J., Chen, S., Scurfield, R.M., and Raskind, M.A. (1990). Severe withdrawal symptoms after discontinuation of alprazolam in eight patients with combat-induced posttraumatic stress disorder. *Journal of Clinical Psychiatry*, **51**, 206–9.

Rodgers, R.J. and Waters, A.J. (1985). Benzodiazepines and their antagonists: a pharmacoethological analysis with particular reference to effects on aggression. *Neuroscience and Biobehavioral Reviews*, **9**, 21–35.

Rosenbaum, J.F., Woods, S.W., Groves, J.E., and Klerman, G.L. (1984). Emergence of hostility during alprazolam treatment. *American Journal of Psychiatry*, **141**, 792–3.

Roy-Byrne, P.P., Cowley, D.S., Greenblatt, D.J., Shader, R.I., and Hommer, D. (1990). Reduced benzodiazepine sensitivity in panic disorder. *Archives of General Psychiatry*, **47**, 534–8.

Salzman, C. (1988). Use of benzodiazepines to control disruptive behaviour in inpatients. *Journal of Clinical Psychiatry*, **49** (suppl.), 13–15.

Salzman, C. Kochansky, G.E., Shader, R.I., Harmhatz, J.S., and Ogletree, A.M. (1975). Is oxazepam associated with hostility? *Disorders of the Nervous System*, **36**, 30–2.

Sellers, E.M. and Busto, U. (1982). Benzodiazepines and ethanol: assessment of the effects and consequences of psychotropic drug interactions. *Journal of Clinical Psychopharmacology*, **2**, 249–62.

Skegg, D.C.G., Richards, S.M., and Doll, R. (1979). Minor tranquillizers and road accidents. *British Medical Journal*, **1**, 917–19.

Smith, J.M. and Misiak, H. (1976). Critical flicker fusion (CFF) and psychotropic drugs in normal human subjects—a review. *Psychopharmacology*, **47**, 175–82.

Tyrer, P. (1974). The benzodiazepine bonanza. *Lancet*, **i**, 709–10.

Wittenborn, J.R., Flaherty, C.F., McGough, W.E., and Nash, R.J. (1979). Psychomotor changes during initial day of benzodiazepine medication. *British Journal of Clinical Pharmacology*, **7**, 69S–76S.

Woods, J.H., Katz, J.L., and Winger, G. (1987). Abuse liability of benzodiazepines. *Pharmacological Reviews*, **39**, 251–413.

Zisook, S. and De Vaul, R.A. (1977). Adverse behavioral effects of benzodiazepines. *Journal of Family Practice*, **5**, 963–6.

4 Historical development of the concept of tranquillizer dependence

Malcolm Lader

The term 'tranquillizer' has become almost synonymous with 'benzodiazepine' as this group of chemical compounds has for so long dominated the scene. However, the use of benzodiazepines and the development over the last 30 years of the concept of normal-dose dependence on these compounds must be set into the context of the earlier widespread use of other sedatives such as the barbiturates and, even further back, related to the use of alcohol-containing beverages.

The widespread use of such substances has almost inevitably provoked considerable concern and comment both within and without the medical profession. Some of this concern reflected a general unease that such extensive usage could not be justified in terms of need and that such usage was dealing superficially and symptomatically with problems arising from socio-economic strains within human societies. The accrual of evidence suggesting that the bulk of long-term usage involved a dependence process, even on normal therapeutic doses, provided the means for those who deprecated the too easy resort to tranquillizers to point to specific rather than unfocused dangers. The controversy continues, particularly as medicolegal aspects become increasingly prominent.

Most of the players in the tranquillizer story are still active in psycho-pharmacology and psychiatry. Any attempt at a disinterested, dispassionate account of the history of the topic would require a non-involved historian to do it justice, rather than myself, one of the players. Many issues are still unresolved and the contributions of various key individuals remain unclear. The archives of the pharmaceutical companies involved remain private property.

This chapter represents my attempt to set down the story of tranquillizer dependence as I see it from my vantage point of being closely involved for about 30 years in the study of the benzodiazepines. That is within one professional lifetime, within one set of skills and experience, within the geographical limitations of concentrating on the UK scene, and within the inescapable biasses that have undoubtedly influenced my judgement. Despite this I hope that I give a reasonably fair account; the reader must decide if I am justified in this hope.

Early history

The present time has been dubbed the 'age of anxiety' (Auden 1946 p.20), 'Then back they come, The fears that we fear.' Despite this, there is no evidence that states of morbid anxiety are either more frequent or more severe than hitherto. Indeed, accounts of the Black Death in the Middle Ages suggest that we live in an age of relative tranquillity—not all chemically-induced! Man, therefore, has always sought ways of lessening his anxiety and of escaping from the realities of daily drudgery.

The use of alcohol stretches back at least 8000 years from the discovery of fermentation possibly in what is now the nation of Georgia. Originally, alcohol had a mostly religious role in primitive societies and its use was highly regulated. Later it was taken medicinally, often as an anxiolytic, and was abused by some. When the Arabs introduced the technique of distillation into Europe in the Middle Ages, the alchemist and his customers hailed alcohol as the long-sought elixir of life. The Gaelic 'usquebaugh', meaning water of life, the term for whisky, was regarded as a panacea. But by the eighteenth century with the introduction of cheap gin, the curses of alcohol had become apparent. We have had an uneasy and ambivalent attitude to alcohol ever since, viz. prohibition in the USA 70 years ago.

Opium also has a history extending over thousands of years and was extolled by Sydenham in 1680 as the most universal and efficacious of 'the remedies which it has pleased Almighty God to give to man to relieve his sufferings'. Like alcohol, opium and its derivatives were taken to relieve anxiety and depression. Like alcohol its addictive properties became increasingly apparent. For example, during the nineteenth century, De Quincey, a habitué, dubbed it 'dread agent of unimaginable pleasure and pain'.

Synthetic chemicals

The nineteenth century also witnessed the effects of the Industrial Revolution, which transformed alchemy into chemistry and old wives' nostrums into pharmaceutical remedies. Nitrous oxide was introduced as a dental and surgical anaesthetic, as were ether and chloroform. The first psychotropic drug to institute that noble tradition of discovery by mistake (serendipity) was bromide. Because potassium bromide was believed to lessen sexual urges and because epilepsy was ascribed to excessive masturbation, bromides were introduced by Locock for the treatment of epilepsy, apparently with gratifying results! By the 1870s bromides were used very widely as sedatives and, again, the dependence potential eventually became apparent, and the drug lapsed into desuetude.

Two organic chemicals were synthesized and introduced as sedatives. Chloral hydrate has retained some usage in its solid derivative forms particularly in the elderly; paraldehyde, however, is obsolete. Both are associated with abuse and dependence.

The most widely used synthetics were the barbiturates. Barbituric acid was prepared by Adolf von Baeyer working in Kekulé's laboratory. The first hypnotic barbiturate, barbitone ('Veronal') was introduced by Fischer and von Mering in 1903, followed by phenobarbitone ('Luminal') in 1912. Amylobarbitone came on the market in 1923. About 2500 barbiturate compounds were synthesized over the succeeding years and about 50 were marketed, of which a dozen or so survive.

It is instructive at this juncture to examine the use of barbiturates in the middle of the present century. A variety of sources suggest that the extent of usage of sedative/tranquillizer/hypnotic medications has remained at much the same level relative to all drug use since the earliest records of prescriptions were available (Woods *et al.* 1987). The percentage of the total has been about 10 per cent until quite recently when it has dropped to about 7.5 per cent. The prescriptions for tranquillizers have dropped proportionately more than those for hypnotics. It must be remembered, however, that overall prescription rates have tended to increase in the past 50 years, so a declining proportion may still mean some absolute increase.

During the peak of their popularity barbiturates were extremely widely prescribed. In the UK production of barbiturates doubled between 1938 and 1946, doubled again by 1950, and then levelled off. However, the abuse and dependence-inducing properties of these compounds became increasingly apparent and, together with alarm over the dangers of overdose, led to a campaign by the UK medical profession in the 1970s to educate prescribing doctors to replace the barbiturates with the benzodiazepines. Other compounds with similar pharmacological properties were introduced but met a similar fate as their dependence potential and toxicity became apparent. They include ethchlorvynol, ethinamate, carbromal, glutethimide, methyprylon, and methaqualone.

In retrospect the story of meprobamate seems like a dress rehearsal for that of the benzodiazepines. This story begins with the discovery of mephenesin in 1946 by Berger and Bradley (Berger 1970). Mephenesin is a muscle relaxant but it has too short a duration of action for practical use in anxiety disorders. Meprobamate (Miltown, Equanil) was developed from it in 1950 as a longer-acting compound. It was widely promoted and widely prescribed as a tranquillizer but was found to have an alarming dependence potential. Thus, by 1964 there existed 'ample evidence that it could induce physical dependence in man' (Essig 1964). Although still available and indeed quite widely used in some countries because of its cheapness (as are the barbiturates), it has largely been supplanted by the benzodiazepines.

Discovery of the benzodiazepines

The story of the benzodiazepines stretches back to Cracow in Poland in the mid-1930s. Dr Leo Sternbach was working on a chemical grouping called the heptoxdiazines (Sternbach 1980). He went to the USA and resumed work on these compounds in the Chemical Research Department of Hoffmann–La Roche USA in Nutley, New Jersey. Disappointingly, they seemed biologically inactive. However, one, Ro#5–0690, was investigated further and in 1957 was found to have hypnotic, sedative, and antistrychnine effects, similar to those of meprobamate (Cohen 1970). To the surprise of the chemists this compound was found to have undergone a spontaneous molecular rearrangement to become a 1:4 benzodiazepine.

The first clinical tests nearly led to the drug (first called methaminodiazepoxide and later chlordiazepoxide) being discarded because it was tested at too large a dose in elderly patients and dysarthria and ataxia were frequent. Quite quickly, however, its clinical effectiveness in appropriate dosage was established, and it was introduced to the market in 1960. Its even more successful congener, diazepam, followed in 1963.

Many other compounds were introduced either as daytime tranquillizers or nighttime hypnotics or both. The most successful have been nitrazepam, flurazepam, temazepam, and triazolam as hypnotics, and diazepam, lorazepam, and alprazolam as tranquillizers. The last is currently the market leader in terms of value. The dates of introduction in the UK of various benzodiazepines are shown in Table 4.1. The tranquillizer market is currently worth US$2 billion worldwide, and is still growing in value as newer, more expensive compounds replace older, cheaper, usually generic compounds.

Dependence potential

A crucial question is why our adverse experiences with the barbiturates and similar drugs did not put us on our guard with respect to similar problems with the benzodiazepines. Although, attempts had been made to distance the benzodiazepines from the barbiturates, both in pharmacological and clinical terms, it was only the safety in overdose of the benzodiazepines compared with barbiturate lethality which truly distinguished them. This aura of safety generalized to side-effects and dependence potential. Furthermore, as we shall soon see, the relative paucity of cases of high-dose dependence seemed reassuring.

High-dose dependence

In the early 1960s two studies explored the capability of the benzodiazepines to induce a physical dependence state when the drugs were given at a high dose for several weeks. In the first, 36 chronically psychotic patients were administered 300 to 600 mg/day of chlordiazepoxide for 2 to 6 months (Hollister *et al.* 1961). These doses are several times the usual recommended clinical dose but the patients managed to tolerate them. Then the drug was abruptly discontinued in 11 patients with single-blind placebo substitution but, because of the long elimination half-lives of some of the active metabolites of

Table 4.1. Year of introduction of benzodiazepines to UK

Generic name	Brand (manufacturer)	Sold since
Chlordiazepoxide	Librium (Roche) *et al.*	1960
Diazepam	Valium (Roche) *et al.*	1963
Nitrazepam	Mogadon (Roche) *et al.*	1965
Oxazepam	Serenid (Wyeth)	1966
Medazepam	Nobrium (Roche)	1971
Lorazepam	Ativan (Wyeth) *et al.*	1972
Clorazepate	Tranxene (Boehringer)	1973
Flurazepam	Dalmane (Roche)	1974
Temazepam	Euhypnos (FCE),	1977
	Normison (Wyeth)	1977
Triazolam	Halcion (Upjohn)	1979
Clobazam	Frisium (Hoechst)	1979
Ketazolam	Anxon (Beecham)	1980
Lormetazepam	Noctamid (Schering)	1981
Flunitrazepam	Rohypnol (Sauter)	1982
Bromazepam	Lexotan (Roche)	1982
Prazepam	Centrax (Warner)	1982
Alprazolam	Xanax (Upjohn)	1983

chlordiazepoxide, bodily concentrations of the benzodiazepines presumably took some time to drop to zero. Depression supervened in six and aggravation of the psychoses in five. Insomnia, agitation, and loss of appetite developed in other patients and major convulsions supervened in three. The symptoms started about 2 days after stopping the benzodiazepine, reached their peak of severity between the fourth and eighth days, and had largely waned by day 10. Parallel data were obtained in the second study involving high doses of diazepam (Hollister *et al.* 1963).

Thus, the development of physical dependence in patients taking high doses of benzodiazepines was established right from the time of introduction of the benzodiazepine tranquillizers. However, as Hollister was to point out later, these studies involved very artificial conditions of forced high-dose use for months on end. Such studies cannot tell us how many patients started on therapeutic courses of benzodiazepines escalate their doses to such high levels that physical dependence becomes inevitable.

During the 1960s and 1970s, the scientific literature became peppered with anecdotal case reports of patients who had escalated their dose of tranquillizer to above the upper recommended therapeutic limit. In one example, Peters and Boeters (1970) documented eight cases of physical dependence on diazepam at an average dose of 60–80 mg/day. In another study of two patients, cessation of 60 and 120 mg/day, respectively, was followed by convulsions and confusional states (Venzlaff 1972). Woody and his colleagues (1975) described two patients taking 100–150 mg of diazepam daily who developed insomnia, tremor, and grand mal seizures on stopping the medication. Bliding (1978) encountered four cases of withdrawal reactions from oxazepam: the most prominent symptoms were anxiety, tension, tremor, and palpitations. Patients within the high-dose category usually take 2–5 times the recommended therapeutic doses of various benzodiazepines.

Notwithstanding, little notice was taken of these reports. During the 1960s the medical profession had perceived the benzodiazepines to be surprisingly safe in overdosage. This awareness coincided with a pandemic of suicidal attempts, particularly in young women. Coupled with many accounts of the safety of benzodiazepines was the claim that the reports on abuse and misuse with escalation of dosage were actually uncommon in view of the extent of usage. Thus, of the several hundred reports in the literature, Marks (1978) concluded that only 118 of those published up to mid-1977 contained fully verified cases of physical dependence with a definite withdrawal syndrome or carefully documented cases of psychological dependence. He concluded reassuringly,

Dependence on benzodiazepines occurs rarely under conditions of clinical use and then usually only after prolonged administration at above average dosage. Clinically it resembles that described as 'barbiturate' or 'alcohol–barbiturate' type . . .[p.1].

The dependence risk with benzodiazepines is very low and is estimated to be approximately one case per 5 million patient months 'at risk' for all recorded cases and probably less than one case per 50 million months in therapeutic use . . .[p.2].

It must be pointed out that this conclusion was almost entirely based on patients who had escalated their dose beyond therapeutic levels, which was why they had come to medical notice. Although Marks' conclusion was criticized at the time, one reviewer pointing out that case reports are a useless epidemiological reference frame (*Lancet* 1979), most prescribers accepted it as consistent with their clinical experience: patients did stay on the same dose indefinitely, tolerance was uncommon, and therefore dependence unlikely.

Contemporaneously, the UK Regulatory Authorities became concerned about the extensive long-term use of benzodiazepines. Following the lead of the Institute of Medicine (USA) and the conclusions of the White House Office of Drug Policy and the National Institute of Drug Abuse (USA), the UK Committee on Review of Medicines (CRM) (1980) published a widely read review that concluded that there was little evidence that hypnotics retained their sleep-promoting properties within 3 to 14 days of continuous use nor that anxiolytics were effective beyond 4 months. However, in the absence of proper epidemiological surveys and the controversy over benzodiazepine dependence, which was just starting, they concurred with Marks' low estimate of dependence risk.

It is worth looking in a little more detail at the references to dependence in the CRM document as it represents one of the earliest attempts anywhere to draw attention to the hazards of long-term prescribing of tranquillizers. Thus, it suggested that addiction occurring in medically supervised treatment was 'comparatively rare and occurred usually in susceptible patients only when high doses (often exceeding the therapeutic range) were used for extended periods'. They continue,

The committee was particularly concerned, however, with the question of withdrawal symptoms. It has been reported that symptoms, including anxiety, apprehension, tremor insomnia, nausea, and vomiting appear on abrupt withdrawal of benzodiazepine therapy. Such symptoms may occur three to ten days following discontinuation of treatment with long-acting benzodiazepines and within 24 hours after abrupt withdrawal of benzodiazepines with a short half life. Although symptoms can occur following even short courses—for example, two weeks—and when given in the recommended therapeutic dosage, such effects are usually associated with abrupt discontinuation of high doses taken habitually. Although the Committee felt that such symptoms when occurring during the course of medically supervised treatment were not necessarily indicative of true dependence (particularly as most were mild and transitory), they were concerned that the similarity of the withdrawal effects to the symptoms of the original illness might suggest to the doctor that previous treatment had proved inadequate and that a further course of benzodiazepines was indicated. Such a phenomenon might contribute to the high number of repeat prescriptions issued, in spite of the lack of satisfactory clinical studies establishing long-term efficacy.

The CRM recommended gradual withdrawal even from therapeutic dosage, that patients receiving benzodiazepine therapy be carefully selected and monitored, and that prescriptions be limited to short-term use.

Thus, although the categorization and discussion of dependence and addition are rather imprecise in the document, the conclusions are clearly stated and prescribing guidelines set out in detail. It is noteworthy, however, that dependence was still being equated with high dosage and a susceptible population.

By the middle of 1981, the number of publications on benzodiazepines had risen substantially and the tally of cases had doubled, and Marks (1983, p.124) partly recanted, 'Nevertheless, it is clear that long-term continuous administration of benzodiazepines, even at therapeutic dosage, can lead to a significant level of dependence.'

Normal-dose dependence

The extensive usage of the benzodiazepines was beginning to raise doubts in a few clinicians' minds by the early 1970s. Astute observers noted an increasing cohort of long-term users. The oft-repeated assertion that this just reflected the chronic nature of anxiety disorders failed to reassure some doubters. However, the alternative explanation was that patients could become physically dependent on therapeutic doses. This was so incompatible with the accepted dogma that tolerance and dependence were inseparable that it was dismissed by most authorities.

One study stands out as being a signpost to the existence of normal-dose dependence. Covi and his colleagues, in this study (1973) and a preceding one (1969), found a minor withdrawal syndrome in anxious patients discontinuing chlordiazepoxide after 20 weeks' use. None of the patients had used more than the prescribed dose. The authors nevertheless raised the possibility that patients who persist with benzodiazepine treatment may represent an 'addictive personality type', although no data were adduced to support this suggestion. These studies, both prospective, should have received more attention. However, Covi and his colleagues themselves stressed the minor nature of the symptoms, did not design their studies specifically to evaluate withdrawal, and wrote up their results in a complex and confusing way. Furthermore, the patients had been treated with other psychotropic drugs, such as phenobarbitone. It was not surprising that the study failed to make an impact.

Other observers were uneasy. A review of the literature on diazepam dependence and a survey of 50 diazepam users was published by Maletzky and Klotter (1976). The review is admirably critical and points out that none of the studies cited used controls sufficient to disprove the possibility that diazepam at therapeutic dose induced dependence. Their own study comprised interviews with 50 patients taking diazepam. The data show clearly that patients tended to increase their dosage, had difficulty discontinuing, experiencing anxiety, tremor, insomnia, and so on. The authors argue persuasively that this constitutes a withdrawal syndrome because sometimes the patient had been free of anxiety when the drug was initially prescribed for some other indication, or the initial anxiety had subsided. Also, many of the patients (17 of 24 who had attempted discontinuation) complained of new symptoms. These data should have had a major impact, setting the alarm bells ringing among the medical profession. They did not. The authors themselves stated (p.111), 'The retrospective, uncontrolled nature of most of the data reported herein makes this study merely suggestive.' They stressed the need for a prospective systematic study, affirmed their intention to do so, but never did. Finally, the report was published in a specialist journal in the addiction field, and did not come to general attention.

By this time two clinicians in the UK had commenced a jeremiad. I wrote a paper entitled 'Benzodiazepines—the opium of the masses?' (Lader 1978) and an ex-associate of mine, Peter Tyrer, drew attention to the 'Benzodiazepine bonanza' (Tyrer 1974). Almost simultaneously we set up studies to explore the possibility that long-term benzodiazepine users might be physically dependent and undergo definite withdrawal reactions of the sedative/hypnotic type, similar to those associated with barbiturate and alcohol use. Tyrer conducted his studies within a clinical context substituting placebo (or propranolol) for diazepam or lorazepam (Tyrer *et al.* 1981). My own studies were laboratory-based, initially with Dr Cosmo Hallström (Hallström and Lader 1981) and subsequently with Dr Hannes Pétursson (Pétursson and Lader 1981, 1984). These studies established unequivocally that normal-dose dependence as manifested by a physical withdrawal syndrome was a definite entity and supervened even if the dosage was tapered off. Tolerance with escalation of dosage was not a prerequisite for physical dependence. Indeed, our initial study compared the withdrawal syndromes in small groups of patients withdrawing from high-dose misuse or low-dose use and found that the syndromes were identical (Hallström and Lader 1981).

Gradually, inexorably, it became accepted that normal-dose benzodiazepine dependence could occur but the frequency of this condition was fiercely contested. Certainly, many of the patients studied were in a way self-selected in that they had tried to stop their medication, had distressing and intolerable withdrawal symptoms, re-instituted their drug, and sought specialist help. It was impossible to know from this provenance whether thousands such patients existed or whether these patients were uncommon. More recent studies such as that by Busto *et al.* (1986) have established that about 15–25 per cent of long-term (over 12 months) users undergo a definite withdrawal syndrome although only a few per cent experience major distress. However, no large-scale prospective studies have been carried out to establish with any precision the precise parameters of the epidemiology of benzodiazepine withdrawal.

A further development has been the realization that withdrawal may be prolonged (Ashton 1984) meriting the term 'post-withdrawal syndrome', or associated with major depressive disorder (Olajide and Lader 1984).

Recently, increasing concern about the hazards of long-term benzodiazepine usage has led to parallel guidelines being issued by the UK Committee on Safety of Medicines and the Royal College of Psychiatrists. These guidelines restrict benzodiazepines to short-term use, stress the need to establish a definite indication, and warn against abrupt withdrawal.

Questions have been raised as to the advisability of withdrawing patients who are apparently stabilized and symptom-free on their regular benzo-diazepine tranquillizer. Neuropsychological impairments can be detected particularly with respect to memory (Pétursson *et al.* 1983; Golombok *et al.* 1988). Furthermore, in the USA Schweizer *et al.* (1989) have averred, 'we have unpublished data which demonstrate that many patients, once they have been withdrawn from their maintenance benzodiazepines, show more improvement on clinical measures of anxiety and depression than they did during their chronically medicated state.'

The widespread usage of the benzodiazepines has inevitably led to thousands of people becoming dependent—perhaps 500 000 in the UK and twice that number in the USA where long-term use is less common. Patients who have become dependent and have either been unable to withdraw or have only succeeded with symptomatic distress feel aggrieved against their doctors and the benzodiazepine manufacturers for not warning them about the risk (Tyrer 1988). In the UK over 10 000 people have started legal proceedings, co-ordinated by about 300 firms of lawyers. It will be the largest civil action ever in the UK.

In the USA a successful initiative in controlling benzodiazepine tranquillizer usage was set up in New York State (Brahams 1990). Triplicate prescription writing was required so that all usage of the tranquillizers could be monitored and the duration of the prescription limited to a 30-day supply. Despite opposition from the manufacturers and local and national medical associations, the regulations were instituted. The prescription rate dropped by up to a half. Overdoses and abuse dropped dramatically. Alcohol usage did not increase to compensate for the lack of tranquillizers, as had been predicted. However, there was a move to return to obsolescent sedatives. Slowly, such measures to restrict tranquillizer use will increase.

The leading benzodiazepine in the USA is now alprazolam which like lorazepam is highly potent and may be associated with more dependence problems than, say, diazepam. Alprazolam has recently been licensed to treat panic disorder. This requires high dosage for long periods and could lead to a major dependence problem. The harbingers are already present. For example, in one study 15 of 17 patients had recurrent or increased panic attacks and nine had significant new withdrawal symptoms (Fyer *et al.* 1987). Rebound anxiety was noted in 22 per cent of patients undergoing a 4-week taper from alprazolam; in 28 per cent rebound panics occurred. Along with withdrawal and rebound at the end of alprazolam treatment, daytime interdose anxiety symptoms may recur with an increasingly short period of drug effectiveness, so-called 'clock watching'. Presumably, tolerance with rebound occurs after each dose: this is characteristic of shorter-acting benzodiazepines. Related to this is early morning 'rebound'—patients wake feeling anxious and shaky until they take their first dose of the day.

Will history repeat itself with alprazolam? Will the last decade of the twentieth century see a major dependence problem in the USA and elsewhere? Perhaps this time we are sufficiently forewarned to limit the duration and the dosage of newly introduced benzodiazepines to the minimum.

References

Ashton, H. (1984). Benzodiazepine withdrawal: an unfinished story. *British Medical Journal*, **288**, 1135–40.
Auden, W.H. (1946). *The age of anxiety. A baroque eclogue*. Random House, New York.
Berger, F.M. (1970). Anxiety and the discovery of tranquillizers. In *Discoveries in biological psychiatry* (ed. F.J. Ayd and B. Blackwell) pp.115–29. Lippincott, Philadelphia.
Bliding, A. (1978). The abuse potential of benzodiazepines with special reference to oxazepam. *Acta Psychiatrica Scandinavica*, **274** (suppl.), 111–16.

Brahams, E. (1990). Medicine and the law. *Lancet*, **336**, 1372–3.

Busto, U., Sellers, E.M., Naranjo, C.A., Cappell, H.D., Sanchez, C.M., and Simpkins, J. (1986). Patterns of benzodiazepine abuse and dependence. *British Journal of Addiction*, **81**, 87–94.

Cohen, I.M. (1970). The benzodiazepines. In *Discoveries in biological psychiatry* (ed. F. J. Ayd and B. Blackwell), pp.130–41. Lippincott, Philadelphia.

Committee on Review of Medicines (1980). Systematic review of the benzodiazepines. *British Medical Journal*, **2**, 719–20.

Covi, L., Park, L.C., Lipman, R.S., Uhlenhuth, E.H., and Rickels, K. (1969). Factors affecting withdrawal response to certain minor tranquillizers. In *Drug abuse: social and psychopharmacological aspects* (ed. J. Cole and J. Wittenborn) pp.93–108. Charles C. Thomas, Springfield, Illinois.

Covi, L., Lipman, R.S., Pattison, J.H., Derogatis, L.R., and Uhlenhuth, E.H. (1973). Length of treatment with anxiolytic sedatives and response to their sudden withdrawal. *Acta Psychiatrica Scandinavica*, **49**, 51–64.

Essig, C.F. (1964). Addiction to nonbarbiturate sedative and tranquillizing drugs. *Clinical Pharmacology and Therapeutics*, **5**, 334–43.

Fyer, A.J., Liebowitz, M.R., Gorman, J.M., Campeas, R., Levin, A., Davies, S.O., Goetz, D., and Klein, D.F. (1987). Discontinuation of alprazolam treatment in panic patients. *American Journal of Psychiatry*, **144**, 303–8.

Golombok, S., Moodley, P., and Lader, M. (1988). Cognitive impairment in long-term benzodiazepine users. *Psychological Medicine*, **18**, 365–74.

Hallström, C. and Lader, M.H. (1981). Benzodiazepine withdrawal phenomena. *International Pharmacopsychiatry*, **16**, 235–44.

Hollister, L.E., Motzenbecker, F.P., and Degan, R.O. (1961). Withdrawal reactions from chlordiazepoxide ('Librium'). *Psychopharmacologia*, **2**, 63–8.

Hollister, L.E., Bennett, J.L., Kimbell, I., Savage, C., and Overall, J.E. (1963). Diazepam in newly admitted schizophrenics. *Diseases of the Nervous System*, **24**, 746–50.

Lader, M.H. (1978). Benzodiazepines—the opium of the masses? *Neuroscience*, **3**, 159–65.

Lancet (1979). Editorial: Benzodiazepine withdrawal. *Lancet*, **i**, 196.

Maletzky, B.M. and Klotter, J. (1976). Addiction to diazepam. *International Journal of Addiction*, **11**, 95–115.

Marks, J. (1978). *The benzodiazepines. Use, overuse, misuse, abuse*. MTP, Lancaster.

Marks, J. (1983). The benzodiazepines—for good or evil. *Neuropsychobiology*, **10**, 115–26.

Olajide, D. and Lader M.H. (1984). Depression following withdrawal from long-term benzodiazepine use: a report of four cases. *Psychological Medicine*, **14**, 937–40.

Peters, U.H. and Boeters, U. (1970). Valium-Sucht. Eine Analyse an hand von 8 Fallen. *Pharmacopsychiatrie-Neuropsychopharmacologie*, **3**, 339–48.

Pétursson, H. and Lader, M. (1981). Withdrawal from long-term benzodiazepine treatment. *British Medical Journal*, **283**, 643–5.

Pétursson, H. and Lader M. (1984). *Dependence on tranquillizers*. Oxford University Press, Oxford.

Pétursson, H., Gudjonsson, G.H., and Lader, M.H. (1983). Psychometric performance during withdrawal from long-term benzodiazepine treatment. *Psychopharmacology*, **81**, 345–9.

Schweizer, E., Case, W.G., and Rickels, K. (1989). Dr. Schweizer and associates reply. *American Journal of Psychiatry*, **146**, 1242.

Sternbach, L.H. (1980). *The benzodiazepine story*. Editiones Roche, Basle.

Tyrer, P. (1974). The benzodiazepine bonanza. *Lancet*, **ii**, 709–10.

Tyrer, P. (1988). Legal repercussions in prescribing benzodiazepines. *Bulletin of the Royal College of Psychiatrists*, **12**, 190.

Tyrer, P., Rutherford, D., and Huggett, T. (1981). Benzodiazepine withdrawal symptoms and propranolol. *Lancet*, **i**, 520–2.

Venzlaff, V. (1972). Valiumsucht. *Internist. Praxis*, **12**, 349.

Woods, J.H., Katz, J.L., and Winger, G. (1987). Abuse liability of benzodiazepines. *Pharmacological Review*, **39**, 254–390.

Woody, G.E., O'Brien, C.P., and Greenstein, R. (1975). Misuse and abuse of diazepam: an increasingly common medical problem. *International Journal of Addiction*, **10**, 843–8.

5 Benzodiazepine dependence syndromes and syndromes of withdrawal

Anna Higgitt and Peter Fonagy

The earlier chapters in this book will have started to provide the reader with a cost–benefit analysis of the use of the benzodiazepine group of drugs. In this chapter we will discuss the variety of ways in which the problematic use of benzodiazepines may come to notice by describing the clinical syndromes of tranquillizer use and withdrawal syndromes.

Clinical syndromes of tranquillizer use

Tranquillizer usage patterns can be divided into short-term (recommended) use, long-term use, and abuse. The currently accepted uses of benzodiazepines have been summarized by the Committee on Safety of Medicines (1988) and circulated widely. Thus the use of these drugs as anxiolytics should be short-term (2–4 weeks only) and restricted to anxiety that is 'severe, disabling or subjecting the individual to unacceptable distress'. Furthermore, benzodiazepines should be used as hypnotics only when insomnia 'is severe, disabling, or subjecting the individual to extreme distress'.

The use of drugs generally is very common and accepted in present-day society. If substances such as aspirin are included, as few as 10 per cent of an American population sample remain totally drug-free over a 1-year period (Uhlenhuth *et al.* 1978). The total numbers of prescriptions for benzodiazepines have fallen since their peak in the mid-1970s (Williams 1983; Muller-Oerlinghausen 1986; Gabe 1990), in particular amongst those fitting the Committee on Safety of Medicine's (1988) guidelines (Williams 1987), but there seems possibly to have been an increase in the numbers of long-term users. Particularly notable is the fact that prescription rates in the elderly population have not fallen as fast as they have for younger people (Sullivan *et al.* 1988; see also Schmidt *et al.* 1989).

The extent of psychotropic drug use in the population was highlighted by a survey conducted in San Francisco on a representative adult sample (Balter *et al.* 1984), in which one-third of the men and almost half of the women had used psychotropic drugs in the previous year—almost a third of these doing so for 6 months or longer. Thus one in 10 adults had taken psychotropic drugs chronically. The extension of this survey to the USA as a whole showed that 13 per cent of men and 29 per cent of women had used psychotropic medication in the previous year and 4 per cent had used them for 6 months or longer on a daily basis. The lack of evidence that benzodiazepines continue to be effective beyond a few weeks (Higgitt *et al.* 1988) makes such prolonged prescribing questionable. In some cases patients undoubtedly continue to take the medication to avoid unpleasant rebound or withdrawal symptoms (see next section). An alternative explanation for the continued intake has been put forward by Schneider-Helmert (1988), using evidence derived from sleep laboratory studies. He showed that the main difference between long-term elderly hypnotic users and their counterparts who were drug-free was in terms of memory function, not in sleep quality. It was argued that patients were unable to recall how poorly they slept after taking the drugs but recalled tossing and turning only too well when deprived of their benzodiazepines. It is possibly the memory of their bad nights that makes them persuade their doctors to continue to prescribe for them.

Women are more likely to be prescribed benzodiazepines both in the long and the short term than are men and there is a tendency for there to be more prescriptions offered to older patients (Skegg *et al.* 1977; Lader 1978; Uhlenhuth *et al.* 1978; Sullivan *et al.* 1988). Patterns of prescribing psychotropic drugs to men and women are different, with women receiving more than twice as many prescriptions for psychotropic drugs, in particular benzodiazepines. There has been a large amount of speculation as to the reasons for this (Chapter 23, this volume). The reasons for the discrepancies are complex and are explored in detail in Chapter 23. Briefly, social pressures and stress may be argued to be greater for women who take responsibility for child care, running the home, and often also holding down a job. Men may be argued to have more outlets for symptom control than do women. There are marked differences in the ways that women seek help and support and in the responses of clinicians to them both in terms of diagnosis and prescriptions issued.

The third type of use of benzodiazepines that requires brief consideration is that of abuse; here we include those patients most typically seen in attendance at Drug Dependence Units. High (often way above therapeutic levels) doses of benzodiazepines are ingested, often in combination with alcohol and other drugs of abuse. The risk of dependence emerging is marked and the frequency of this sort of problem, once dismissed as a rarity, is now recognized as a major issue (Lader 1989).

Withdrawal syndromes

Benzodiazepine dependence syndromes may probably most usefully be considered as comprising two main types: therapeutic (or low-dose) dependence and high-dose abuse, though we will argue below for separate consideration of those with particularly prolonged withdrawal reactions. Laux and Puryear (1984) divided benzodiazepine dependence not only into primary high-dose (abuse of benzodiazepines only) and primary low-dose (therapeutic) dependency but considered secondary (multiple drug abuse) dependence separately. Ingestion of other drugs in addition to the benzodiazepines does to some extent cloud the clinical picture but multiple drug abusers have enough in common with the high-dose abusers (for example, in terms of personality and psychiatric history) for them to be considered together.

Estimates of the proportion of long-term benzodiazepine users who are in fact dependent upon their medication vary widely. Some studies claim that none of the patients whose drugs they withdrew showed any withdrawal symptoms (Laughren *et al.* 1982) whilst other workers have reported a prevalence much nearer to 100 per cent (Péturrson and Lader 1984). The latter workers, in a tertiary referral centre, would be expected to see a larger proportion of more severe cases. The likelihood of a withdrawal reaction emerging is generally accepted to increase with the length of drug use, the history of psychotropic drug and alcohol use, age, the extent of social problems affecting the patient, and speed of withdrawal. Rickels *et al.* (1983) noted that patients with 8 or more months of prior sedative/benzodiazepine therapy were more than eight times as likely to experience a withdrawal reaction as those with no such history (43 versus 5 per cent). A review by Noyes *et al.* (1988) concluded that nearly half of those who had taken benzodiazepines for an average of 3 years experienced a withdrawal reaction when medication was stopped. A similar conclusion was reached by Hanin and Marks (1988) in a very extensive literature survey.

The existence of rebound reactions (an increase in the severity of the original symptoms beyond pre-treatment levels), presumed to indicate receptor readjustment after abrupt cessation of short-term intake of benzodiazepines, is well accepted (e.g. Lader and Lawson 1987, a review of rebound insomnia; Fontaine *et al.* 1984 and Power *et al.* 1985—rebound anxiety after short-term treatment). It has been cogently argued that rebound and withdrawal differ only quantitatively from each other (Lader and File 1987) and the issue will not be considered further here. Whether the difference in withdrawal reactions according to the particular drug under consideration is of relevance remains a moot point.

An alternative subdivision of the types of benzodiazepine dependence has been offered by Kraupl-Taylor (1989). He suggests that one can consider both a therapeutic and a morbid dependence. The therapeutic dependence would be acceptable to both physician and patient as it mitigates the suffering of patients with longstanding and fluctuating anxious–depressive symptoms. He argued that such 'dependence' is of no more concern than the 'dependence' of a diabetic on insulin. He held that the morbid dependence was an unfortunate complication with patients escalating their dosage in order to avoid unpleasant withdrawal symptoms on attempts at drug reduction.

Normal-dose dependence

There have now been several studies investigating the response of therapeutic-dose benzodiazepine users to withdrawal of their medication. The typical withdrawal symptoms have been delineated and outcome monitored. Unfortunately, almost every study has used its own definition of what constitutes a withdrawal symptom, and an almost infinite range of symptoms have been claimed to form part of the withdrawal syndrome. Thus, the development of two or more new symptoms, an increase in self-ratings of symptoms of 50 per cent or more above baseline followed by a return to lower values, and a combination of these two approaches have all been advocated. The present authors defined a severe benzodiazepine withdrawal syndrome as being made up of three criteria, all of which had to be met (see Higgitt *et al.* 1988).

1. There must be a record of at least three of the following new complaints emerging in association with the withdrawal of benzodiazepines: (a) impairment of memory; (b) impaired concentration; (c) insomnia; (d) lack of energy; (e) metallic taste in mouth; (f) blurred vision; (g) eye soreness; (h) light/touch/noise sensitivity; (i) derealization; (j) cramps; (k) pins and needles; (l) severe pains.

2. At least two of these symptoms should be reported to persist for 4 weeks following the last dose.

3. At least one of these symptoms should be of sufficient intensity to clearly interfere with the person's daily life.

Ashton *et al.* (1990) monitored 49 symptoms in their withdrawal study allocating a score of 0–3 according to intensity. Schweizer *et al.* (1990) used a 34-item withdrawal check-list. Tyrer and his colleagues have tended to use the Comprehensive Psychopathological Rating Scale (CPRS) of Asberg *et al.* (1978) and reported on any extra unusual symptoms while the work from the Institute of Psychiatry has focused on the 12 items mentioned above. Recently an empirically based 22-item self-report scale, the clinical institute withdrawal assessment—benzodiazepines (CIWA-B) has been put forward (see Busto *et al.* 1989). There is thus not a great deal of consistency across the studies performed in this area. Table 5.1 provides a useful grouping of typically reported withdrawal symptoms.

The clinical picture found varies from patient to patient. The early reports referred to withdrawal fits and hallucinations and perhaps were close to the confusional states of delirium tremens. Schneiderian first-rank symptoms have even been reported in benzodiazepine withdrawal, again in an abuser (Roberts and Vass 1986). As acknowledged below, these patients were generally taking high doses of benzodiazepines and were very abruptly withdrawn. The typical

Table 5.1. Withdrawal symptoms

Class of symptom	Symptom
General debility	Lethargy, tiredness, weakness, unwell
Affective changes	Irritability, panics, mood swings, depression, anxiety
Abnormal sensations	Migraines, 'jelly-legs', headaches, tinnitus, paraesthesiae, hypersensitivity
Cardiovascular	Palpitations, racing pulse
Abdominal	Borborygmi
Disturbed consciousness	Derealization, memory problems, light-headedness, insomnia

benzodiazepine withdrawal syndrome has been eloquently described by its sufferers on a number of occasions (see, for example Ashton 1984).

It is clear from examining Table 5.1 that many of the symptoms could be interpreted as a return of a pre-existing anxiety state. This led some workers early on to argue against the existence of normal-dose benzodiazepine dependence. In the counterargument certain of the reported symptoms were held to be specific to benzodiazepine withdrawal (perceptual disturbances including hypersensitivity to sound, light, and smell) but surveys of even the mildly anxious (pre-exam students) reveal their presence in a significant proportion of the sample (Rodrigo and Williams 1986). The typical withdrawal reaction contains both a recrudescence of symptoms of anxiety and the onset of new, distinct symptoms such as persistent tinnitus, involuntary movements, paraesthesiae, perceptual changes, and confusion. Further examination of some of the relevant studies should clarify the issue.

A typical study of the normal-dose withdrawal syndrome is reported by Busto *et al.* (1986). This study concerned patients who had received benzodiazepines daily for at least 3 months in doses in the therapeutic range. Those with multiple drug abuse problems were excluded. The study was double-blind and placebo-controlled with 40 patients either undergoing abrupt withdrawal or a tapering of their drug dosage. The patients were either switched to placebo or to diazepam in a dose roughly equivalent to their regular benzodiazepine intake. In the latter case the diazepam was reduced gradually over an 8-week period. Patients who received placebo (and hence an abrupt withdrawal) reported more, as well as more severe, symptoms than those withdrawn gradually. For example, 90 per cent of the placebo group reported symptoms above 7 on the 10-point scale in comparison with 28 per cent of the diazepam group. The worse symptoms in the placebo group no doubt contributed to their markedly greater drop-out rate (37 per cent as compared with 5 per cent in the diazepam group). The onset of symptoms was also much earlier in the placebo than in the diazepam group. Symptoms gradually reduced in both groups and were absent by the first follow-up 4 weeks after the end of the study. The authors felt that they had unequivocally demonstrated a withdrawal reaction to therapeutic doses of benzodiazepines, which, however, was not severe as can be the case with withdrawal from higher dosages.

A study of 57 patients with a minimum of 12 months continuous intake of benzodiazepines examined the effect of abrupt withdrawal (Rickels *et al.* 1990). Depending on the outcome criteria employed, withdrawal syndrome was detected in 58–100 per cent. Withdrawal symptoms reached a maximum level sooner in those subjects who had been on short- as opposed to long-half-life benzodiazepines (2 as opposed to 4–7 days). In the latter case the plasma levels of the drugs would be expected to take longer to fall. The most severe withdrawal syndromes were found in those who had been on high doses of short-half-life drugs (lorazepam and alprazolam), who had higher baseline levels of anxiety and depression, and who were assessed as high in neuroticism and dependency. The follow-up period was short at only 5 weeks, but it emerged that more of those who had been on the short-half-life drugs resumed taking their benzodiazepines again.

A companion study (Schweizer *et al.* 1990) examined the effect upon the withdrawal reaction of tapering the dose in comparison with an abrupt withdrawal (see also Cantopher *et al.* 1990 concerning the effect of tapering). Sixty-three patients took part in this study. The vast majority of patients still experienced a withdrawal reaction despite the tapering dose. The rate of reduction was initially set at 25 per cent of the dose per week, although this proved too rapid a reduction for some. It was noted that withdrawal symptoms were worse in the second half of the taper and it seems that one can reduce initially at a more rapid rate than is possible later as drug dosage falls. Symptoms were less severe than was the case for an abrupt withdrawal and no significant difference could be detected between the long- and short-half-life drugs, but 42 per cent of those on short and 32 per cent of those on long-half-life benzodiazepines either did not withdraw or relapsed. Personality factors (see below) were major outcome predictors.

The difficulty of helping patients to withdraw from benzodiazepines is highlighted by a study reported by Hallström and colleagues (1988). Of 44 people taken into their 10-week study only 23 complied fully with the treatment. Of these, eight were fully withdrawn and 11 reduced their intake by 50 per cent or more. The finding by Higgitt *et al.* (1987) that, once a pattern of reduction in intake was started, patients frequently continued the reduction after the end of a formal treatment programme may make us more optimistic about these findings.

The actual incidence of withdrawal reactions, the speed of onset of symptoms, and their severity have all been linked to the particular types of benzodiazepines. Early work considered purely the half-life of the different benzodiazepines. Busto *et al.* (1986) reported that the time course of the withdrawal reaction following placebo substitution was different according to whether a short- or a long-acting benzodiazepine had been used. In the former situation (five on lorazepam and three on oxazepam; half-life in both cases of about 15 hours) withdrawal symptoms emerged within 1 day, whereas for those on long-acting drugs (10 on diazepam and one on flurazepam; half-life around 70 hours) over 4 days elapsed before symptoms were noted. In the same study the drop-outs were all patients who had been on short-half-life drugs. These findings are backed up by the Schweizer *et al.* (1990) study. However, a recent study comparing withdrawal reactions from lorazepam, diazepam, and bromazepam (Murphy and Tyrer 1991) reports the greatest drop-out rate for those randomized to lorazepam. Since both lorazepam and bromazepam have similar half-lives (12–14 hours), the explanation for this difference must be sought elsewhere (e.g. potency). The two short-half-life benzodiazepines concerned in the Schweizer *et al.* study are both high-potency (lorazepam and alprazolam).

Within most reports of benzodiazepine dependence there is a notable heterogeneity of diagnoses for the subjects under consideration. Thus the diagnoses for Busto *et al.*'s (1986) group of 40 patients included anxiety (74 per cent), insomnia (17 per cent), panic attacks (5 per cent), back pain, and restless legs. Others make note of the presence of those with manic depressive disorder, major depression, dysthymia, posttraumatic stress disorder, childhood sexual abuse, alcohol abuse, and even no psychiatric diagnosis. The presence of an affective disorder diagnosis may be of particular importance in that it may make the patient at a high risk of developing a severe depression on withdrawal of the benzodiazepines. Frequent mention is made of coexistent personality disorder and this issue seems to be of major relevance to prognosis.

Peter Tyrer and his colleagues argue that, along with showing a poorer response to treatment of anxiety disorders, patients who have a personality disorder diagnosis are likely to report the most severe withdrawal reaction (Tyrer 1989; Murphy and Tyrer 1991). This applies in particular to those who received a diagnosis of passive-dependent personality disorder using the Personality Assessment Schedule (Tyrer and Alexander 1988) when one is considering normal-dose dependence. There is a high likelihood of diagnosing high-dose abusers as possessing a borderline personality disorder (see Tarnopolsky and Berelowitz 1987; Tyrer 1989). Ashton (1989) points to the likelihood of normal-dose-dependent patients scoring highly on the Eysenck Neuroticism scale whilst those who abuse can be expected to be high P (psychoticism) scorers. She, however, reported no relationship between the possession of a personality disorder diagnosis and success in withdrawal from this group of drugs (Ashton *et al.* 1990). Hers appears to be a minority view with Schweizer *et al.* (1990, p. 908) concluding that 'personality factors contribute significantly to the patient's difficulties with gradual discontinuation of therapeutic doses of benzodiazepines'.

The prolonged benzodiazepine withdrawal syndrome

It is generally assumed that, in response to benzodiazepine administration, compensatory changes take place in the central nervous system which do not immediately re-equilibrate upon drug withdrawal resulting in rebound or withdrawal symptoms. If one were to employ just a pharmacokinetic and pharmacodynamic explanation for the occurrence of benzodiazepine withdrawal symptoms, then the onset of the symptoms within 1 day to 1 week of cessation of intake or reduction in dosage, depending on the half-life of the drug concerned, would be predicted. This, of course, has been found to be the case (e.g. Rickels *et al.* 1990). Furthermore, it could be stated with some certainty that the withdrawal syndrome would have a limited life span. Once the drug had been totally eliminated from the body and the receptors had readjusted to a drug-free state, then withdrawal symptoms should settle. For the majority of patients who suffer from a benzodiazepine withdrawal syndrome, this latter prediction is also true with a cessation of symptoms within a matter of weeks. However, a substantial minority of those who can be diagnosed as suffering from the benzodiazepine withdrawal syndrome suffer a far more protracted course.

The extent of persistence of the withdrawal syndrome is considerable. About one-third of patients report significant symptoms 10 months to 3.5 years following withdrawal (Ashton 1987; Golombok *et al.* 1987; Holton and Tyrer 1990). We argue that it is not possible to explain such chronicity without making use of cognitive and behavioural explanatory models. Elsewhere (Higgitt and Fonagy 1991), we provide a detailed exposition of our views and put forward a cognitive-behavioural model to account for the persistence of this syndrome in certain cases. We will present a brief summary here.

A comprehensive explanatory model for the clinical picture presented by those suffering persistent benzodiazepine withdrawal symptoms must include a psychological component, including cognitive aspects. Research into animal addictions (for a review see Corfield-Sumner and Stolerman 1978) has demonstrated the central role of learning in their development. The focus has so far been on behavioural factors in both human and animal addiction research but we argue for attention to the cognitive abnormalities that we hypothesize play a part in the benzodiazepine dependence syndrome.

In our work with patients whose benzodiazepine withdrawal symptoms persist we have been struck by the resemblance our patients show to those often diagnosed as suffering from somatization disorder (APA 1987). Our patients also show: fear of serious disease; lack of evidence of organic pathology commensurate with their concern about their symptoms; frequent requests for medical referrals along with a certain selectivity in the appraisal of medical advice; a tendency to treat as catastrophic most bodily signs and symptoms; and, finally, constant requests for reassurance and information concerning their symptoms.

We have used the resemblance of our patients to those diagnosed as suffering from hypochondriasis to suggest a different approach to conceptualizing their problems: there may be common underlying cognitive mechanisms. In both cases one can hypothesize a perceptual and/or cognitive style where certain bodily symptoms are amplified or augmented, mislabelled, and consequently misinterpreted.

This group of patients seems to experience withdrawal symptoms more intensively than those whose withdrawal syndrome settles rapidly. Five mechanisms are suggested as contributing to this amplification. First, such patients may have irrational beliefs concerning the action of drugs that may lead them to experience withdrawal intensely. For example, patients continue to believe that drugs are still helping them despite accumulated evidence to the contrary. Dose reductions cause them to expect an increase in anxiety, so they will be sensitized to anxiety and anxiety-like manifestations. Second, the most obvious explanation to the patient for any interoceptive experiences is naturally the drug dose reduction; at the time of drug reduction any and every bodily change, generally easily ignored, will be linked to the drug. Third, the patient is generally all too aware that withdrawal is occurring and this itself induces apprehension, which is itself associated with the physical symptoms of arousal that will be added to the bodily experiences these patients experience as withdrawal. The loss of the ability to discriminate between symptoms of withdrawal and apprehension concerning withdrawal may be the primary deficit in prolonged benzodiazepine withdrawal syndrome. Fourth, these individuals often use their medication to regulate their autonomic arousal and have no other coping mechanisms available to them once the drug is withdrawn. Finally, in line with patients with somatization disorder, we suggest that patients with a prolonged benzodiazepine withdrawal syndrome have a personality trait that leads them to attend more intensely to bodily sensations than is normal. Reports that withdrawal severity is more closely linked to personality and psychopathology than to pharmacokinetic factors (e.g. Schweizer *et al.* 1990; see also Tyrer 1989) lend weight to our explanatory model.

The prolonged nature of the symptoms in this group of patients may in part at least be explained by the following hypotheses, which also lend themselves to treatment interventions. Using the terminology of Beck, continued drug intake, and hence dependence, will be fostered by 'catastrophic' interpretations of experience (Beck *et al.* 1979). If a patient believes: 'Taking the pill is the only way I can cope' why should they stop doing so? The systematic identification of such cognitions, and their replacement by more adaptive ones, can prove a highly effective and simple intervention (Higgitt *et al.* 1987). However, one needs at times to work hard to alter the quite fixed beliefs some patients have developed. For instance, some patients use quite specific physical symptoms such as an ear infection as further evidence and many obsessionally collect evidence from the media to strengthen their belief in the cause of their symptoms. Also, these patients have little confidence in themselves (sometimes termed low self-efficacy; Bandura 1978), which leads to increased anxiety about the performance of tasks without their medication.

Our model thus suggests that an individual with little confidence about being able to manage without tranquillizers will make catastrophic assumptions concerning the impact of dose reduction; this will result in a greatly enhanced emotional reaction with associated bodily symptoms. These in turn may, through mislabelling, be magnified further and lead to severe and relatively intractable withdrawal symptoms.

High-dose dependence

Early reports of benzodiazepine dependence concerned patients ingesting large quantities of the drugs, well above the current therapeutic range. Thus Hollister and colleagues as early as 1961 described a physical dependence syndrome being induced by the administration of chlordiazepoxide in doses that were six to ten times higher than the recommended anxiolytic dose. The pioneering research work carried out in Professor Lader's department at the Institute of Psychiatry at first included many with high-dose dependence and the added complication of alcohol use. The early stress upon the risks of withdrawal fits and psychosis can be traced back to this particular patient group and the fact that early withdrawal studies tended to impose a very abrupt withdrawal of the benzodiazepines.

Experience in drug dependence units is revealing a substantial number of high-dose abusers of benzodiazepines. The extent of the problem is hinted at by the fact that about 60 per cent of attenders at a London drug dependence unit had benzodiazepines detected in their routine urine drug screens on at least one occasion (Beary *et al.* 1987) with benzodiazepines being the second most common drugs abused, after methadone (see also Perera *et al.* 1987). In some cases this is sporadic use—both of benzodiazepines alone and in a polydrug abuse context. It has been reported that benzodiazepines serve to boost the effects of opiates as well as to cushion the depression as cocaine effects wear off (Preston *et al.* 1984). Where there is sustained high-dose use there is an extremely high risk of dependence. Most of this drug abuse is oral but there are reports of intravenous administration of temazepam, drawn up from the capsules (Farrell and Strang 1988; Sakol *et al.* 1989). This area has been recently reviewed (Seivewright 1990) and the lack of clear management guidelines highlighted, in contrast to the situation with the low-dose-dependent patients. It is likely that in-patient detoxification may well be needed in some cases, in part because of the risk of withdrawal fits related to the high doses being used. Furthermore, insufficient attention to benzodiazepine withdrawal may lead to poor outcome with opiate detoxification attempts (Huws 1989).

References

APA(American Psychiatric Association) (1987). *Diagnostic and statistical manual of mental disorders*, (3rd edn, revised). American Psychiatric Press, Washington, DC.

Asberg, M., Montgomery, S.A., Perris, C., Schalling, D., and Sed vall, G. (1978). A comprehensive psychopathological rating scale, *Acta Psychiatrica Scandinavica*, **271** (suppl.), 5–27.

Ashton, H. (1984). Benzodiazepine withdrawal: an unfinished story. *British Medical Journal*, **288**, 1135–40.

Ashton, H. (1987). Benzodiazepine withdrawal: outcome in 50 patients. *British Journal of Addiction*, **82**, 665–91.

Ashton, H. (1989). Risks of dependence on benzodiazepine drugs: a major problem of long term treatment. *British Medical Journal*, **298**, 103–4.

Ashton, C.H., Rawlins, M.D. and Tyrer, S.P. (1990). A double-blind placebo-controlled study of buspirone in diazepam withdrawal in chronic benzodiazepine users. *British Journal of Psychiatry*, **157**, 232–8.

Balter, M.B., Manheimer, D.I., Mellinger, G.D., and Uhlenhuth, E.H. (1984). A Cross-national comparison of anti-anxiety sedative drug use, *Current Medical Research and Opinion*, **8** (suppl.), 5–20.

Bandura, A. (1978). Reflections on self efficacy. In *Advances in behaviour research and therapy*, (1st edn) (ed. S. Rachman), pp.139–66. Pergamon Press, Oxford.

Beary, M.D., Christofides, J., Fry, D., Ghodse, A.H., Smith, H., and Smith, V. (1987). The benzodiazepines as substances of abuse. *Practitioner*, **231**, 19–20.

Beck, A.T., Rush, A.J., Shaw, B.F., and Emery, G. (1979). *Cognitive therapy of depression*. Guildford Press, New York.

Busto, U., Sellers, E.M., Naranjo, C.A., Cappell, H., Sanchez-Craig, M., and Sykora, K. (1986). Withdrawal reaction after long-term use of benzodiazepines. *New England Journal of Medicine*, **315**, 854–9.

Busto, U.E., Sykora, K., and Sellers, E.M. (1989). A clinical scale to assess benzodiazepine withdrawal. *Journal of Clinical Psychopharmacology*, **9**, 412–16.

Cantopher, T., Olivieri, S., Cleave, N., and Guy Edwards, J. (1990). Chronic benzodiazepine dependence: a comparative study of abrupt withdrawal under propranolol cover versus gradual withdrawal. *British Journal of Psychiatry*, **156**, 406–11.

Committee on Safety of Medicines (1988). Benzodiazepines, dependence and withdrawal symptoms. *Current Problems*, **21**, 1–2.

Corfield-Sumner, P.K. and Stolerman, I.P. (1978). Behavioural tolerance. In *Contemporary research in behavioural pharmacology* (ed. D.E. Blackman and D.J. Sanger). Plenum Press, New York.

Farrell, M. and Strang, J. (1988). Misuse of temazepam. *British Medical Journal*, **297**, 1402.

Fontaine, R., Chouinard, G., and Annable, L. (1984). Rebound anxiety in anxious patients after abrupt withdrawal of benzodiazepine treatment. *American Journal of Psychiatry*, **141**, 848–52.

Gabe, J. (1990). Towards a sociology of tranquillizer prescribing. *British Journal of Addiction*, **85**, 41–8.

Golombok, S. Higgitt, A., Fongay, P., Dodds, S., Saper, J., and Lader, M. (1987). A Follow up study of patients treated for benzodiazepine dependence. *British Journal of Medical Psychology*, **60**, 141–9.

Hallström, C., Crouch, G., Robson, M., and Shine, P. (1988). The treatment of tranquillizer dependence by propranolol. *Postgraduate Medical Journal*, **64** (suppl. 2), 40–4.

Hanin, B. and Marks, J. (1988). Dépendance aux benzodiazepines et syndrome de sevrage. Revue de la littérature. *Psychiatrie et Psychobiologie*, **3**, 347–64.

Higgitt, A. and Fonagy, P. (1991). Withdrawal from benzodiazepines and the persistent benzodiazepine dependence syndrome. In *Recent advances in psychiatry* (ed. K. Granville Grossman), pp.45–59. Churchill Livingstone, London.

Higgitt, A., Golombok, S., Fonagy, P., and Lader, M. (1987). Group treatment of benzodiazepine dependence. *British Journal of Addiction*, **82**, 517–32.

Higgitt, A., Fonagy, P., and Lader, M. (1988). *The natural history of tolerance to the benzodiazepines*, Psychological Medicine Monograph, Supplement 13. Cambridge University Press, Cambridge.

Holton, A. and Tyrer, P. (1990). Five year outcome in patients withdrawn from long-term treatment with diazepam. *British Medical Journal*, **300**, 1241–2.

Huws, R. (1989). Benzodiazepine addiction in heroin addicts. *British Journal of Psychiatry*, **154**, 886.

Kraupl-Taylor, F. (1989). The damnation of benzodiazepines. *British Journal of Psychiatry*, **154**, 697–704.

Lader, M. (1978). Benzodiazepines—the opium of the masses? *Neuroscience*, **3**, 159–65.

Lader, M. (1989). Benzodiazepine dependence. *International Review of Psychiatry*, **1**, 149–56.

Lader, M. and File, S. (1987). The biological basis of benzodiazepine dependence. *Psychological Medicine*, **17**, 539–47.

Lader, M. and Lawson, C. (1987). Sleep studies and rebound insomnia: methodological problems, laboratory findings and clinical implications. *Clinical Neuropharmacology*, **10**, 291–312.

Laughren, T.P., Battey, Y., Greenblatt, D.J., and Harrop, D.S. (1982). A controlled trial of diazepam withdrawal in chronically anxious outpatients. *Acta Psychiatrica Scandinavica*, **65**, 171–9.

Laux, G. and Puryear, D.A. (1984). Benzodiazepines—misuse, abuse and dependency. *American Family Physician*, **30**, 139–47.

Muller-Oerlinghausen, B. (1986). Prescription and misuse of benzodiazepines in the Federal Republic of Germany. *Pharmacopsychiatry*, **19**, 8–13.

Murphy, S.M. and Tyrer, P.T. (1991). A double-blind comparison of the effects of gradual withdrawal of lorazepam, diazepam and bromazepam in benzodiazepine dependence. *British Journal of Psychiatry*, **158**, 511–16.

Noyes, R., Garvey, M.J., Cook, B.L., and Perry, P.J. (1988). Benzodiazepine withdrawal: a review of the evidence. *Journal of Clinical Psychiatry*, **49**, 382–9.

Perera, K.M.H., Tulley, M., and Jenner, F.A. (1987). The use of benzodiazepines among drug addicts. *British Journal of Addiction*, **82**, 511–15.

Péturrson, H. and Lader, M. (1984). *Dependence on tranquillizers*, Maudsley Monograph, no. 28. Oxford University Press, Oxford.

Power, K.G., Jerrom, D.W.A., Simpson, R.J., and Mitchell, M. (1985). Controlled study of withdrawal symptoms and rebound anxiety after six week course of diazepam for generalised anxiety. *British Medical Journal*, **290**, 1246–8.

Preston, K.L., Griffiths, R.R., Stitzer, M.S., Bigelow, G.E., and Liebson, A. (1984). Diazepam and methadone interactions in methadone maintenance. *Clinical Pharmacology and Therapeutics*, **36**, 534–41.

Rickels, K., Case, G., and Downing, R.W. (1983). Long-term benzodiazepine therapy and clinical outcome. *Journal of the American Medical Association*, **250**, 767–71.

Rickels, K., Schweizer, E., Case, W.G., and Greenblatt, D.J. (1990). Long-term therapeutic use of benzodiazepines. 1. Effects of abrupt discontinuation. *Archives of General Psychiatry*, **47**, 899–907.

Roberts, K. and Vass, N. (1986). Schneiderian first rank symptoms caused by benzodiazepine withdrawal. *British Journal of Psychiatry*, **148**, 593–4.

Rodrigo, E.K. and Williams, P. (1986). Frequency of self-reported 'anxiolytic withdrawal' symptoms in a group of female students experiencing anxiety. *Psychological Medicine*, **16**, 467–72.

Sakol, M.S., Stark, C., and Sykes, R. (1989). Buprenorphine and temazepam abuse by drug takers in Glasgow—an increase. *British Journal of Addiction*, **84**, 439–41.

Schmidt, L.G., Grohman, R., Muller-Oehleringhausen, B., Otto, M., Ruther, E., and Wolf, B. (1989). Prevalence of benzodiazepine abuse and dependence in psychiatric in-patients with different nosology: an assessment of hospital-based drug surveillance data. *British Journal of Psychiatry*, **154**, 839–43.

Schneider-Helmert, D. (1988). Why low-dose benzodiazepine-dependent insomniacs can't escape their sleeping pills. *Acta Psychiatrica Scandinavica*, **78**, 706–11.

Schweizer, E., Rickels, K., Case, W.G., and Greenblatt, D.J. (1990). Long-term therapeutic use of benzodiazepines. 2. Effects of gradual taper. *Archives of General Psychiatry*, **47**, 908–15.

Seivewright, N. (1990). Treatment and outcome of drug dependence. *Current Opinion in Psychiatry*, **3**, 403–7.

Skegg, D.G., Doll, R., and Perry, J. (1977). Use of medicines in general practice. *British Medical Journal*, **1**, 1561–3,

Sullivan, C.F., Copeland, J.R.M., Dewey, M.E., Davidson, I.A., McWilliam, C., Saunders, P., Sharma, V.K., and Voruganti, L.N.P. (1988). Benzodiazepine usage among the elderly: Findings of the Liverpool Community Survey. *International Journal of Geriatric Psychiatry*, **3**, 289–92.

Tarnopolsky, A. and Berelowitz, M. (1987). Borderline personality: A review of recent research. *British Journal of Psychiatry*, **151**, 724–34.

Tyrer, P. (1989). Risks of dependence on benzodiazepine drugs: the importance of patient selection, *British Medical Journal*, **298**, 102–5.

Tyrer, P. and Alexander, J. (1988) Personality Assessment Schedule. In *Personality disorders: diagnosis, management and course*. (ed. P. Tyrer), pp.43–62. Wright, London.

Uhlenhuth, E.H., Balter, M.B., and Lipman, R.S. (1978). Minor tranquilizers: clinical correlates of use in an urban population, *Archives of General Psychiatry*, **35**, 350.

Williams, P. (1983). Patterns of psychotropic drug use. *Social Science and Medicine*, **17**, 845–51.

Williams, P. (1987). Long-term benzodiazepine use in general practice. In *Benzodiazepines in current clinical practice* (ed. H. Freeman and Y. Rue), pp.19–31. Royal Society of Medicine Services, London.

6 The role of the benzodiazepine receptor in anxiety

Paul Glue, Susan J. Wilson, and David Nutt

Since the synthesis of the first benzodiazepine, chlordiazepoxide, in 1955 this class of drugs has become one of the most widely used ever. Although the anxiolytic, sedative, and anticonvulsant properties of these drugs were discovered early on, advances in the pharmacology of benzodiazepines were made only relatively recently. In 1975 a number of biochemical, pharmacological, and electrophysiological studies indicated that the actions of benzodiazepines were associated with the inhibitory neurotransmitter gamma-aminobutyric acid (GABA) (Costa *et al.* 1975; Fuxe *et al.* 1975; Haefely *et al.* 1975). Subsequently, specific benzodiazepine receptors were identified in brain (Mohler and Okada 1977; Squires and Braestrup 1977). These binding sites for the benzodiazepines are now known to be part of the GABA-A molecular complex, a chloride ionophore produced by the amalgamation of five protein subunits, one of which (the gamma) is an absolute requirement for benzodiazepine binding (see Nutt 1990*b* for review).

The benzodiazepine receptor modulates GABA receptor function in a unique way (reviewed in Nutt 1990*b*; Roy-Byrne and Nutt 1991; Zorumski and Isenberg 1991). It is now known that there are three classes of drugs that bind to the benzodiazepine receptor (see Fig. 6.1). Agonists are drugs such as diazepam that are anxiolytic and sedating due to their ability to potentiate the actions of the natural transmitter GABA. Drugs that have the opposite action (to reduce GABA function) are called inverse agonists, and these are anxiogenic and arousing. The third class of drugs are antagonists, which have few effects but potently antagonize all the actions of agonists and inverse agonists. To date only one antagonist, flumazenil (Anexate—Roche), is available for clinical use, although others have been synthesized and shown to be active in animal studies (see Nutt 1990*b*). The basic pharmacology of benzodiazepines is described in greater detail in Chapter 7, and will not be discussed further here. This chapter will concentrate on human studies examining the role of benzodiazepine receptors in anxiety.

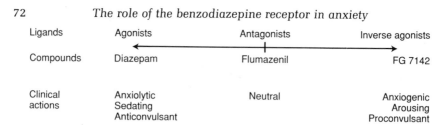

Fig. 6.1. Spectrum of activity of benzodiazepine receptor ligands.

How might benzodiazepine receptors be involved in anxiety?

The unique pharmacology of the benzodiazepine receptor makes for at least three hypotheses, which are outlined in Table 6.1. The possibility of an endogenous anxiolytic benzodiazepine was first suggested by animal studies with the antagonist flumazenil (File *et al.* 1982). At low doses a paradoxical anxiogenic effect was observed in rats during the social interaction test. One explanation for this is the presence of an endogenous anxiolytic agonist ligand whose actions are blocked by flumazenil. Evidence for such a compound came later with the elegant work of de Blas and colleagues who raised selective antibodies to the benzodiazepine desmethyldiazepam (Sangameswaran and de Blas 1985). These and other investigators have used this technique to demonstrate the occurrence of this drug and diazepam in brain tissue from rats, cows, humans, and a range of other species (Sangameswaran and de Blas 1985; Sangameswaran *et al.* 1986; Wildmann *et al.* 1987; Unseld *et al.* 1989). Since this somewhat iconoclastic discovery several groups have discovered these and other benzodiazepine agonists in a range of vegetables and other products including rat chow (reviewed in Klotz 1991). The current thinking is that the origins of the benzodiazepines may be from fungi such as *Aspergillus*, cultures of which have been demonstrated to produce drugs

Table 6.1. Possible mechanisms for benzodiazepine receptor involvement in anxiety

Hypothesis	Evidence
Excess of endogenous inverse agonist	Putative ligands—tribulin, butyl-β-carboline, DBI
Deficit of endogenous agonist	Benzodiazepine agonists (diazepam, desmethyldiazepam) in brain; ingested from food source
Shift of receptor function towards inverse agonism	Chronic benzodiazepine treatment leads to decreased agonist and increased inverse agonist efficacy

with benzodiazepine structure such as cholecystokinin analogues (Chang *et al.* 1985; Snyder 1986). Although these benzodiazepines are present probably in every brain, it has not yet been demonstrated that they are capable of being released. However, it is possible that a deficiency of such could predispose to anxiety, despite the content being low and variable.

The possibility of an endogenous anxiogenic benzodiazepine has been approached by several groups following on from the revelation that the β-carboline β-CCE was anxiogenic in animal studies (File *et al.* 1982). Early suggestions centred on the conjugation of tryptophan and formalhydyde, which will produce β-carbolines by a non-enzymatic process (reviewed by Nutt 1983). Subsequently, this line of argument has quieted down due to the great propensity for artefactual condensation products, although it has been recently suggested that butyl-β-carboline might be produced in the brain (Medina *et al.* 1989). Other approaches have involved the discovery of peptides that can modulate GABA function such as diazepam binding inhibitor (DBI) (Alho *et al.* 1985). This is a large peptide with micromolar affinity for the benzodiazepine receptor that, in some behavioural tests, is inverse agonist-like (Guidotti *et al.* 1983). Now it appears that, if it has any relevance, it is likely to be in the field of steroidogenesis and the peripheral benzodiazepine receptor (McCauley and Gee 1991). A less well characterized candidate is tribulin. This was discovered as a natural inhibitor of benzodiazepine receptor binding in urine extracts (Sandler 1982; Clow *et al.* 1983). A role in anxiety is suggested by findings of increased excretion in conditions such as lactate-induced panic, alcohol withdrawal, and generalized anxiety disorder (GAD) (Bhattacharya *et al.* 1982; Clow *et al.* 1988*a,b*). Tribulin has been shown to consist of at least two substances, one of which has monoamine oxidase inhibitory activity and has been identified as isatin (Glover *et al.* 1988); the nature of the compound that binds to the benzodiazepine receptor is still unknown.

The third possibility is that the nature of the spectrum of benzodiazepine receptor function may alter. This has been conceptualized as an ability to modulate the position of the neutral or set point. Such a change can be clearly demonstrated after chronic treatment with benzodiazepine agonists in that their efficacy is reduced whereas that of the inverse agonists is increased (see Nutt 1990*a,b*); moreover the neutral status of antagonists is changed in that they become somewhat inverse agonist in nature (Little *et al.* 1987). In this paradigm anxiety is construed as a shift in the receptor set point in the inverse agonist direction. This is thought to lead to a general reduction in GABA inhibition that predisposes to the sudden paroxysmal surges of anxiety called panic attacks (see below).

How can we assess benzodiazepine receptor function in anxious humans?

Because the brain is a relatively inaccessible organ, a number of indirect techniques for investigating receptor systems in man have been developed.

Established methods are listed in Table 6.2. However, not all of these approaches can be used in the study of benzodiazepine receptors in man.

One method of assessing central receptor function is to assay levels of associated neurotransmitter(s) in blood or cerebrospinal fluid (CSF) samples. This is not yet possible for benzodiazepines, as there is still no definitive evidence of endogenous benzodiazepine ligands to date. Recent reports have suggested an elevation of benzodiazepines in the CSF and brain tissue of patients with hepatic encephalopathy (for review see Basile *et al.* 1991) and idiopathic recurring stupor (Tinuper *et al.* 1992). These findings, coupled with the observation that flumazenil can reverse some of the signs of these conditions (Grimm *et al.* 1988; Tinuper *et al.* 1992), suggest that benzodiazepine agonists may contribute to the lowering of consciousness in such patients.

Another investigational technique is to examine those receptors on peripheral tissues that also exist in the brain (e.g. α- and β-adrenoceptors on platelets and lymphocytes) as these may act as models of central receptors (see Elliott 1985). Unfortunately, it is not possible to obtain benzodiazepine receptors from peripheral tissue, as they only exist in the central nervous system associated with GABA-A receptors. A so-called peripheral benzodiazepine receptor has been described. However, this is not GABA receptor-linked, and is actually a mitochondrial transport protein that has no relevance to the therapeutic actions of these drugs, since it is only sensitive to a subpopulation of clinically used benzodiazepines (see Nutt 1990*b*).

A further method for investigating brain receptors is to examine brain tissue obtained post-mortem in order to measure receptor numbers or

Table 6.2. Methods for assessment of receptor function in man

Central	Peripheral
CSF neurotransmitter concentrations	Plasma/urine transmitter concentrations
Brain tissue receptor binding post-mortem	Platelet/lymphocyte receptor binding
Neurotransmitter concentrations post-mortem	
Receptor challenge tests (effects on endocrine/ biochemical/physiological/ psychological variables)	
PET/SPECT studies	

neurotransmitter concentrations. While depressive and schizophrenic disorders have been extensively studied in this way, such studies are almost impossible to carry out in anxiety disorders in that patients tend to be younger and to commit suicide less frequently. A direct study of benzodiazepine receptors in focal epilepsy did not show altered receptor numbers (Sherwin *et al.* 1986), although a more recent positron emission tomography (PET) study using [^{11}C] flumazenil has demonstrated a localized reduction in one case of focal epilepsy (Savic *et al.* 1988; see below).

Post-mortem tissue has also been used to demonstrate the presence of the benzodiazepine agonists diazepam and desmethyldiazepam in human brain, even in those stored in paraffin since the 1940s (Sangameswaran *et al.* 1986). However, this approach has not so far been applied to patients with psychiatric disorders. It should be emphasized that as yet there is no evidence that these endogenous benzodiazepine agonists can be released or have physiological functions, so the relevance of any findings would be uncertain.

To date, the best method for assessing benzodiazepine receptors in man is by the use of challenge paradigms. In this technique, drugs are administered and subsequent physiological, psychological, biochemical, or endocrine changes provide indices of receptor sensitivity. However, interpretation of any changes may be complicated. For instance, stress associated with the unfamiliarity of test procedures may alter hormone levels or psychological ratings. Challenges that produce peripheral symptoms (e.g. nausea, tachycardia) may cause secondary mood, cognitive, or hormonal changes that will complicate interpretation of drug effects. Despite these caveats, challenge testing provides the best available information on the involvement of benzodiazepine receptors in the anxiety disorders. Another promising area is in the use of PET or SPECT to examine benzodiazepine receptors *in vivo*. This chapter will concentrate on responses to benzodiazepine challenge paradigms in patients with anxiety disorders and in normal subjects, and briefly review PET studies of benzodiazepine receptors.

Receptor challenge studies

Responses to benzodiazepine challenge paradigms in normal subjects are summarized in Table 6.3. A comparison of responses in normal subjects and patients with anxiety disorders is summarized in Table 6.4.

Endocrine effects

In normal subjects, diazepam and other benzodiazepine agonists reduce plasma cortisol and tend to increase growth hormone levels (Butler *et al.* 1968; Syvälahti and Kanto 1975; Koulu *et al.* 1979; Ajlauni and El-Khateeb 1980; Kannan 1981; Shur *et al.* 1983; Gram *et al.* 1984; Charney *et al.* 1986; Hommer *et al.* 1986; Risby *et al.* 1989). Vasopressin and prolactin are unaltered by alprazolam or diazepam (Shur *et al.* 1983; Risby *et al.* 1989).

Table 6.3. Responses to challenge doses of benzodiazepine ligands in normal controls

	Responses*	Agonist	Antagonist	Inverse agonist†
Endocrine	cortisol	↓/nc	nc	↑
	ACTH	↓		
	Growth hormone	↑		↑
	Prolactin	nc	nc	↑
	Vasopressin	nc		
Biochemical	Noradrenaline	↓/nc	nc	
	Adrenaline	↓		
Physiological	Systolic BP	↓/nc	↓	↑
	Diastolic BP	↓/nc	↓	↑
	Heart rate	nc	↓	↑
	SEM	↓	↓	
Wake EEG	Fast activity	↑	nc	
Sleep EEG	Sleep time	↑	nc/↓	↓↓
	Sleep latency	↓	↑	
	No. wakenings	↓	↑	
	Stage 2%	↑	nc	
	Spindles	↑	nc	
	SWS %	↓↓	↓	
Psychological	VAS sleepy	↑	↑	↓
	VAS anxious	↓	nc	↑↑(?)
	Cognitive tasks	↓	↓/nc	?↑

* VAS, Visual analogue self-rating scale; SEM, saccadic eye movements; BP, blood pressure; SWS, slow wave sleep.
† ↓, fall; nc, no change; ↑, increase.

The benzodiazepine antagonist flumazenil has no effect on plasma cortisol or prolactin (Noderer *et al.* 1988). Increases in plasma growth hormone, prolactin, and cortisol were reported in two normal subjects who developed severe anxiety after taking the inverse agonist FG 7142 (Dorow *et al.* 1983).

From the above studies, it appears that changes in plasma cortisol can distinguish between the effects of benzodiazepine ligands. Whether these differ from responses in untreated anxious patients is unknown, as no comparative studies have been reported.

Biochemical effects

The benzodiazepine agonists, diazepam, alprazolam, lormetazepam, and flunitrazepam, reduce plasma noradrenaline (NA) or the metabolite 3-methoxy-4-hydroxyphenylethylene glycol in normal subjects (Hossman *et* al. 1980; Charney *et al*. 1986; Duka *et al*. 1986; Marty *et al*. 1986; Risby *et al*. 1989). However, this finding has not been universally replicated (Kumar *et al*. 1978; Picotti *et al*. 1982). Plasma adrenaline is reduced by midazolam but not by diazepam perhaps as midazolam is more potent (Marty *et al*. 1986). The antagonist flumazenil has no effect on plasma NA levels in normal subjects, but does reverse the agonist-induced fall in plasma NA levels (Duka *et al*. 1986).

Recently, a more sophisticated technique to measure sympathetic nervous system activity has been developed, where the plasma NA appearance rate is calculated using a tritiated NA isotope dilution technique and 'arterialized' venous plasma. Using this technique, the finding that diazepam reduces NA appearance rates in normal subjects has been confirmed, and a reduction in adrenaline also shown (Roy-Byrne *et al*. 1988). In contrast to control subjects, the effects of diazepam on reducing NA appearance rates are diminished in patients with panic disorder, although adrenaline responses are not different (Roy-Byrne *et al*. 1989; see Table 6.4).

Psychological responses
Self-rating scales

Benzodiazepine agonists increase self-ratings of sedation, tiredness, and calmness, with minimal effects on anxiety ratings because of low baseline values (Hossman *et al*. 1980; Bond and Lader 1983; Charney *et al*. 1986; Higgit *et al*. 1986; Hommer *et al*. 1986; Roy-Byrne *et al*. 1988; Risby *et al*.

Table 6.4. Responses to challenge doses of benzodiazepine ligands in patients with anxiety disorders compared with normal controls. All comparisons are between patients with panic disorders and controls unless indicated

Responses*	Agonist†	Antagonists†
Noradrenaline	↓	
Systolic BP		↑
Diastolic BP		↑
Heart rate		↑
SEM	↓/=‡	=
VAS sleepy	↓/=	=
VAS anxious	NA	↑ ↑
Cognitive tasks	↓/=	

* VAS, Visual analogue self-rating scale; SEM, saccadic eye movements; BP, blood pressure.
† ↓, Reduced response; = similar response; ↑, increased response; NA, not applicable due to basal differences.
‡ ↓, in panic disorder; =, generalized anxiety disorder.

1989; Ball *et al.* 1991). The antagonist flumazenil increases self-ratings of dizziness and sleepiness in normal subjects (Nutt *et al.* 1990), and other studies have reported increases in self-ratings of inner tension, anxiety, withdrawal, discontentedness, sadness, antagonism, and other items (Darragh *et al.* 1983; Duka *et al.* 1986; Higgitt *et al.* 1986).

The paucity of published reports on the effects of inverse agonists is undoubtedly because their unpleasant anxiogenic effects make such investigations so ethically difficult that as yet none have been deliberately carried out. The first accidental exposure was to FG7142, which was assumed to be an agonist since at that time the concept of antagonists, let alone inverse agonists, had not been formulated. The two subjects who received FG 7142 described psychological and behavioural symptoms of severe anxiety that were not amenable to psychological interventions and yet could be rapidly reversed by intravenous (i.v.) administration of the agonist lormetazepam (Dorow *et al.* 1983).

Another study in which normal subjects were given the partial inverse agonist RO 15–3505 was done on the supposition that it was an antagonist. This illusion was shattered when all the subjects reported unpleasant or fearful symptoms, including restlessness, irritability, anxiety, weakness, dizziness, hyperalertness, and flushing (Gentil *et al.* 1990). In a study of the antagonist β-carboline ZK 93426 subjects reported increased alertness, restlessness, mild apprehension, and other unpleasant physical symptoms (Duka *et al.* 1988). This suggested that this compound may have slight inverse agonist properties, and led to the suggestion that this or similar compounds may have utility as memory-enhancing agents (Sarter and Stephens 1989).

Surprisingly, despite the classic reports of Shagass and colleagues that barbiturate sensitivity is reduced in anxious patients (Shagass 1954; Shagass and Naiman 1956), there are few studies comparing subjective responses to benzodiazepines in anxious patients and controls. There is only one attempt to evaluate sensitivity to sedation with benzodiazepines; this found no significant difference between panic patients and controls despite a trend for patients to be less sedated (Roy-Byrne *et al.* 1989, 1990). This contrast with the earlier work probably reflects the use of subjective reports in the benzodiazepine study in contrast to the harder end point of electroencephalogram (EEG) changes and speech slurring used by Shagass. We have found that subjective ratings of sedation can be unreliable in patients and would suggest that more definite dependent variables such as the slowing of saccadic eye movements (discussed later) may offer a better means of assessing this question.

In contrast to the findings with diazepam, subjective responses to flumazenil differ considerably between panic patients and controls. Compared with controls, panic patients report significant increases in self-ratings of anxiety, dizziness, tremor, tachycardia, gastrointestinal symptoms (butterflies and stomach churning), headache, and skin flushing (Nutt *et al.* 1990, 1993; see Table 6.4). In other words flumazenil provokes many of the symptoms of panic in panic patients, and is the first panicogen yet discovered with a proven action on a receptor in the brain. Symptom responses to flumazenil are diminished after successful treatment with imipramine (Ball, unpublished data). In several patients with GAD, symptom responses to flumazenil were similar to those of controls (Ball *et al.* 1992), and symptom responses in normal subjects with high (>16) and low (<5) *N*-scores on the Eysenck Personality Questionnaire are also identical (Glue *et al.*, manuscript in preparation). The anxiogenic effects of flumazenil in panic disorder resemble the effects of inverse agonists in normal subjects; this has been interpreted as indicating a shift in receptor function in panic patients (Nutt *et al.* 1990). This anxiogenic effect appears to be specific to panic disorder rather than to GAD or trait anxiety, and it will be of considerable interest to carry out flumazenil challenges in other conditions associated with anxiety or panic attacks (e.g. major depression, alcohol withdrawal). The reduced anxiogenic effects after imipramine treatment may indicate that flumazenil sensitivity is a state marker for panic disorder and that imipramine treatment normalizes receptor sensitivity. However, it has been difficult to persuade panic patients to agree to a repeat challenge with flumazenil, and further studies in drug-free remitted panic patients are required.

Effects on performance and cognitive tasks

Diazepam and other benzodiazepine agonists produce impairment in a range of cognitive and performance tasks (Ghoneim *et al.* 1984*a*,*b*; Golombok and Lader 1984; Lister 1985; Brosan *et al.* 1986; Higgitt *et al.* 1986; Roy-Byrne *et al.* 1987; Gentil *et al.* 1990). Early studies reported that flumazenil had no effect on psychomotor performance or behaviour (Darragh *et al.* 1983; Emrich *et al.* 1984), although a more recent study demonstrated slowing of tapping rate and reaction time, and impaired performance in a symbol-copying task (Higgitt *et al.* 1986), possibly due to the large doses used having partial agonist actions. Although partial inverse agonist drugs have been reported to enhance memory in animal studies (see Sarter and Stephens 1989; Izquierdo and Medina 1991) this has not been specifically examined in man (see Dorow *et al.* 1987).

There is a general clinical impression that benzodiazepine-induced performance impairments are less apparent in anxious patients than in controls. This is supported by some comparative studies (Malpas *et al.* 1974; Melo de Paula 1977; Oblowitz and Robins 1983) but not others (Linnoila *et al.* 1983). The main problem with these investigations has been the lack of diagnostic specificity in subject selection. Recently, there has been a more rigorous assessment of this question in panic patients. A preliminary report demonstrated reduced diazepam-induced cognitive impairment in word-identification and word-recall memory tasks in these subjects following a single 15-mg dose of diazepam (Roy-Byrne *et al.* 1989). However, the significance of this difference did not hold up in a larger study, although a similar but non-significant trend was observed in a modified experimental paradigm in which incremental doses of diazepam were given (Roy-Byrne *et al.* 1990). An interesting possibility is that anxious subjects develop acute tolerance less rapidly than controls so that the slower rate of diazepam infusion obscures a possible difference in sensitivity.

Physiological effects

Cardiovascular

Systolic and diastolic blood pressure are slightly reduced by benzodiazepine agonists, with a minimal effect on heart rate (Hossman *et al.* 1980; Charney *et al.* 1986; Duka *et al.* 1986; Higgitt *et al.* 1986 Roy-Byrne *et al.* 1988, 1989; Risby *et al.* 1989). More substantial falls in blood pressure occur after anaesthetic doses of diazepam or midazolam (Marty *et al.* 1986). In normal subjects flumazenil slightly lowers systolic and diastolic blood pressure and heart rate (Higgitt *et al.* 1986; Nutt *et al.* 1990). Blood pressure and heart rate were increased in one subject who received the inverse agonist FG 7142, during a period of intense agitation. The weak partial inverse agonist/antagonist β-carboline ZK 93426 has been shown not to affect blood pressure or heart rate (Duka *et al.* 1988).

Blood pressure and heart rate changes after diazepam are of similar magnitude in panic patients and controls (Roy-Byrne *et al.* 1989). Associated with the severe anxiety provoked by flumazenil, patients with panic disorder have significant increases in systolic and diastolic blood pressure and heart rate compared with controls (Nutt *et al.* 1990; see Table 6.4).

Body sway

Body sway is a measure of the corrective mechanisms that maintain upright posture while standing and is increased by sedative drugs. Benzodiazepine agonists increase body sway (Swift *et al.* 1981; Campbell and Somerton 1982; Swift 1984; Patat and Foulhoux 1985) in a dose-dependent manner (Robin *et al.* 1991). However, it has not been demonstrated to be as sensitive as visual analogue ratings of drug effects (Robin *et al.* 1991).

Saccadic eye movements

Saccadic eye movements (SEM) are rapid eye movements that centre objects of visual interest on the fovea. Once initiated, SEM are independent of conscious control, but can be influenced by centrally acting drugs. Drug-induced changes in SEM therefore offer a means of assessing central drug effects on a reliable physiological measure that is independent of conscious control (for review see Glue 1991). There is a large body of work showing that benzodiazepines slow peak saccade velocity (Glue 1991). This slowing is dose-dependent, in that administration of small incremental doses of benzodiazepines produces progressive stepwise slowing of saccades (Hommer *et al.* 1986; Ball *et al.* 1991). Changes in saccadic eye movements are highly significantly correlated with other benzodiazepine-induced changes (e.g. increases in plasma growth hormone and self-ratings of sedation, or falls in cortisol and saccade parameters) and with plasma benzodiazepine levels (Hommer *et al.* 1986; Van Steveninck *et al.* 1990; Ball *et al.* 1991). Flumazenil produces a slight but significant slowing of peak saccade deceleration in normal subjects with a similar but non-significant trend in peak saccade velocity, similar to the effect expected from a weak partial agonist (Wilson *et al.* 1991). When administered after midazolam or diazepam, it reverses agonist-induced slowing of saccades, restoring peak velocity and other parameters to baseline levels (Ball *et al.* 1991).

Patients with panic disorder are more resistant to diazepam-induced reductions in peak saccade velocity than controls (Roy-Byrne *et al.* 1990; see Table 6.4). This has been interpreted as indicating reduced benzodiazepine receptor sensitivity in this disorder. Benzodiazepine sensitivity in patients with GAD, as measured by diazepam-induced falls in peak saccade velocity, is of intermediate magnitude compared with that of patients with panic disorder and normal controls (Cowley *et al.* 1991). Normal subjects with high and low *N*-scores (see above) have identical midazolam-induced slowing of saccadic eye movements (Glue *et al.* 1991). Saccadic eye movement responses to flumazenil in patients with panic disorder are similar to those of normal volunteers (Wilson *et al.* 1992), which is in sharp contrast to the marked anxiogenic effects of flumazenil in panic patients (see above). It might be hypothesized that inverse agonists would increase rather than decrease saccadic eye movements, based on their opposite effects to those of benzodiazepine agonists. However, it may not be possible to speed up saccadic eye movements under normal conditions (Glue 1991), and further testing using partial inverse agonists is required to clarify this area.

Awake and asleep EEG

The effect of benzodiazepines on the EEG has been extensively investigated by many laboratories using a range of different experimental methods. The EEG is a very sensitive measure of state of awareness and small changes in a subject's level of vigilance will produce large changes in the amount of theta and alpha activity recorded. Control of vigilance is difficult to standardize and this may account for the widely varying reports of EEG effects on activity in the alpha and slow-frequency wavebands. Each laboratory uses its own method of computer analysis, usually based on time series or period analysis, and uses different methods of comparison within and between subjects. Other problems may occur; for instance, a convincing dose–response relationship may be reported for slow activity in the power spectrum of normal subjects for a psychotropic drug, which is a little difficult to interpret since normal subjects do not commonly show any slow activity in the waking EEG. An explanation may be that eye movement artefacts appearing in the reference lead can be reduced after administration of the drug and, unless these have been carefully eliminated from the data, they may suggest spurious EEG changes or obscure actual cerebral effects.

However, there are effects of benzodiazepines on the waking EEG which are universally agreed and these appear to be independent of small changes in state of awareness. Beta activity is nearly always increased by benzodiazepine agonists (Hermann and Schaerer 1986), particularly in frontal areas, and indeed may appear for the first time after administration of these drugs. Its frequency varies from subject to subject and may be related to the subjects' intrinsic activity such as alpha frequency. The evolution of beta activity seems to follow the plasma levels of these agents fairly consistently, and can therefore be used as a measure of duration of effect. Only the barbiturate drugs have a similar effect on the EEG which is not related directly to state of awareness. Drowsiness effects on the EEG, such as increased theta activity and decreased alpha amplitude and frequency, have been widely reported (Saletu 1982; Laurian et al. 1984; Hermann and Schaerer 1986), as have non-specific effects on the cortical evoked response (Saletu 1974). To our knowledge there have been no studies directly comparing these actions of benzodiazepine agonists in anxious patients and controls.

The benzodiazepine antagonist flumazenil does not produce the same increase in fast activity in the EEG as is seen with agonists (Schopf et al. 1984). However it does reduce or abolish the agonist-induced fast activity described above (Laurian et al. 1984) and also has an alerting effect on the EEG when given after an agonist, in line with the subjective reports. Changes noted after administration of flumazenil alone, such as increased alpha activity and theta changes, are difficult to separate from the direct effects on vigilance produced by the side effects of flumazenil. Attempts have been made to differentiate these effects (Schopf et al. 1984) but further investigation is needed. Interestingly, the changes in the amplitude of various components of the evoked potential are similar to those produced by diazepam (Higgitt et al. 1986).

Benzodiazepine agonists have anticonvulsant effects on interictal spikes in the EEG of epileptic patients in varying degrees according to dose and type of epilepsy (Binnie 1982; Milligan et al. 1982; Gorman and Marciani 1985). However, when flumazenil is infused over a dose range of 0.5 to 3 mg i.v., it also reduces interictal spiking (Hart et al. 1991; Savic et al. 1991) and a single dose has reduced photic stimulation-evoked seizures for up to 3 days (Binnie 1991, personal communication). The observation by Hart et al. (1991) that the effects of flumazenil and diazepam were additive argues that it is not acting as a partial agonist but is either blocking the actions of an endogenous convulsant inverse agonist or is having a receptor 'resetting' action (see Nutt 1990b). The inverse agonist FG 7142 was reported to show no convulsant effect on the EEG in normal subjects who experienced severe anxiety (Dorow et al. 1983).

A more revealing measure of the effects of the various benzodiazepine agents has been the study of sleep. Using the changes in the EEG to classify the recordings into the various stages of sleep in a standardized manner according to agreed criteria (Rechtschaffen and Kales 1968) provides a sensitive measure of drug effects with few of the problems of artefact and variability of waking pharmacoEEG studies.

Benzodiazepine agonists, whether primarily used as hypnotic or as anxiolytic agents, produce similar changes in the sleep EEG, both in normal subjects and in insomniacs. The timing, duration, and degree of these changes vary with the pharmacokinetic properties of these agents, but the qualitative effect is similar. They have sleep-promoting effects, i.e. there is a decreased time to the onset of sleep and a tendency for longer total sleep time, with reduced awakenings in the insomniac patients (Gillin and Byerley 1990). In addition, there are changes in sleep architecture, the most widely described of which is increased amount of stage 2 sleep and, within this, an increase in the number of sleep spindles (Adam and Oswald 1984). Less consistently, a decrease in amount of stage 4 or total slow-wave sleep has been reported, particularly after the first night, and this is said to persist after the drug is stopped. Increased latency to rapid eye movement (REM) onset has been described mostly with higher benzodiazepine doses. There has been a recent study of sleep following administration of bretazenil, a partial benzodiazepine agonist. Bretazenil had the effects on sleep architecture of full agonists but without their sleep-promoting effects (Guldner *et al.* 1991). Nevertheless, despite the many studies in insomnia, there has been no direct comparison of the sensitivity of these subjects with normals to the actions of the benzodiazepines.

Flumazenil also has effects on sleep (Gaillard and Blois 1989). In general these are in the opposite direction to the agonists' effects, with increased time to sleep onset and more waking during the night. However there is a transient but significant decrease in slow-wave sleep, like the agonist effect. When flunitrazepam and flumazenil are administered together, some agonist effects were abolished, notably the sleep-promoting effects and the increase in spindles. Intriguingly, there was an additive effect on the slow-wave sleep, such that it was reduced more markedly by the drug combination than by each drug individually. This is exactly the same finding as for interictal spiking (Hart *et al.* 1991) and suggests the blockade of some endogenous slow-wave sleep-promoting factor.

The β-carboline antagonist/inverse agonist ZK 93426 has been shown to wake control subjects from lormetazepam-induced sleep within 10 min of i.v. administration (Duka *et al.* 1988) and also to prevent the normal decrease in vigilance and short periods of sleep observed in normal subjects left lying relaxed for long periods (Dorow *et al.* 1987).

Thus, within the limits of experimental techniques, waking and sleep EEG responses to benzodiazepine ligands offer another means of distinguishing between agonists, antagonists, and inverse agonists, and of monitoring the time course of their action within the central nervous system. It would now be timely to begin to compare such responses across different diagnostic groups.

In vivo receptor studies

One of the most promising methods for studying benzodiazepine receptors in the human brain is PET. This technique provides quantitative measurements of physiological or biochemical processes in the human brain. Earlier studies examined changes in local neuronal activity (e.g. cerebral blood flow or glucose utilization) associated with anxiety, while more recent studies have directly visualized benzodiazepine receptors. For instance, anticipatory anxiety in normal subjects and lactate-induced panic in patients with panic disorder both produce bilateral increases in cerebral blood flow in the temporal poles (Reiman *et al.* 1989). Patients with GAD have elevated glucose metabolic rates in parts of the occipital, temporal, and frontal lobes (Wu *et al.* 1991). The benzodiazepine agonist clorazepate reduces glucose metabolic rate in patients with GAD, with the greatest changes occurring in brain areas with the highest density of benzodiazepine receptors (Buchsbaum *et al.* 1987; Wu *et al.* 1991). Direct measurements of benzodiazepine receptor numbers in human brain have been made using radiolabelled benzodiazepine ligands (usually [^{11}C]flumazenil) (Pappata *et al.* 1988; Savic *et al.* 1988; Persson *et al.* 1989; Abadie *et al.* 1991). Using this technique, reduced benzodiazepine binding has been demonstrated in epileptic foci (Savic *et al.* 1988), but there are still no published studies in anxious patients. Unfortunately, the propensity of flumazenil to produce fear and anxiety (Nutt *et al.* 1990) may limit its suitability for PET studies in panic disorder. Another imaging technique that is beginning to be applied to the study of benzodiazepine receptors is SPECT (single-photon emission computerized tomography). Compounds containing ^{123}I such as iomazenil ([^{123}I]flumazenil) have been used to quantify benzodiazepine receptors in normal subjects (Woods *et al.* 1992) and in patients with focal epilepsy (Cordes *et al.* 1992).

Investigating benzodiazepine tolerance

Tolerance to benzodiazepines has been examined using a number of challenge paradigms. Shur *et al.* (1983) demonstrated reduced growth hormone responses to diazepam in subjects on long-term benzodiazepine treatment compared with controls. Growth hormone responses increased after 4 days of benzodiazepine withdrawal. Unfortunately, because of the lack of clinical details about the subjects and the small numbers who had repeat tests, it is not possible to determine whether growth hormone responses to diazepam are different in anxious patients and controls. Subjective (Shur *et al.* 1983; Roy-Byrne *et al.* 1991) and cognitive (Roy-Byrne *et al.* 1991) effects of benzodiazepines are diminished in benzodiazepine-tolerant subjects compared with those in controls.

Benzodiazepine tolerance has also been investigated using SEM. A preliminary report showed that the reduction in peak velocity after a single dose of nitrazepam disappeared after 6 days of treatment with this drug, despite much higher serum concentrations (Griffiths *et al.* 1983). Using a similar experimental design, this group also showed cross-tolerance between nitrazepam and diazepam (Griffiths *et al.* 1984). Using incremental doses of diazepam, reduced slowing of saccadic eye movements has been demonstrated in patients with panic disorder after chronic alprazolam treatment compared with untreated panic patients (Roy-Byrne *et al.* 1991). This does not appear to be due to alprazolam-treated patients having slower baseline peak saccade velocities, values of which were similar to those of the untreated patients. Our group is presently using a similar paradigm to quantify levels of tolerance in benzodiazepine-dependent subjects. In these studies, benzodiazepine-dependent subjects are administered incremental doses of midazolam, and subsequent changes in eye movements are compared with control subjects. Figure 6.2 is an example of marked tolerance to midazolam in a female subject who had been taking

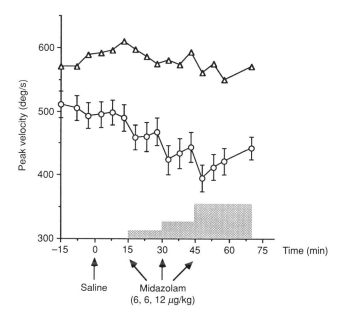

Fig. 6.2. Effects of consecutive infusions of saline placebo and madazolam (6, 6, and 12 μg/kg i.v.) on peak saccade velocity in (open triangles) a female subject tolerant to benzodiazepines and in (open circles) a drug-free control group (μ=14; mean $\pm$ SEM). Reproduced with permission from Glue (1991).

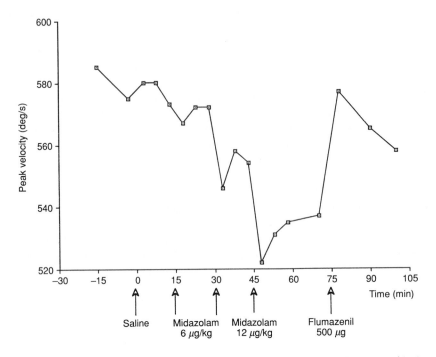

Fig. 6.3. Effects of consecutive infusions of saline placebo and midazolam (6, 6, and 12 μg/kg i.v.) on peak saccade velocity in a male healthy volunteer, suggesting acute tolerance to midazolam.

the equivalent of 20 mg diazepam daily for several years. Not only is there no effect of midazolam on peak velocity, but this patient's baseline peak velocity is also clearly not reduced by her regular benzodiazepine treatment.

In contrast to chronic tolerance, there is little known about acute tolerance to benzodiazepines. This phenomenon is well described and has clinical importance in that patients who have taken an overdose of benzodiazepine agonist sufficient to result in coma commonly regain consciousness despite plasma levels even higher than on admission (Greenblatt *et al.* 1978). Acute tolerance to three different benzodiazepines was studied in the classic report of Ellinwood *et al.* (1985). They demonstrated that triazolam and diazepam produced more acute tolerance than lorazepam. Our own studies on the effects of i.v. midazolam (Ball *et al.* 1991) revealed that, within 15 min of administration of each midazolam dose, peak saccade velocities tend to increase towards baseline values, and that this trend becomes more marked after subsequent doses of midazolam. This effect in a single subject is illustrated in Fig. 6.3. Over such a short time period, these changes are unlikely to be due to drug metabolism, although drug distribution may be involved.

Conclusions

Advances in pharmacological and other sciences have increased our understanding of the benzodiazepine receptor and its important role in the production and alleviation of anxiety. Benzodiazepine receptor challenge paradigms produce reliable changes in a number of endocrine, physiological, and psychological variables. Changes in some variables (e.g. cortisol, self-ratings of anxiety) appear to distinguish between agonist, antagonist, and inverse agonist drugs. However, knowledge about the effects of inverse agonists and antagonists is incomplete, and changes in other variables (e.g. noradrenaline, adrenaline, sleep EEG parameters) may also be useful in distinguishing between these ligands.

Despite the considerable body of knowledge about the effects of agonists and antagonists in normal subjects, there are relatively few studies comparing benzodiazepine-induced changes in controls with those of anxious patients (Table 6.4). Hopefully, this deficiency will be rectified soon in spite of complications such as differences in baseline values and the effects of anxiety. For example, the observation that diazepam reduces self-ratings of anxiety in anxious patients but not in controls is due to elevated baseline ratings in the former group. Similarly, different response in cognitive or performance tasks may be due to the effects of anxiety rather than to true pharmacological differences (see Lister 1991).

The best established facts to date implicating abnormal benzodiazepine receptor sensitivity in anxiety are the recent findings in panic disorder. These studies have shown abnormal biochemical, physiological, and subjective responses of panic patients to diazepam and flumazenil. Perhaps the best evidence is that of the SEM testing abnormalities which provide the most direct challenge of central benzodiazepine receptors while minimizing potentially confounding variables such as cognitive or emotional factors. Future prospects include the study of benzodiazepine receptor sensitivity in other anxiety states (e.g. GAD, normal anticipatory anxiety) or conditions associated with anxiety (e.g. agitated depression, alcohol withdrawal). Although of considerable theoretical interest, the ethical problems associated with challenges using inverse agonist drugs mean this line of investigation will probably be unfulfilled.

References

Abadie, P., Bisserbe, J.C., Boulenger, J.P., Travere, J.M., Barre, L., Petit, M.C., Zarifian, E., and Baron, J.C. (1991). Central benzodiazepine receptors: quantitative positron emission tomography study in healthy subjects and anxious patients. In *New concepts in anxiety* (ed. M. Briley and S.E. File), pp.203–10. Macmillan Press, London.

Adam, K. and Oswald, I. (1984). Effects of lormetazepam and of flurazepam on sleep. *British Journal of Clinical Pharmacology*, **17**, 531–8.

Ajlauni, K. and El-Khateeb, M. (1980). Effect of glucose on growth hormone, prolactin and thyroid-stimulating hormone response to diazepam in normal subjects. *Hormone Research*, **13**, 160–6.

Alho, H. Costa, E., Ferrero, P., Fujimoto, M., Cosenza-Murphy, P., and Guidotti, A. (1985). Diazepam-binding inhibitor: a neuropeptide located in selected neuronal populations of rat brain. *Science* **229**, 179–82.

Ball, D.M., Glue, P., Wilson, S., and Nutt, D.J. (1991). Pharmacology of saccadic eye movements in man (1): effects of the benzodiazepine receptor ligands midazolam and flumazenil. *Psychopharmacology*, **105**, 361–7.

Ball, D.M., Wilson, S., Glue, P., Lawson, C., and Nutt, D.J. (1992). Alteration in benzodiazepine receptor function underlying panic disorder. In *Handbook of anxiety*, Vol. 5 (ed. G. Burrows, M. Roth, and R. Noyes), Ch. 22. Elsevier, Amsterdam.

Basile, A.S., Jones, E.A., and Skolnick, P. (1991). The pathogenesis and treatment of hepatic encephalopathy: evidence for the involvement of benzodiazepine receptor ligands. *Pharmacological Reviews*, **43**, 27–71.

Bhattacharya, S.K., Glover, V., Sandler, M., Clow, A., Topham, A., Bernadt, M., and Murray, R. (1982). Raised endogenous monoamine oxidase inhibitor output in post withdrawal alcoholics: effects of l-dopa and ethanol. *Biological Psychiatry*, **17**, 687–94.

Binnie, C.D. (1982) The use of the interictal EEG in the study of antiepileptic drugs. In Kyoto symposia (ed. P.A. Buser, W.A. Cobb, and T.Okuma). *Electroencephalography and Clinical Neurophysiology*, **36** (suppl.), 504–12.

Bond, A. and Lader, M. (1983). Correlations among measures of response to benzodiazepines in man. *Pharmacology, Biochemistry and Behavior*, **18**, 295–8.

Brosan, L., Broadbent, D., Nutt, D., and Broadbent, M. (1986). Performance effects of diazepam before and after prolonged administration. *Psychological Medicine*, **16**, 561–71.

Buchsbaum, M.S., Wu, J., Haier, R., Hazlett, E., Ball, R., Katz, M., Sokolski, K., Lagunas-Solar, M., and Langer, S. (1987). Positron emission tomography assessment of effects of benzodiazepines on regional glucose metabolic rate in patients with anxiety disorder. *Life Sciences*, **40**, 2393–400.

Butler, P.W.P., Besser, G.M., and Steinberg, H. (1968). Changes in plasma cortisol induced by dexamphetamine and chlordiazepoxide given alone and in combination in man. *Journal of Endocrinology*, **40**, 391–2.

Campbell, A.J. and Somerton, D.T. (1982). Benzodiazepine drug effect on body sway in elderly subjects. *Journal of Clinical and Experimental Gerontology*, **4**, 341–7.

Chang, R.S.L., Lotti, V.J., Monaghan, R.L., Birnbaum, J., Stapley, E.O., Goetz, M.A., Albers-Schonberg, G., Patchett, A.A., Liesch, J.M., Hensens, O.D., and Springer, J.P. (1985). A potent nonpeptide cholecystekinin antagonist selective for peripheral tissues isolated from *Aspergillus alliaceus*. *Science*, **230**, 177–9.

Charney, D.S., Breier, A., Jatlow, P.I., and Heninger, G.R. (1986). Behavioral, biochemical and blood pressure responses to alprazolam in healthy subjects: interactions with yohimbine. *Psychopharmacology*, **88**, 133–40.

Clow, A., Glover, V., Armando, I., and Sandler, M. (1983). New endogenous benzodiazepine receptor ligand in human urine: identity with endogenous monoamine oxidase inhibitor? *Life Sciences*, **33**, 735–41.

Clow, A., Glover, V., Sandler, M., and Tiller, J. (1988a). Increased urinary tribulin output in generalised anxiety disorder. *Psychopharmacology*, **95**, 378–80.

Clow, A., Glover, V., Weg, M.W., Walker, M.P., Sheehan, D.V., Carr, D.B., and

Sandler, M. (1988*b*). Urinary catecholamine metabolite and tribulin output during lactate infusion. *British Journal of Psychiatry*, **152**, 122–6.

Cordes, M., Henkes, H., Ferstl, F., Schmitz, B., Hierholzer, J., Schmidt, D., and Felix, R. (1992). Evaluation of focal epilepsy: a SPECT scanning comparison of 123I-iomazenil versus HM-PAO. *American Journal of Neuroradiology*, **13**, 249–53.

Costa, E., Guidotti, A., and Mao, C.C. (1975). Evidence for involvement of GABA in the actions of benzodiazepines: studies on rat cerebellum. In *Mechanism of action of benzodiazepines* (ed. E. Costa and P. Greengard), pp. 113–30. Raven Press, New York.

Cowley, D.S., Roy-Byrne, P.P., Hommer, D., Greenblatt, D.J., Nemeroff, C., and Ritchie, J. (1991). Benzodiazepine sensitivity in anxiety disorders. *Biological Psychiatry*, **29**, 57A.

Darragh, A., Lambe, R., O'Boyle, C., Kenny, M., and Brick, I. (1983). Absence of central effects in man of the benzodiazepine antagonist Ro 15-1788. *Psychopharmacology*, **80**, 192–5.

Dorow, R., Horowski, R., Paschelke, G., Amin, M., and Braestrup, C. (1983). Severe anxiety induced by FG 7142, a β-carboline ligand for benzodiazepine receptors. *Lancet*, **ii**, 98–9.

Dorow, R., Duka, T., Holler, L., and Sauerbrey, N. (1987). Clinical perspectives of β-carbolines: from first studies in humans. *Brain Research Bulletin*, **19**, 319–26.

Duka, T., Ackenheil, M., Noderer, J., Doenicke, A., and Dorow, R. (1986). Changes in noradrenaline plasma levels and behavioural responses induced by benzodiazepine agonists with the benzodiazepine antagonist Ro 15-1788. *Psychopharmacology*, **90**, 351–7.

Duka, T., Goerke, D., Dorow, R., Holler, L., and Fichte, K. (1988). Human studies on the benzodiazepine receptor antagonist β-carboline ZK 93–426: antagonism of lormetazepam's psychotropic effects. *Psychopharmacology*, **95**, 463–71.

Ellinwood, E.H., Heatherly, D.G., Nikaido, A.M., Bjornsson, T.D., and Kilts, C. (1985). Comparative pharmacokinetics and pharmacodynamics of lorazepam, alprazolam and diazepam. *Psychopharmacology*, **86**, 392–9.

Elliott, J.M. (1985). Platelet receptor binding studies in affective disorders. *Journal of Affective Disorders*, **6**, 219–39.

Emrich, H.M., Sonderegger, P., and Mai, N. (1984). Action of the benzodiazepine antagonist Ro 15-1788 in humans after sleep withdrawal. *Neuroscience Letters*, **47**, 369–73.

File, S.E., Lister, R.G., and Nutt, D.J. (1982). The anxiogenic action of benzodiazepine antagonists. *Neuropharmacology*, **21**, 1022–37.

Fuxe, K., Agnatil, L.F., Bolme, P., Hikfelt, J., Lidbrink, P., Ljungdahl, A., Pesez de la Mora, M., and Ogren, S.O. (1975). The possible involvement of GABA mechanism on the action of benzodiazepines on central catecholamine neurons. *Pychopharmacology Bulletin*, **11**, 55–6.

Gaillard, J-M and Blois, R. (1989). Differential effects of flunitrazepam on human sleep in combination with flumazenil. *Sleep*, **12**, 120–32.

Gentil, V., Tavares, S., Gorenstein, C., Mathias, L., Gronich, G., and Singer, J. (1990). Acute reversal of flunitrazepam effects by Ro 15–1788 and Ro 15–3505: inverse agonism, tolerance and rebound. *Psychopharmacology*, **100**, 54–9.

Ghoneim, M.M., Hinrichs, J.V., and Mewaldt, S.P. (1984*a*). Dose–response analysis of the behavioural effects of diazepam: 1. learning and memory. *Psychopharmacology*, **82**, 291–5.

Ghoneim, M.M., Mewaldt, S.P., and Hinrichs, J.V. (1984*b*). Dose–response analysis of the behavioural effects of diazepam: 2. psychomotor performance, cognition and mood. *Psychopharmacology*, **82**, 296–300.

Gillin, J.C. and Byerley, W.F. (1990). The diagnosis and management of insomnia. *New England Journal of Medicine*, **322**, 239–48.

Glover, V., Halket, J.M., Watkins, P.J., Clow, A., Goodwin, B.L., and Sandler, M. (1988). Isatin: identity with the purified endogenous monoamine oxidase inhibitor tribulin. *Journal of Neurochemistry*, **51**, 656–9.

Glue, P. (1991). The pharmacology of saccadic eye movements. *Journal of Psychopharmacology*, **5**, 377–87.

Golombok, S. and Lader, M. (1984). The psychopharmacological effects of premazepam, diazepam and placebo in healthy human subjects. *British Journal of Clinical Pharmacology*, **18**, 127–33.

Gorman, J. and Marciani, M.G. (1985). EEG spiking activity, drug levels and seizure occurrence in epileptic patients. *Annals of Neurology*, **17**, 597–603.

Gram, L.F., Christensen, L., Kristensen, C.B., and Kragh-Sorensen, P. (1984). Suppression of plasma cortisol after oral administration of oxazepam in man. *British Journal of Clinical Pharmacology*, **17**, 176–8.

Greenblatt, D.J., Woo, E., Allen, M.D., Orsulak, P.J., and Shader, R.I. (1978). Rapid recovery from massive benzodiazepine overdose. *Journal of the American Medical Association*, **240**, 1872–4.

Griffiths, A.N., Tedeschi, G., Smith, A.T., and Richens, A.T. (1983). The effect of repeated doses of temazepam and nitrazepam on human psychomotor performance. *British Journal of Clinical Pharmacology*, **15**, 615–16.

Griffiths, A.N., Marshall, R.W., and Richens, A. (1984). Saccadic eye movement analysis as a measure of drug effects on human psychomotor performance. *British Journal of Clinical Pharmacology*, **18**, 73s–82s.

Grimm, G., Ferenci, P., Katzenschlager, R., Madl, C., Schneeweiss, B., Laggner, A.N., Lenz, K., and Gangl, A. (1988). Improvement of hepatic encephalopathy treated with flumazenil. *Lancet*, **ii**, 1392–4.

Guidotti, A., Forchetti, C.M., Corda, M.G., Konkel, D., Bennett, C.D., and Costa, E. (1983). Isolation, characterization, and purification to homogeneity of an endogenous polypeptide with agonistic action on benzodiazepine receptors. *Proceedings of the National Academy of Sciences, USA*, **80**, 3531–5.

Guldner, J., Rothe, B., Sterger, A., and Holsboer, F. (1991). Influence of the benzodiazepine partial agonist bretazenil on sleep EEG and nocturnal secretion of cortisol and growth hormone. *Biological Psychiatry*, **29**, 466s.

Haefely, W., Kulscar, A., Mohler, H., Pieri, L., Polc, P., and Schaffner, R. (1975). Possible involvement of GABA in the central actions of benzodiazepines. In *Mechanism of action of benzodiazepines* (ed. E. Costa and P. Greengard), pp. 1131–52. Raven Press, New York.

Hart, Y.M., Meinardi, H., Sander, J.W.A.S., Nutt, D.J., and Shorvon, S.D. (1991). The effect of intravenous flumazenil on interictal electroencephalographic epileptic activity: results of a placebo-controlled study. *Journal of Neurology, Neurosurgery and Psychiatry*, **54**, 305–9.

Hermann, W.M. and Schaerer, E. (1986). Pharmaco-EEG: Computer EEG analysis to describe the projection of drug effects on a functional cerebral level in humans. In *Handbook of EEG and clinical neurophysiology*, Vol. 2, *Clinical applications of computer analysis of EEG and other neurophysiological signals* (ed. F.H. Lopes da Silva, W. Storm van Leeuwen, and A. Remond), pp.385–445. Elsevier, Amsterdam.

Higgitt, A., Lader, M., and Fonagy, P. (1986). The effects of the benzodiazepine antagonist Ro 15–1788 on psychophysiological performance and subjective measures in normal subjects. *Psychopharmacology*, **89**, 395–403.

Hommer, D.W., Matsuo, V., Wolkowitz, O., Chrousos, G., Greenblatt, D.J., Weingartner, H., and Paul, S.M. (1986). Benzodiazepine sensitivity in normal human subjects. *Archives of General Psychiatry*, **43**, 542–51.

Hossman, V., Maling, T.J.B., Hamilton, C.A., Reid, J.L., and Dollery, C.T. (1980). Sedative and cardiovascular effects of clonidine and diazepam. *Clinical Pharmacology and Therapeutics*, **28**, 167–76.

Izquierdo, I. and Medina, J.H. (1991). GABA-A receptor modulation of memory: the role of endogenous benzodiazepines. *Trends in Pharmacological Sciences*, **12**, 260–5.

Kannan, V. (1981). Diazepam test of growth hormone secretion. *Hormone and Metabolic Research*, **13**, 390–4.

Klotz, U. (1991). Occurrence of 'natural' benzodiazepines. *Life Sciences*, **46**, 209–15.

Koulu, M., Lammintausta, R., Kangas, L., and Dahlstrom, S. (1979). The effect of methysergide, pimozide and sodium valproate on diazepam-stimulated growth hormone secretion in man. *Journal of Clinical Endocrinology and Metabolism*, **48**, 119–26.

Kumar, S.M., Kothary, S.P., and Zsigmond, E.K. (1978). Plasma free norepinephrine and epinephrine concentrations following diazepam-ketamine induction in patients undergoing cardiac surgery. *Acta Anaesthesiologica Scandinavica*, **22**, 593–600.

Laurian, S., Gaillard, J-M., Le, P.K., and Schopf, J. (1984). Effects of a benzodiazepine antagonist on the diazepam-induced electrical brain activity modifications. *Neuropsychobiology*, **11**, 55–8.

Linnoila, M., Erwin, C.W., Brendle, A., and Simpson, D. (1983). Psychomotor effects of diazepam in anxious patients and healthy volunteers. *Journal of Clinical Psychopharmacology*, **3**, 88–96.

Lister, R.G. (1985). The amnestic action of benzodiazepines in man. *Neuroscience and Biobehavioral Reviews*, **9**, 87–94.

Lister, R.G. (1991). Anxiety and cognition. In *New concepts in anxiety*, (ed. M. Briley and S.E. File) pp. 406–17 Macmillan Press, London.

Little, H.J., Nutt, D.J., and Taylor, S.C. (1987). Kindling and withdrawal changes at the benzodiazepine receptor. *Journal of Psychopharmacology*, **1**, 35–46.

Malpas, A., Legg, N.J., and Scott, D.F. (1974). Effects of hypnotics on anxious patients. *British Journal of Psychiatry*, **124**, 482–4.

Marty, J., Gauzit, R., Lefevre, P., Couderc, E., Farinotti, R., Henzel, C., and Desmonts, J.M. (1986). Effects of diazepam and midazolam on baroreflex control of heart rate and on sympathetic activity in humans. *Anesthesia Analgesia*, **65**, 113–19.

McCauley, L.D., and Gee, K.W. (1992). Peripheral-type benzodiazepine receptors and modulation of steroidogenesis in rat brain mitochondria. In *GABAergic synaptic transmission: molecular, pharmacological and clinical aspects*, Vol. 47, *Advances in biochemical psychopharmacology*. (ed. G. Biggio, A. Concas, and E. Costa), pp.143–8. Raven Press, New York.

Medina, J.H., Levi de Stein, M., and De Robertis, E. (1989). n-[^{3}H]butyl-β-carboline-3-carboxylate, a putative endogenous ligand, binds preferentially to subtype 1 of central benzodiazepine receptors. *Journal of Neurochemistry*, **52**, 665–70.

Melo de Paula, A.J. (1977). Intravenous lorazepam and diazepam in the treatment of acute anxiety states in the neurotic: a controlled study. *Clinical Therapeutics*, **1**, 125–34.

Milligan, N., Dhillon, S., Oxley, J. and Richens, A. (1982). Absorption of diazepam from the rectum and its effect on interictal spikes in the EEG. *Epilepsia*, **23**, 323–31.

Mohler, H. and Okada, T. (1977). Demonstration of benzodiazepine receptors in the central nervous system. *Science*, **198**, 849–51.

Noderer, J., Duka, T., and Dorow, R. (1988). Benzodiazepin-antagonisierung mit Ro 15-1788: psychometrische, hormonelle und biophysikalische Parameter. *Anaesthetist*, **37**, 535–42.

Nutt, D.J. (1983). Pharmacological and behavioural studies on benzodiazepine antagonists and contragonists. In *Benzodiazepine recognition site ligands: biochemistry and pharmacology* (ed. G. Biggio and E. Costa), pp.153–73. Raven Press, New York.

Nutt, D.J. (1990*a*). The pharmacology of human anxiety. *Pharmacological Therapeutics*, **47**, 233–66.

Nutt, D.J. (1990*b*). Selective ligands for benzodiazepine receptors: recent developments. In *Current aspects of the neurosciences*, Vol. 2, (ed. N.N. Osborne), pp. 259–93. MacMillan Press, London.

Nutt, D.J., Glue, P., Lawson, C., and Wilson, S. (1990). Evidence for altered benzodiazepine receptor sensitivity in panic disorder: effects of the benzodiazepine antagonist flumazenil. *Archives of General Psychiatry*, **47**, 917–25.

Nutt, D.J., Glue, P., Lawson, C.W., Wilson, S.J., and Ball, D.M. (1993). Do benzodiazepine receptors have a causal role in panic disorder? In *Psychopharmacology of panic*, British Association for Psychopharmacology Monograph (ed. S.A. Montgomery). Oxford University Press.

Oblowitz, H. and Robins, A.H. (1983). The effect of clobazam and lorazepam on the psychomotor performance of anxious patients. *British Journal of Clinical Pharmacology*, **16**, 95–9.

Pappata, S., Samson, Y., Chavoix, C., Prenant, C., Maziere, M. and Baron, J.C. (1988). Regional specific binding of ^{11}C-Ro 15–1788 to central type benzodiazepine receptors in human brain: quantitative evaluation by PET. *Journal of Cerebral Blood Flow Metabolism*, **8**, 304–13.

Patat, A., and Foulhoux, P. (1985). Effect on postural sway of various benzodiazepine tranquillizers. *British Journal of Clinical Pharmacology*, **20**, 9–16.

Persson, A., Pauli, S., Swahn, C.G., Halldin, C., and Sedvall, G. (1989). Cerebral uptake of ^{11}C-Ro 15–1788 and its acid metabolite ^{11}C-Ro 15–3890; PET study in healthy volunteers. *Human Psychopharmacology*, **4**, 215–20.

Picotti, G.B., Corli, O., Galva, M.D., Bondiolotti, G.P., and Carruba, M.O. (1982). Effects of oral chlormethyldiazepam on plasma adrenaline and noradrenaline and cardiovascular reactivity in preoperative patients. *European Journal of Clinical Pharmacology*, **23**, 383–8.

Rechtschaffen, A. and Kales, A. (ed.) (1968). *A manual of standardized terminology, techniques and scoring system for sleep stages of human subjects*, Public Health Service Publication no, 204. US Government Printing Office, Washington, DC.

Reiman, E.M., Fusselman, M.J., Fox, P.T., and Raichle, M.E. (1989). Neuroanatomical correlates of anticipatory anxiety. *Science*, **243**, 1071–4.

Risby, E.D., Hsiao, J.K., Golden, R.N., and Potter, W.Z. (1989). Intravenous alprazolam challenge in normal subjects: biochemical, cardiovascular and behavioural effects. *Psychopharmacology*, **99**, 508–14.

Robin, D.W., Hasan, S.S., Lichtenstein, M.J., Shiavi, R.G., and Wood, A.J.J. (1991). Dose-related effect of triazolam on body sway. *Clinical Pharmacology and Therapeutics*, **49**, 581–8.

Roy-Byrne, P.P., and Nutt, D.J. (1991). Benzodiazepines: biological mechanisms. In *Benzodiazepines in clinical practice: risks and benefits* (ed. P.P. Roy-Byrne and D.S. Cowley), pp.3–18. American Psychiatric Press, Washington, DC.

Roy-Byrne, P.P., Uhde, T.W., Holcomb, H., Thompson, K., King, A.K., and Weingartner, H. (1987). Effects of diazepam on cognitive processes in normal subjects. *Psychopharmacology*, **91**, 30–3.

Roy-Byrne, P.P., Lewis, N., Villacres, E., Diem, H., Greenblatt, D.J., Shader, R.I., and Veith, R. (1988). Suppression of norepinephrine appearance rate in plasma by diazepam in humans. *Life Science*, **43**, 1615–23.

Roy-Byrne, P.P., Lewis, N., Villacres, E., Diem, H., Greenblatt, D.J., Shader, R.I., and Veith, R. (1989). Preliminary evidence of benzodiazepine subsensitivity in panic disorder. *Biological Psychiatry*, **26**, 744–8.

Roy-Byrne, P.P., Cowley, D.S., Greenblatt, D.J., Shader, R.I., and Hommer, D. (1990). Reduced benzodiazepine sensitivity in panic disorder. *Archives of General Psychiatry*, **47**, 534–8.

Roy-Byrne, P.P., Cowley, D.S., Ritchie, J., Nemeroff, C., and Hommer, D. (1991). Benzodiazepine sensitivity in panic disorder: effects of alprazolam treatment. *Biological Psychiatry*, **29**, 55A.

Saletu, B. (1974). Classification of psychotropic drugs based on human evoked potentials. In *Modern problems of pharmacopsychiatry*. Vol. 8. *Psychotropic drugs and the human EEG* (ed. T.M. Itil), pp.258–85. Karger, Basle.

Saletu, B. (1982). The use of pharmaco-EEG in drug profiling. In *EEG in drug research* (ed. W.M. Hermann), pp.173–200. Fischer, Stuttgart.

Sandler, M. (1982). The emergence of tribulin. *Trends in Pharmacological Sciences*, **3**, 471–2.

Sangameswaran, L. and De Blas, A.L. (1985). Demonstration of benzodiazepine-like molecules in the mammalian brain with a monoclonal antibody to benzodiazepines. *Proceedings of the National Academy of Sciences, USA*, **82**, 5560–4.

Sangameswaran, L., Fales, H.M., Friedrich, P. and De Blas, A.L., (1986). Purification of a benzodiazepine from bovine brain and detection of benzodiazepine-like immunoreactivity in human brain. *Proceedings of the National Academy of Sciences, USA*, **83**, 9236–40.

Sarter, M. and Stephens, D.N. (1989). Disinhibitory properties of β-carboline antagonists of benzodiazepine receptors: a possible therapeutic approach for senile dementia? *Biochemical Society Transactions*, **17**, 81–3.

Savic, I., Persson, A., Roland, P., Pauli, S., Sedvall, G., and Widen, L. (1988). In-vivo demonstration of reduced benzodiazepine receptor binding in human epileptic foci. *Lancet*, **ii**, 863–6.

Savic, I., Widen, L., and Stone-Elander, S. (1991). Feasibility of reversing benzodiazepine tolerance with flumazenil. *Lancet*, **i**, 133–7.

Schopf, J., Laurian, S., Le, P.K., Gaillard, J.-M. (1984). Intrinsic activity of the benzodiazepine antagonist Ro 15-1788 in man: an electrophysiological investigation. *Pharmacopsychiatry*, **17**, 79–83.

Shagass, C. (1954). The sedation threshold. A method for measuring tension in psychiatric patients. *Electroencephalography and Clinical Neurophysiology*, **6**, 221–33.

Shagass, C. and Naiman, J. (1956). The sedation threshold as an objective index of manifest anxiety in psychoneurosis. *Journal of Psychosomatic Research*, **1**, 49–57.

Sherwin, A., Matthew, E., Blain, M., and Guevremont, D. (1986). Benzodiazepine receptor binding is not altered in human epileptogenic cortical foci. *Neurology*, **36**, 1380–2.

Shur, E., Peturrson, H., and Checkley, S. (1983). Long-term benzodiazepine administration blunts growth hormone response to diazepam. *Archives of General Psychiatry*, **40**, 1105–8.

Snyder, S.H. (1986). Virtuoso design of drugs. *Nature*, **323**, 292–3.

Squires, R.F. and Braestrup, C. (1977). Benzodiazepine receptors in rat brain. *Nature*, **266**, 732–4.

Swift, C.G. (1984). Postural instability as a measure of sedative drug response. *British Journal of Clinical Pharmacology*, **18**, 87S–90S.

Swift, C.G., Haythorne, J.M., Clarke, P., and Stevenson, I.H. (1981). The effect of ageing on measured responses to single doses of oral temazepam. *British Journal of Clinical Pharmacology*, **11**, 413P–414P.

Sylvälahti, E. and Kanto, J. (1975). Serum growth hormone, serum immunoreactive insulin and blood glucose responses to oral and intravenous diazepam in man. *International Journal of Clinical Pharmacology*, **12**, 74–8.

Tinuper, P., Montagna, P., Cortelli, P., Avoni, P., Lugaresi, A., Schoch, P., Bonetti, E.P., and Gallarsi, R. (1992). Idiopathic recurring stupor: a case with possible involvement of the gamma-aminobutyric acid (GABA) ergic system. *Annals of Neurology*, **31**, 503–6.

Unseld, E., Krishna, D.R., Fischer, C., and Klotz, U. (1989). *Biochemical Pharmacology*, **38**, 2473–8.

van Steveninck, A.L., Verver, S., Kroon, J.M., Schoemaker, H.C., Breimer, D.D., and Cohen, A.F. (1990). Relationships between plasma concentration of temazepam and effects of saccadic peak velocity in individual subjects. *British Journal of Clinical Pharmacology*, **30**, 310P.

Wildmann, J., Mohler, H., Vetter, W., Ranalder, U., Schmidt, K., and Maurer, R. (1987). Diazepam and N-desmethyldiazepam are found in rat brain and adrenal and may be of plant origin. *Journal of Neural Transmission*, **70**, 383–98.

Wilson, S., Glue, P., and Nutt, D.J. (1991). Flumazenil and saccadic eye movements in patients with panic disorder and normal subjects. *Human Psychopharmacology*, **7**, 45–50.

Woods, S.W., Serbyl, J.P., Goddard, A.W., Dey, H.M., Zoghbi, S.S., Germine, M., Baldwin, R.M., Smith, E.O., Charney, D.S., Heninger, G.R., Hoffer, P.B., and Innu, R.B. (1992). Dynamic imaging after injection of the benzodiazepine receptor ligand [123I]-iomazenil in healthy human subjects. *Psychiatry Research and Neuroimaging*, **45**, 67–77.

Wu, J.C., Buchsbaum, M.S., Hershey, T.G., Hazlett, E., Sicotte, N., and Johnson, J.C. (1991). PET in generalized anxiety disorder. *Biological Psychiatry*, **29**, 1181–99.

Zorumski, C.F. and Isenberg, K.E. (1991). Insights into the structure and function of GABA–benzodiazepine receptors: ion channels and psychiatry. *American Journal of Psychiatry*, **148**, 162–73.

7 The biology of benzodiazepine dependence

Sandra E. File

There are two ways in which benzodiazepine dependence has been assessed in animal experiments. One is by measuring the development of tolerance to the behavioural effects of the benzodiazepines; the second is by measuring the incidence of physical symptoms on the withdrawal of benzodiazepine treatment. Whether or not the same adaptive changes underlie both phenomena is not known for certain, and will be discussed at the end of this chapter. The first section of this chapter will discuss the climate into which the benzodiazepines were introduced. The second section will review the evidence from behavioural studies in animals for the development of tolerance to the effects of benzodiazepines and for the occurrence of behavioural changes on drug withdrawal. The final section will focus on studies of the neurochemical mechanisms underlying the development of benzodiazepine dependence.

Introduction of the benzodiazepines

The benzodiazepines were introduced as sedating and anxiolytic agents and rapidly replaced as drug of choice meprobamate, which had in its turn largely replaced the barbiturates. The abuse and dependence risks from barbiturates and meprobamate were well known when the benzodiazepines were introduced and the withdrawal syndrome in humans was characterized by insomnia, weight loss, tremor, anxiety, and seizures—very similar to the alcohol withdrawal syndrome.

Although the mechanism of action of the benzodiazepines was not initially known, in the earliest animal tests they were compared with meprobamate and the barbiturates and the pharmacological profile of the benzodiazepines was that they were sedative, increased food intake, and decreased anxiety and seizures. Since the characteristics of the withdrawal syndrome seen with other sedative anxiolytics were insomnia, weight loss, increased anxiety, and seizures (i.e. the complete opposite of the pattern of effects seen with benzodiazepine administration), it would not have been unreasonable to wonder whether, upon their removal from chronic treatment, the benzodiazepines might also produce this pattern of withdrawal effects. The notion that the pattern of responses seen during drug withdrawal was the opposite to the pattern seen originally upon drug administration was certainly current at the time. However, there seem to have been no animal studies into whether there were withdrawal responses after chronic treatment with benzodiazepines, in spite of the report of an abstinence syndrome in experimental human subjects that persisted for 9 days after withdrawal from high doses of chlordiazepoxide (Hollister et al. 1961).

There was no technical reason why the behavioural effects of withdrawing animals from chronic benzodiazepine treatment could not have been assessed in animals prior to the clinical use of benzodiazepines. All of the tests had been used for assessing the potentially beneficial effects of the benzodiazepines and had been used to measure changes in the opposite direction with drugs such as amphetamine and convulsants. However, the use of animal tests to test dependence on sedative–anxiolytics was not common in the early 1960s. Animal investigations into the alcohol withdrawal syndrome did not really progress until the late 1960s with studies by Freund (1969), and, in general, the studies concentrated on the incidence of seizures (e.g. Essig and Lam 1968). Some animal studies had been published on barbiturate withdrawal (e.g. Fraser and Isbell 1954; Essig and Flanary 1959), but these were rare. Withdrawal convulsions had been reported in dogs following chronic meprobamate treatment (Essig 1958) but, again, animal studies were rare.

Although there were no studies on the development of benzodiazepine dependence, there were early studies on the effects of chronic treatment. Randall et al. (1961) reported studies in which rats were administered large doses of diazepam for several weeks. In one experiment, rats were given 1000, 100, or 10 mg/kg body weight for 6 weeks; a reduction in food intake and impaired weight gain was reported with the highest dose, but no effects with other doses. Although the benzodiazepines were known to generally *increase* food intake, this reduction occasioned no comment and, indeed, 1000 mg/kg is an enormous dose. In a second study rats were given 240, 80, or 20 mg/kg for 42 weeks and it was reported that they showed no signs of sedation or ataxia. This is extraordinary, since diazepam at 0.5 mg/kg will reduce motor activity in rats. It therefore means either that tolerance had developed to the sedative effects, or that the authors used exceptionally insensitive tests. In a third study, rats were given diazepam (320, 80, or 20 mg/kg) for more than 24 weeks and no effects detected. These experiments would have been ideal for assessing whether diazepam caused physical dependence, but no such measurements seem to have been made and the studies were viewed only as toxicity testing. Randall et al. (1961) also reported a study in which dogs were given diazepam (40, 10, or 2.5 mg/kg) for 35 days or 3–6 months. The highest dose was reported to cause sedation, but it was not specified whether this was after acute administration or throughout the period of treatment. However, one dog died from major seizures after 22 weeks of diazepam treatment. Unfortunately, the onset of seizures in relation to the diazepam administration was not reported, so it is impossible to determine whether this could have been an example of a withdrawal seizure. Marmosets were also treated with diazepam (40, 20, or 5 mg/kg) for 3 months and no untoward responses noted. Once again, these studies would have been ideal for assessing physical dependence, but this possibility does not seem to have been considered.

Behavioural evidence for the development of tolerance and withdrawal responses

Studies from 1963 to 1974

Development of tolerance to sedative effects

There were clinical reports of rapid development of tolerance to the sedative effects (Warner 1965; Kaplan *et al.* 1973). There was no evidence that pharmacokinetic changes contributed to the development of tolerance in man, but two animal papers did provide evidence for some metabolic tolerance to very high doses of chlordiazepoxide (Hoogland *et al.* 1966; Christensen 1973). Acute tolerance to the reduction in electroencephalogram (EEG) amplitude was reported in cats and it was speculated (probably incorrectly) that this might be due to the action of a metabolite (Barnett and Fiore 1973). However, there were several reports from animal studies where the tolerance to sedative effects was clearly functional. For example, tolerance to the reduction in lever-pressing was reported after 3–5 days of treatment in rats (Margules and Stein 1968; Stein and Berger 1971; Wise *et al.* 1972); tolerance to the reduction of spontaneous locomotor activity was reported after 14 days of treatment in mice and rats (Goldberg *et al.* 1967); tolerance to the prolongation of barbiturate sleeping time was reported after 3–14 days of chlordiazepoxide treatment (Goldberg *et al.* 1967; Jori *et al.* 1969; Orme *et al.* 1972).

Tolerance to anticovulsant effects

Goldberg *et al.* (1967) reported tolerance to the anticonvulsant effects of chlordiazepoxide in rats and mice against seizures evoked by maximal electroshock. Killam *et al.* (1973) reported the development of tolerance to the anticonvulsant effects of several benzodiazepines against seizures evoked in photosensitive baboons. Browne and Penry (1973) reported tolerance in human patients to the anti-epileptic actions of benzodiazepines.

Changes in seizure activity upon benzodiazepine withdrawal

Killam *et al.* (1973) reported epileptic-like responses that lasted from a few days to a few weeks after withdrawal from benzodiazepine administration. Yanagita and Takahashi (1973) reported withdrawal symptoms in monkeys after two 4-week periods of diazepam administration (10–20 mg/kg); in two of the four monkeys tested there were severe withdrawal responses including convulsions. Withdrawal from 4 weeks of chlordiazepoxide (75 mg/kg/day) produced withdrawal responses of moderate intensity, but, after 4 weeks of a higher dose (113 mg/kg/day), three of the four monkeys had convulsions. The authors also noted that the withdrawal symptoms in monkeys were very long-lasting and recommended that testing should be extended to 7 days after benzodiazepine withdrawal.

Studies from 1974 to 1980

Tolerance to sedative, anxiolytic, and anticonvulsant effects

Sansone (1979) reported that after 5 days of treatment, tolerance developed to the sedative effects of chlordiazepoxide in mice, but not to the locomotor stimulant effect of lower doses. Reports continued that there was rapid (3–5 days) tolerance to the sedative effects of the benzodiazepines (measured by their depressant effect on unpunished lever-pressing), which contrasted with the increase in anxiolytic effects over 5 days (measured by the increase in punished lever-pressing), e.g. the reports of Cook and Sepinwall (1975) and Cannizzaro et al. (1972). In the social interaction test of anxiety, File and Hyde (1978) reported that there was rapid (5 days) development of tolerance to the sedative effects of chlordiazepoxide (measured by the decrease in spontaneous motor activity), whereas after 5 days of treatment an anxiolytic effect (measured by a selective increase in social interaction) could be detected. However, after 25 days of treatment with chlordiazepoxide in the rat, tolerance to its anxiolytic effect in the social interaction test was reported (Vellucci and File 1979).

This seemed to be in contrast to the results from the Geller–Seifter conflict test, although in most cases the period of chronic treatment did not extend past 5 days. There were two exceptions (Margules and Stein 1968; McMillan and Leander 1978) where chronic treatment led to a further increase in punished responding, but in both cases after 10 days this increase was accompanied by an increase in unpunished responding, i.e. there seemed to be a non-specific stimulant effect. However, there was evidence that the anxiolytic effects lasted for at least 10 days (McMillan and Leander 1978). Shearman et al. (1979) also reported that the anxiolytic effects of chlordiazepoxide and diazepam persisted after 10 days of treatment in a drug discrimination test in which the benzodiazepines were antagonizing the stimulus cue of the convulsant pentylenetetrazole. Interestingly though, partial tolerance was found in this test since, on acute administration of the benzodiazepines, only 17 per cent selected the lever associated with pentylenetetrazole, whereas, after 10 days of treatment, twice as many did so.

Tolerance was reported to the anticonvulsant action of benzodiazepines against seizures induced by strychnine and bicuculline (Lippa and Regan 1977), but not to those induced by pentylenetetrazole (Juhasz and Dairman 1977; Lippa and Regan 1977). This conclusion was based on only a single dose of pentylenetetrazole (PTZ) and it was therefore difficult to determine whether this dose was equivalent to the doses of the other convulsants. The duration of treatment was only 4–7 days and, again, a longer treatment time might have led to the development of tolerance. However, these reports (one in abstract form only) led to the widespread and oft-repeated belief that tolerance did not develop to the anti-PTZ effects of the benzodiazepines. This, by some strange reasoning, led to the belief that the action of benzodiazepines against seizures induced by PTZ (but not by other agents) reflected their anxiolytic activity.

Studies of physical dependence

Three studies reported the development of physical dependence on benzo-diazepines by administering them in the diet. Yanaura *et al.* (1975) fed diazepam to rats (0.5, 1, or 2 mg/g of food) for 1 week and, on withdrawal, there was a significant decrease in body weight; cross-dependence between phenobarbital and diazepam was also demonstrated by this method. McMillan and Leander (1978) administered chlordiazepoxide (50 mg/kg) in the drinking water for 7 weeks; on withdrawal of the drug there was a significant hyperac-tivity (reflected in an increase in unpunished responding) that began on the second day and lasted for 14 days of withdrawal. Sadly, it was not possible to assess any anxiogenic responses during withdrawal, since the control animals made virtually no punished responses and further decreases would have been impossible to reach. Suzuki *et al.* (1980) administered diazepam in the food of rats in doses increasing from 1 mg/g of food to 8mg/g over a 5-week period; upon drug withdrawal significant decreases in body weight were detected from 24–72 h after withdrawal and these were exacerbated by administration of a drug that inhibits the synthesis of serotonin (5-HT).

Rastogi *et al.* (1976) administered diazepam (10 mg/kg) or bromazepam (10 mg/kg) to rats for 22 days and examined effects in the chronically treated group and in a group withdrawn from benzodiazepines for 48 h. There were no significant changes in body weight, but there was a significant hyperactivity in both the withdrawal groups.

Studies from 1981 to 1990
Tolerance to the sedative effects

Studies into the development of tolerance to the sedative effects of benzo-diazepines continued. File (1981) reported the rapid development of tol-erance, even to the short-acting benzodiazepines such as lorazepam and triazolam; it was clear that the continuous presence in the brain of the drug was not necessary for the development of tolerance. File (1984) reported that, in chronically treated rats, the plasma concentrations of chlordiazepoxide and its metabolites did not correlate with the behavioural effect and that pharmacokinetic changes could not explain the development of tolerance to the sedative effects of most doses. Lister *et al.* (1983*a,b*) found similar results with reference to the concentrations of lorazepam in the brain.

More analytical questions were asked, such as whether the benzodiazepine receptor was involved in mediating the development of tolerance (File 1982*a*). The roles of associative conditioning (File 1982*b*; Greeley and Cappell 1985; Griffiths and Goudie 1986; King *et al.* 1987) and instrumental learning (Herberg and Montgomery 1987) were examined. The duration of tolerance was assessed. There was relatively rapid (a few days) recovery from tolerance to a benzodiazepine's sedative effects when the duration of treatment was only a few days (File 1982*a,b*; Rosenberg *et al.* 1983). When treatment was continued for 21 days, complete recovery from tolerance to the sedative effects had not occurred 2 weeks after the end of treatment in that the scores were still significantly above the acute treatment group (see Fig. 7.1). Extrapolating the curve in Fig. 7.1 suggests that it might take about 5 weeks for the response to diazepam to fully recover to the level shown by the group given a single acute injection.

Tolerance that developed after only a single dose was demonstrated to the hypnotic effects of diazepam in mice, and pharmacokinetic explanations were excluded (Yoong *et al.* 1986). Single-dose tolerance to diazepam-induced rotarod impairment (Henauer *et al.* 1984) and to the lorazepam-induced

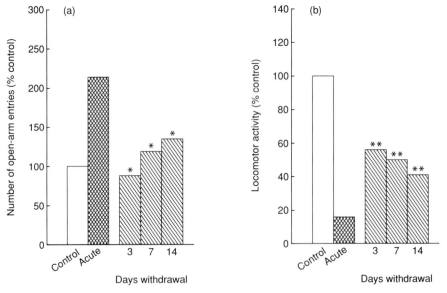

Fig. 7.1. Responses, shown as a percentage of the control score, of rats to a test dose of diazepam (5 mg/kg) after a single administration (acute) and 3, 7, and 14 days after the last of 21 daily diazepam injections (withdrawal days). All rats were tested with the same dose of diazepam. *$p<0.05$, **$p<0.01$, compared with the response to acute treatment. (a) The anxiolytic response to diazepam is shown by an increase in the percentage of entries on to open arms in the plus maze. (b) The sedative response to diazepam is shown by the decrease in locomotor activity in the holeboard. Taken from unpublished data of Hitchcott and File.

reductions in locomotor activity (File *et al.* 1988) and anticonvulsant effects (Lister and Nutt 1986) were reported.

Surprisingly little cross-tolerance was found between the benzodiazepines and pentobarbital (Cesare and McKearney 1980; Lister *et al.* 1983*b*; Rosenberg *et al.* (1983). These results are in contrast to the many reports of cross-dependence between barbiturates and benzodiazepines.

In contrast to the rapid development of tolerance to the sedative effects, there appeared to be no tolerance to the locomotor stimulant effects of chlordiazepoxide and diazepam even after 20 days (File and Pellow (1985) or to the stimulant effects on electrical self-stimulation after 40 injections of chlordiazepoxide (Herberg and Montgomery 1987).

Tolerance to anticonvulsant effects

The myth that tolerance did not develop to the anti-PTZ effects of benzo-diazepines was exploded. File (1983*a*) demonstrated that tolerance *did* develop to the anticonvulsant effects of diazepam against seizures induced by PTZ and that it could be demonstrated after 5 or 20 days, depending on the test dose of PTZ. The rate of development of tolerance to PTZ-induced seizures was also shown to depend on the strain of mice used and the behavioural measure of convulsions (File 1983*b*). Gent *et al.* (1985) reported the development of tolerance to PTZ-induced seizures after 4 days of treatment with clobazam in mice. Frey *et al.* (1984) reported that tolerance developed after 4 days to the anticonvulsant action of diazepam in dogs against PTZ-induced seizures. Scherkl *et al.* (1988) reported that tolerance developed to PTZ-induced seizures in mice after 4 days of clonazepam treatment and 7 days of clorazepate. Gonsalves and Gallager (1986) reported that tolerance to PTZ-induced seizures had developed after 3 weeks of continuous release of diazepam from silastic capsules implanted subcutaneously in rats. Acute tolerance to anti-PTZ effects has also been reported after diazepam administration in dogs (Frey *et al.* 1984) and clobazam in mice (Feely *et al.* 1986).

Tolerance to anxiolytic effects

Tolerance was reported to the anxiolytic effect of benzodiazepines in the rat neophobia test (Cooper *et al.* 1981), the Vogel conflict test (Brown *et al.* 1984; Gonzalez *et al.* 1984; Soderpalm 1987), the mouse punished crossing test (Stephens and Schneider 1985; Fritz *et al.* 1986), the defensive burying test (Treit 1985), the Geller–Seifter conflict test (Rock and Barrett 1987), the social interaction and elevated plus-maze tests (Baldwin *et al.* 1987; File *et al.* 1987; File 1989; File and Baldwin 1989), and a drug-discrimination paradigm (Emmett-Ogelsby *et al.* 1983). Thus, there remains little doubt from the animal literature that tolerance does develop to the effects of benzodiazepines in animal tests of anxiety.

The duration of tolerance to diazepam's anxiolytic effects in the plus-maze was examined. Tolerance had developed after 21 days of treatment with diazepam (4 mg/kg/day). The rats were then retested with diazepam 3 days or 1 or 2 weeks after the end of the chronic treatment. It can be seen from Fig. 7.1 that there was still partial tolerance at the 2-week test point, in that the scores were still significantly below those of the acute treatment group.

Withdrawal responses
Since the introduction of benzodiazepine antagonists and inverse agonists there have been several studies in which withdrawal was precipitated by the administration of a drug that could antagonize the action of the benzodiazepines. This is analogous to precipitating morphine withdrawal with naloxone. These studies are complex to interpret because the results depend on the precise timing of the administration of the antagonist, the particular antagonist used, the dose of the antagonist, the withdrawal response measured, and the species used. These have been extensively reviewed by Woods *et al.* (1987), who counselled against interpreting all antagonist-elicited responses as evidence of withdrawal responses. For a theoretical discussion of benzodiazepine-precipitated withdrawal see File and Hitchcott (1990).

Increased anxiety during withdrawal
Behavioural changes indicating increased anxiety during withdrawal have been reported in a drug-discrimination paradigm following 7 or 11 days of diazepam (60 mg/kg/day; Emmett-Ogelsby *et al.* 1983), in the social interaction test after withdrawal from 21 days of chlordiazepoxide (5–20 mg/kg/day; Baldwin *et al.* 1987) or diazepam (40 mg/kg/day; Oakley *et al.* 1988), and in the elevated plus-maze tests after withdrawal from 21 days of chlordiazepoxide (5–20 mg/kg/day; File *et al.* 1987), 21, 14, or 7 days of diazepam (1, 2.5, or 4 mg/kg/day; File 1989; File *et al.* 1989), or 21 days of lorazepam (1 mg/kg/day; File 1990).

Physical signs of withdrawal
The studies in which physical signs of withdrawal have been recorded have been summarized in File (1990). The doses used in these studies were generally extremely high and the results provide no more than a qualitative description of the withdrawal syndrome in animals. However, it is clear that the symptoms persist for up to 2 weeks after drug withdrawal. Even after treatment with low doses of diazepam (4 mg/kg/day for 21 days) there was an elevation of plasma corticosterone concentrations that lasted for 2 weeks after diazepam was discontinued (Table 7.1). It is difficult to know whether this long-lasting corticosteroid elevation is truly a withdrawal response since the concentrations were also elevated in the 21-day diazepam group. However, long-lasting elevations in corticosteroids could well contribute to some of the very long-lasting symptoms experienced by some patients on withdrawal from benzodiazepines. In contrast to the effects on corticosterone, the group treated with diazepam for 21 days showed reduced plasma prolactin

Table 7.1. Mean (± SEM) plasmas concentrations of prolactin and corticosterone (measured by radioimmunoassay) in rats handled and injected with water for 21 days (control) or with diazepam (4 mg/kg/day for 21 days) and tested 30 min, 42 h, or 2 weeks after the last dose. All the rats had been tested in the plus maze before sacrifice*

	Mean (± SEM) plasmas concentrations (ng/ml)			
	Controls	Diazepam day 21	42 h after withdrawal	2 weeks after withdrawal
Prolactin	50.3 ± 8.2	29.0 ± 6.4[†]	42.0 ± 6.8	52.4 ± 11.0
Corticosterone	35.1 ± 6.3	161.9 ± 29.4[‡]		113.5 ± 15.9

* Unpublished data from File, Andrews, and Townsend.   † p <0.05 compared with control group.
‡ p <0.01 compared with control group.

concentrations, but these were not changed either 42 h or 2 weeks after diazepam withdrawal.

Neurochemical mechanisms of dependence

Benzodiazepine binding

The existence of benzodiazepine-binding sites in the central-nervous system (CNS) was discovered in 1977 (Braestrup and Squires 1977) and an obvious question was whether chronic treatment would change benzodiazepine binding. Rosenberg and Chiu found a decrease in benzodiazepine binding 14 h after 7–10 days with high doses of flurazepam (up to 150 mg/kg/day intraperitoneally (i.p.); Chiu and Rosenberg 1978; Rosenberg and Chiu 1979) and after 4 weeks when flurazepam was added to the drinking water (Rosenberg and Chiu 1981). This was due to a decrease in the number of benzodiazepine receptors, but it is unclear whether the rats were drug-free (i.e. in a withdrawal state) at the time of the experiment. Using lower benzodiazepine doses, decreased benzodiazepine receptor binding has also been reported after 10–14 days treatment with diazepam (5–10 mg/kg/day; Grimm and Hershkowitz 1981), and after 3 weeks treatment with chlordiazepoxide or clonazepam (1–7.5 mg/kg/day; Crawley et al. 1982). Similar results have been found in fetal mouse cortical and spinal cord cultures after in vitro exposure to clonazepam and diazepam (Prezioso and Neale 1983; Sher 1983, 1986; Sher et al. 1983). Mele et al. (1984) found that after 5 days of diazepam treatment there was a small, but significant decrease in the dissociation constant K_D for diazepam binding. After 10 days of treatment, diazepam was withdrawn, but the decreased K_D persisted for 7 days.

Not all studies have found decreases in benzodiazepine-receptor binding following chronic treatment. Twenty-four to 28 h after drug withdrawal,

Mohler *et al.* (1978) found no change in benzodiazepine binding in rats that had been treated daily with diazepam (3 mg/kg) or phenobarbital (30 mg/kg) for 30 days. Braestrup *et al.* (1979) found that 8 weeks of treatment with high doses of diazepam (90 mg/kg/day) or lorazepam (60 mg/kg/day) failed to affect [³H] diazepam binding. Results of studies in which rats have been injected with lower, more clinically relevant doses of benzodiazepines, or where rats were implanted with diazepam-releasing capsules have also found benzodiazepine-receptor binding to be unchanged (Mohler *et al.* 1978; Gallager *et al.* 1984; Heninger and Gallager 1988). Also, in fetal cortical cells exposed *in vitro* to a low concentration of diazepam, no change in [³H]diazepam binding was found (Shibla *et al.* 1981). Miller *et al.* (1988) found no change in *in vitro* benzodiazepine binding in brain cortical membranes taken from mice 24 h after 7 days of lorazepam treatment (2 mg/kg/day). However, 12 h after this treatment they did find a decrease in *in vivo* binding, although this is difficult to interpret because at this time there was still residual lorazepam in the brain and there would still be a considerable receptor occupancy (File *et al.* 1989).

In general, it is difficult to interpret these changes in benzodiazepine binding since there is no general consensus and different experimenters have used widely different doses of different benzodiazepines and differing time intervals after the end of treatment. It is therefore difficult to be certain whether the changes reflect an effect of the chronic treatment *per se* or whether they represent changes that would occur in a drug-free withdrawal state. However, in one recent study the binding changes could be more definitely linked to a withdrawal state because the binding studies were conducted at a time when

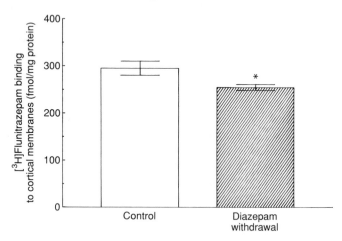

Fig. 7.2. Mean (± SEM) [³H]flunitrazepam binding (fmol/mg protein) at 25°C to cortical membranes from rats 24 h after the last of 21 days of injections of water/Tween (control) or diazepam (2 mg/kg/day). $*p < 0.05$. Taken from unpublished data of Andrews and File.

the rats were displaying behavioural signs of increased anxiety (File *et al.* 1991). In extensively washed cortical membranes taken from rats 24 h after the last of 21 days of diazepam treatment (2 mg/kg/day) there was a decrease in benzodiazepine binding (Fig. 7.2). It is therefore possible that this decreased binding contributed to the behavioural change of increased anxiety.

In contrast to this decreased binding, Miller *et al* (1988) found an increase in benzodiazepine receptors 4 days after the end of lorazepam (2 mg/kg/day) treatment and Lopez *et al.* (1990) found increased benzodiazepine receptors 2 and 4 days after the end of alprazolam treatment. These binding changes coincided with a period of increased locomotor activity, but there is no obvious reason why the binding and behavioural changes should be linked. It is possible that this late occurring up-regulation of benzodiazepine receptors reflects an adaptive, compensatory mechanism that leads to recovery from the increased anxiety that occurs during the acute withdrawal state. It is important in attempting to link behavioural and biochemical changes to realize that there are three possible types of relationship between the two. They may be completely independent, albeit occurring at the same time; they may be causally linked; or the biochemical change may reflect a compensatory mechanism that serves to limit the extent of the behavioural change. This notion that some of the neurochemical changes may reflect compensatory, rather than causal, mechanisms will be returned to when changes in neurotransmitter release are discussed.

GABA

The effect of chronic benzodiazepine treatment on GABA binding also seems to be dependent on the precise time at which the binding was performed in relation to the last dose. Marangos and Crawley (1982) found that 2 h after withdrawal from clonazepam treatment (3 weeks with doses increasing from 2 to 15 mg/kg/day) there was an increase in muscimol binding, reflecting an increase in GABA receptors, in the mouse forebrain and cerebellum. These increases were no longer detectable in the forebrain at 26 h, but in the cerebellum they remained significant until 50 h after withdrawal. A similar up-regulation in GABA receptors was indicated by the enhanced responsivity to GABA of cortical slices taken from mice after 14 days of treatment with 2 mg/kg/day clorazepam (Mally *et al.* 1990). After treatment with the less potent benzodiazepine, chlordiazepoxide, increased binding was only significant in the cerebellum 2 h after the last dose.

At a longer time interval after the last dose (24–28 h after withdrawal of diazepam, 3 mg/kg/day for 30 days) when the animals would be manifesting signs of increased anxiety or decreased seizure thresholds, Mohler *et al.* (1978) found a significant decrease in GABA binding (due to a reduction in the number of receptors) in the striatum. The ability of GABA and muscimol to enhance benzodiazepine binding has also been reported to be reduced after chronic benzodiazepine treatment (Gallager *et al.* 1984; Mele *et al.* 1984;

Schiller and Farb 1986), as was muscimol-stimulated chloride flux, 24 h but not 48 or 96h after withdrawal from 5 days of diazepam treatment (Lewin *et al.* 1989).

In keeping with decreased benzodiazepine and/or GABA binding and/or a decrease in GABA–benzodiazepine coupling, Gallager and colleagues have found that 3 weeks of treatment with diazepam (5 mg/kg/day) results in a decreased sensitivity of the rat dorsal raphe (but not substantia nigra) neurone to GABA (Gallager *et al.* 1984; Wilson and Gallager 1987). This effect was shown to persist for up to 96 h after diazepam treatment was terminated (Gallager *et al.* 1984). It therefore seems that a decreased functioning of the GABA–benzodiazepine receptor complex is most likely to correspond with the period of withdrawal when there are behavioural changes of increased anxiety and sensitivity to seizures, but may also correspond to the time at which tolerance to diazepam's behavioural effects can be demonstrated. Thus, after 3 weeks of exposure to diazepam, released from subcutaneously implanted silastic capsules, Heninger *et al.* (1990) found decreases in the mRNA for the cortical α_1 subunits of the GABA receptor.

Hitchcott *et al.* (1990) found increased release of GABA from the hippocampus of rats treated for 21 days with diazepam (4 mg/kg) and tested 30 h or 1 week after drug withdrawal. However, the change in hippocampal GABA release was not significant following 21 days of treatment with a lower dose of diazepam (2 mg/kg; see Fig. 7.3). Interestingly, the behavioural indications of anxiety are *more* marked after 21 days of treatment with the *lower* dose of diazepam, thus suggesting that treatment with the higher dose might lead more rapidly to an adaptive, compensatory increase in GABA release. The enhanced GABA release was regionally specific, and

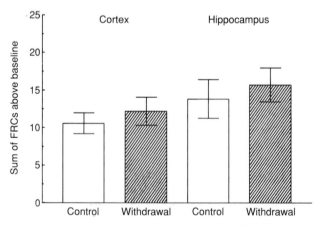

Fig. 7.3. Mean (±SEM) K+-stimulated release of [14C]GABA from cortical and hippocampal slices taken from rats 24 h after the last of 21 days of water/Tween injections (control) or diazepam (2 mg/kg/day, withdrawal). Taken from unpublished data of Andrews and File. (FRC, fractional rate coefficient)

no significant changes were found in the cortex following 21 days of treatment with diazepam (2 or 4 mg/kg/day); see Fig. 7.3. and Hitchcott et al. (1990). Regional changes have also been found in the mRNA for GAD (glutamic acid decarboxylase, which catalyses the synthesis of GABA from glutamate). This is unchanged in the cortex, but increased in the CA4 and granule cell layers of the dentate gyrus in the hippocampus in brain slices taken 24 h after the last of 21 injections of 2 mg/kg diazepam (Rattray et al. 1993).

While an increase in GABA release is unlikely to underlie the increased anxiety seen during benzodiazepine withdrawal, the decreased release found 2 weeks after withdrawal from diazepam (4 mg/kg) treatment (Hitchcott et al. 1990) could account for some of the very long-lasting problems seen in some patients. The functional significance of this very long-lasting change in release remains to be established, but it is clear that changes in both binding and release can be detected for some considerable time after the end of benzodiazepine treatment.

Monoamines

Acute treatment with benzodiazepines increases concentrations of 5-HT in the frontal cortex and hippocampus (e.g. Jenner et al. 1975; Lister and File 1983); after 5 and 10 days of treatment the elevations were no longer significant, although they had not returned to control levels. Lister and File (1983) suggested that the benzodiazepines induced changes in both synthesis and turnover of 5-HT and that tolerance developed to these two effects at different rates. The relationships between changes in 5-HT synthesis and turnover and the development of tolerance to particular behavioural effects of benzodiazepines has not yet been established.

Changes in monoamines have also been reported during benzodiazepine withdrawal. In addition to the physical signs of withdrawal observed by Rastogi et al. (1976), the group of rats that had been withdrawn from diazepam or bromazepam had decreased concentrations of noradrenaline and dopamine in several brain areas. Rastogi et al. (1978) also reported that, in rats withdrawn for 48 h from 22 days of diazepam treatment, there were significant increases of tyrosine hydroxylase (the rate-limiting enzyme in the synthesis of dopamine) in the striatum, decreases in brain tryptophan hydroxylase and 5-HT, and increases in the metabolite of 5-HT, 5-hydroxyindoleacetic acid. Bantutova et al. (1978) reported apparently contradictory results for noradrenaline and dopamine: they found significant increases in whole brain noradrenaline and dopamine concentrations. They agreed, however, that there were decreases in 5-HT in rats withdrawn for 3 days after 60 days of diazepam treatment. Andrews et al. (1993) found decreases in cortical and hippocampal 5-HT and decreased hippocampal noradrenaline concentration in rats withdrawn 24 h from 21 days of diazepam treatment (2 mg/kg/day).

Hitchcott et al. (1990) found that the release of 5-HT from the cortex was decreased after 5 days of treatment with diazepam (4 mg/kg/day) and this decrease was maintained after 21 days of treatment and for up to 1 week after diazepam withdrawal. These changes are unlikely to underlie the changes in anxiety, but may relate to other behavioural effects of the benzodiazepines. The release of 5-HT from the hippocampus was increased 30 h after withdrawal from diazepam (4 mg/kg/day for 21 days) and stayed elevated for 1 week (Hitchcott *et al.* 1990). An increase in 5-HT release from the hippocampus was also found 24 h after withdrawal from diazepam (2 mg/kg/day; see Fig. 7.4).

Withdrawal from diazepam (4 mg/kg/day for 21 days) did not change the release of noradrenaline from the hippocampus; noradrenaline release was increased (by 32 and 48 per cent at 20 and 40 mM potassium, respectively) in the cortex 30 h after the last dose of diazepam (Fig. 7.5), but this increase just failed to reach significance. With higher doses of diazepam this change in noradrenaline release may become significant and this could account for the hyperactivity and some of the physical symptoms seen during benzodiazepine withdrawal.

Treatment of benzodiazepine withdrawal responses

Evidence is accumulating that the different withdrawal responses may be mediated by changes in different neurotransmitter systems. For example, clonidine reversed the hyperactivity and diarrhoea seen during withdrawal from diazepam (Kunchandy and Kulkarni 1986), but did not reverse the increased anxiety (Baldwin *et al.* 1989). The calcium channel antagonist nitrendipine can decrease the incidence of seizures induced by FG 7142

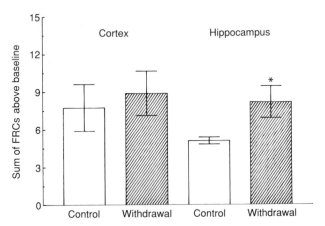

Fig. 7.4. Mean (±SEM) K$^+$-stimulated release of ^{3}[H]5HT from cortical and hippocampal slices taken from rats 24 h after the last of 21 days of water/Tween injections (control) or diazepam (2 mg/kg/day, withdrawal). *$p<0.05$ compared with control data. Taken from unpublished data of Andrews and File. For further details see Andrews *et al.* (1992). (FRC, fractional rate coefficient.)

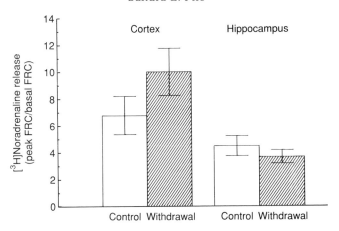

Fig. 7.5. Mean (±SEM) K^+-stimulated release of ^{3}[H]noradrenaline from cortical and hippocampal slices taken from rats 40 h after the last of 21 days of vehicle injections (control) or diazepam (4 mg/kg/day, withdrawal). Taken from unpublished data of Hitchcott and File.

when mice were withdrawn from 7 days of flurazepam treatment (Dolin *et al.* 1990). However, this reversal may reflect a specific interaction with FG 7142 and may not be applicable to spontaneous seizures or those induced by other agents.

Flumazenil (the benzodiazepine antagonist) can both reverse the increased anxiety seen during withdrawal and, with intermittent administration, can prevent the development of dependence as evidenced by increased anxiety (Baldwin and File 1988; Baldwin *et al.* 1989, 1990) or physical signs of withdrawal (Gallager *et al.* 1986). Flumazenil can also reverse the decrease in bicuculline seizure threshold seen 24 h after withdrawal from 3 weeks of diazepam treatment (Hitchcott *et al.* 1989) and the GABA subsensitivity of dorsal raphe neurones seen after withdrawal from 3 weeks of diazepam (Gonsalves and Gallager 1985, 1988). There is a some evidence that flumazenil may also have beneficial clinical effects in patients who have been treated chronically with benzodiazepines. Lader and Morton (1991) have reported alleviation by flumazenil of very long-lasting benzodiazepine withdrawal symptoms and Savik *et al.* (1991) reported that flumazenil restored the therapeutic response to clonazepam in epileptics who had become tolerant to its anti-epileptic effects.

In considering the evidence for reversal of benzodiazepine withdrawal symptoms, it is important to realize that this can be achieved at several levels. The first is a temporary, functional reversal. For example, the increased anxiety that can be detected 24 h after 21 days of diazepam (0.5 or 2 mg/kg/day) can be completely reversed by giving the normal daily diazepam dose (File *et al.* 1991). This is probably a functional reversal, with the anxiolytic action of diazepam counteracting the anxiogenic withdrawal response, but it is also a treatment that serves to maintain the dependence mechanism. Functional reversals that may not maintain the dependence state are illustrated by recent studies by Costall *et al.* (1989, 1990). They showed that injections of the 5-HT$_3$ receptor antagonist ondansetron reversed the anxiogenic response seen in the social interaction test on withdrawal from diazepam, but ondansetron also increased social interaction in control animals. When ondansetron was injected into the amygdala or dorsal raphe nucleus it reversed the decrease in light–dark transitions shown by mice 48 h after withdrawal from diazepam (20 mg/kg/day for 14 days) but it also resulted in an increase in transitions in control-treated mice. Low doses of another 5-HT$_3$ receptor antagonist, zacopride, reversed the anxiogenic response detected in the social interaction test on withdrawal from diazepam, but did not increase social interaction in control animals (Andrews and File 1991). Similarly, ondansetron has been found to reduce the decrease in body weight and food intake seen in rats withdrawn from diazepam, without having any effect in control animals (Goudie and Leathley 1990). Treatment with 5-HT$_3$ receptor antagonists is unlikely to actively reverse the dependence process, but may provide symptomatic cover during the period of diazepam withdrawal, and thus may be of therapeutic use.

The reversal of the increased anxiety detected in rats 24 h after withdrawal from diazepam (2 mg/kg/day for 21 days) by the GABA$_B$ agonist baclofen (File *et al.* 1991) may provide more information about the neurochemical mechanisms mediating this withdrawal response. Baclofen was without effect in control-treated animals and it was speculated that it may have been acting by decreasing transmitter release, e.g. by counteracting the increased hippocampal 5-HT release. This interpretation receives support from the effects of 5-HT$_{1A}$ agonists in benzodiazepine withdrawal. Goudie and Leathley (1991) reported that a high dose of ipsapirone potentiated the decrease in food intake and weight loss seen on withdrawal from chlordiazepoxide. File and Andrews (1991) found that a high dose of buspirone potentiated the anxiogenic responses detected on withdrawal from diazepam. These effects to potentiate withdrawal responses may reflect action at postsynaptic 5-HT$_{1A}$ receptors. However, a presynaptic action of lower doses is suggested by the finding that very low doses of buspirone reverse the anxiogenic responses detected on withdrawal from diazepam (File and Andrews 1991). However, although these experiments may provide more information about the neurochemical mechanisms underlying withdrawal responses, baclofen administration may simply be counteracting some of the changes. Perhaps most fundamental of all is the action proposed for the benzodiazepine antagonist flumazenil. It has been suggested that, as well as reversing the symptoms of benzodiazepine withdrawal, flumazenil actively restores the GABA–benzodiazepine complex to a drug-naîve state (Gallager *et al.* 1986; File and Hitchcott 1990).

Conclusions

In considering the biological basis of benzodiazepine dependence we are still unable to determine whether the same mechanisms underlie the development of tolerance to the behavioural actions of the benzodiazepines and the occurrence of behavioural changes when these drugs are withdrawn. It would be parsimonious to suggest (e.g. Lader and File 1987) that the adaptive changes that are triggered by repeated drug are examples of the development of tolerance without the occurrence of withdrawal responses, and vice versa, and, for a theoretical discussion of the possible independence of the two phenomena, see File and Hitchott (1991). Progress on this issue cannot be made until the timings of biochemical studies are precisely defined in terms of continued benzodiazepine receptor occupancy and, more importantly, with respect to behavioural studies. In order to interpret the biochemical changes it is necessary to know whether there is indeed tolerance to the behavioural actions of the drug and whether specific responses can be detected on drug withdrawal. Ideally, one should search for treatment regimes that lead to one phenomenon and not the other and then should seek a biochemical change showing the same dissociation.

Although little progress has been made on the separation of the phenomena of tolerance and withdrawal, evidence is certainly growing that different neurochemical changes underlie different behavioural changes. The primary change seems to occur at the GABA–benzodiazepine receptor complex, but this then triggers changes in other neurotransmitters. As already discussed, not all the biochemical changes will be causally linked to the behavioural changes detected during benzodiazepine dependence, and some may even be compensatory changes acting to limit or reduce the impact of others.

It is too soon to give a definitive list of which neurochemical changes underlie which signs of benzodiazepine dependence. However, it is clear from the animal work reviewed in this chapter that evidence for benzodiazepine dependence clearly exists and that this is independent from any drug-seeking behaviour or influence of media pressures to produce certain behavioural symptoms. Perhaps most intriguing of all are the findings of very long-lasting biochemical changes following withdrawal from benzodiazepine treatment. This certainly suggests that some of the long-lasting problems reported clinically might also have a biological basis.

References

Andrews, N. and File, S.E. (1991). Serotonergic mediation of the anxiogenic effects of diazepam withdrawal. *Society of Neuroscience Abstracts*, **17**, 152.
Andrews, N., Zharkovsky, A., and File, S.E. (1992). Raised [^{3}H]-5-HT release

and $^{45}Ca^{2+}$ uptake in diazepam withdrawal inhibition by baclofen. *Pharmacology Biochemistry and Behavior*, **41**, 695–9.

Andrews, N., Barnes, N.M., Steward, L.J., West, K.E., Cunningham, J., Wu, P-Y., Zangrossi, H., and File, S.E. (1993). A comparison of rat brain amino acid and monoamine content in diazepam withdrawal and after exposure to a phobic stimulus. *British Journal of Pharmacology*, (In press).

Baldwin, H.A. and File, S.E. (1988). Reversal of increased anxiety during benzodiazepine withdrawal: evidence for an anxiogenic endogenous ligand for the benzodiazepine receptor. *Brain Research Bulletin*, **20**, 603–6.

Baldwin, H.A. and File, S.E. (1989). Flumazenil prevents the development of chlordiazepoxide withdrawal in the social interaction test of anxiety. *Psychopharmacology*, **97**, 424–6.

Baldwin, H.A., Aranko, K., and File, S.E. (1987). Evidence that the incidence of withdrawal responses to benzodiazepines is linked to the development of tolerance. *Society of Neuroscience Abstracts*, **13**, 452.

Baldwin, H.A., Hitchcott, P.K., and File, S.E. (1989). Evidence that the increased anxiety detected in the elevated plus-maze during chlordiazepoxide withdrawal is not due to enhanced noradrenergic activity. *Pharmacology, Biochemistry and Behavior*, **34**, 931–9.

Baldwin, H.A., Hitchcott, P.K., and File, S.E. (1990). The use of flumazenil in prevention of diazepam dependence in the rat. *Human Psychopharmacology*, **5**, 57–61.

Bantutova, I., Ovcharov, R., and Koburova, K. (1978). Changes in the convulsion threshold and in the level of brain biogenic amines in rats chronically treated with phenobarbital or diazepam. *Acta Physiologica et Pharmacologica Bulgarica*, **4**, 26–9.

Barnett, A. and Fiore, J.W. (1973). Acute tolerance to diazepam in cats. In *The benzodiazepines*. (ed. S. Garattini, E. Mussini, and L.O., Randall), pp.545–58. Raven Press, New York.

Braestrup, C. and Squires, R.F. (1977). Specific benzodiazepine receptors in rat brain characterized by high-affinity [^{3}H] diazepam binding. *Proccedings of the National Academy of Sciences, USA*, **74**, 3805–9.

Braestrup, C., Nielsen, M., Nielsen, E.B., and Lyon, M. (1979). Benzodiazepine receptors in the brain as affected by different experimental stresses: the changes are small and not unidirectional. *Psychopharmacology*, **65**, 273–7.

Brown, C.L., Jones, B.J., and Oakley, N.R. (1984). Differential rate of tolerance development to the sedative, anxiolytic and anticonvulsant effects of benzodiazepines. CINP Congress Abstracts, p. 243.

Browne, T.R. and Penry, J.K. (1973). Benzodiazepines in the treatment of epilepsy. A review. *Epilepsia*, **14**, 277–310.

Cannizzaro, G., Nigito, S., Provenzano, P.M., and Vitikowa, T. (1972). Modification of depressant and disinhibitory action of flurazepam during short term treatment in the rats. *Psychopharmacologia*, **26**, 173–84.

Cesare, D.A. and McKearney, J.W. (1980). Tolerance to suppressive effect of chlordiazepoxide on operant behavior: Lack of cross tolerance to pentobarbital. *Pharmacology, Biochemistry and Behavior*, **13**, 545–8.

Chiu, T.H. and Rosenberg, H.C. (1978). Reduced diazepam binding following chronic benzodiazepine treatment. *Life Sciences*, **23**, 1153–8.

Christensen, J.D. (1973). Tolerance development with chlordiazepoxide in relation to the plasma levels of the parent compound and its main metabolite in mice. *Acta Pharmacologica et Toxicologica*, **33**, 262–72.

Cook, L. and Sepinwall, J. (1975). Behavioral analysis of the effects and mechanisms of action of benzodiazepines. In *Mechanisms of action of benzodiazepines* (ed. E. Costa and P. Greengard), pp.1–28. Raven Press, New York.

Cooper, S.J., Burnett, G., and Brown, K. (1981). Food preference following acute or chronic chlordiazepoxide administration: Tolerance to a antineophobic action. *Psychopharmacology*, **73**, 70–4.

Costall, B., Jones, B.J., Kelly, M.E., Naylor, R.J., Oakley N.R., Onaivi E.S., and Tyers, M.B. (1989). The effects of ondansetron (GR 38032F) in rats and mice treated subchronically with diazepam. *Pharmacology, Biochemistry and Behavior*, **34**, 769–78.

Costall, B., Jones, B.J., Kelly, M.E., Naylor, R.J., Onaivi, E.S., and Tyers, M.B. (1990). Sites of action of ondansetron to inhibit withdrawal from drugs of abuse. *Pharmacology, Biochemistry and Behavior*, **36**, 97–104.

Crawley, J.N., Marangos, P.J., Stivers, J., and Goodwin, F.K. (1982). Chronic clonazepam administration induces benzodiazepine receptor subsensitivity. *Neuropharmacology*, **21**, 85–9.

Dolin, S.J., Patch, T.L., Rabbani, M., Siarey, R.J., Bowhay, A.R., and Little, H.J. (1990). Nitrendipine decreases benzodiazepine withdrawal seizures but not the development of benzodiazepine tolerance or withdrawal signs. *British Journal of Pharmacology*, **101**, 691–7.

Emmett-Ogelsby, M.W., Spencer, D.G., Elmesallamy, F., and Lal, H. (1983). The pentylenetetrazol model of anxiety detects withdrawal from diazepam in rats. *Life Sciences*, **33**, 161–8.

Essig, C.F. and Flanary, H.G. (1959). Convulsions in cats following withdrawal of barbital sodium. *Experimental Neurology*, **1**, 529–33.

Essig, C.F. and Lam, R.C. (1968). Convulsions and hallucinatory behaviour following alcohol withdrawal in the dog. *Archives of Neurology*, **18**, 626–32.

Essig, C.F. (1958) Withdrawal convulsions in dogs following chronic meprobamate intoxication. *Archives of Neurological Psychiatry*, **80**, 414–17.

Feely, M., Gent. J.P., Haigh, J.R.M., and Peaker, S. (1986). Acute clobazam administration induces anticonvulsant tolerance to N-desmethylclobazam in mice. *British Journal of Pharmacology*, **89**, 643.

File, S.E. (1981). Rapid development of tolerance to the sedative effects of lorazepam and triazolam in rats. *Psychopharmacology*, **73**, 240–5.

File, S.E. (1982a). Recovery from lorazepam tolerance and the effects of a benzodiazepine antagonist (RO 15-1788) on the development of tolerance. *Psychopharmacology*, **77**, 284–8.

File, S.E. (1982b). Development and retention of tolerance to the sedative effects of chlordiazepoxide: role of apparatus cues. *European Journal of Pharmacology*, **81**, 637–43.

File, S.E. (1983a). Tolerance to the anti-pentylenetetrazole effects of diazepam in the mouse. *Psychopharmacology*, **79**, 284–6.

File, S.E. (1983b). Strain differences in mice in the development of tolerance to the antipentylenetetrazole effects of diazepam. *Neuroscience Letters*, **42**, 95–8.

File, S.E. (1984). Behavioural Pharmacology of benzodiazepines. *Progress in Neuro-Psychopharmacology and Biological Psychiatry*, **8**, 19–31.

File, S.E. (1989). Chronic diazepam treatment: effect of dose on development of tolerance and incidence of withdrawal in an animal test of anxiety. *Human Psychopharmacology*, **3**, 59–64.

File, S.E. (1990). The history of benzodiazepine dependence: a review of animal studies. *Neuroscience and Biobehavioral Reviews*, **14**, 135–146.

File, S.E., and Andrews, N. (1991). Low, but not high doses of buspirone reduce the anxiogenic effects of diazepam withdrawal. *Psychopharmacology*, **105**, 578–82.

File, S.E. and Baldwin, H.A. (1989). Changes in anxiety in rats tolerant to, and withdrawn from, benzodiazepines: behavioural and biochemical studies. In *Psychopharmacology of anxiety* (ed. P. Tyrer), pp.28–51. Oxford University Press, Oxford.

File, S.E. and Hitchcott, P.K. (1990). A theory of benzodiazepine dependence that can explain whether flumazenil will enhance or reverse the phenomena. *Psychopharmacology*, **101**, 525–32.

File, S.E. and Hitchcott, P.K. (1991). Benzodiazepine dependence. In *New concepts in anxiety* (ed. M. Briley and S.E. File), pp.397–421. MacMillan Press, London.

File, S.E. and Hyde, J.R.G. (1978). Can social interaction be used to measure anxiety? *British Journal of Pharmacology*, **62**, 19–24.

File, S.E. and Pellow, S. (1985). No cross-tolerance between the stimulatory and depressant actions of benzodiazepines in mice. *Behavioural Brain Research*, **17**, 1–7.

File, S.E., Baldwin, H.A., and Aranko, K. (1987). Anxiogenic effects from benzodiazepine withdrawal are linked to the development of tolerance. *Brain Research Bulletin*, **19**, 607–10.

File, S.E., Wilks, L.J., and Mabbutt, P.S. (1988). Withdrawal, tolerance and sensitization after a single dose of lorazepam. *Pharmacology, Biochemistry and Behavior*. **31**, 937–40.

File, S.E., Baldwin, H.A., and Hitchcott, P.K. (1989). The effect of flumazenil on levels of anxiety in rats after one week of chronic diazepam treatment. *Neuroscience Letters*, S36, S63.

File, S.E., Mabbutt, P.S., and Andrews, N. (1991). Diazepam withdrawal responses measured in the social interaction test of anxiety and their reversal by baclofen. *Psychopharmacology*, (In press).

Fraser, H.F. and Isbell, H. (1954). Abstinence syndrome in dogs after chronic barbiturate medication. *Journal of Pharmacology and Experimental Therapeutics*, **112**, 261–7.

Freund, G. (1969). Alcohol withdrawal syndrome in mice. *Archives of Neurology*, **21**, 315–20.

Frey, H.H., Philippin, H.P., and Scheuler, W. (1984). Development of tolerance to the anticonvulsant effect of diazepam in dogs. *European Journal of Pharmacology*, **104**, 27–38.

Fritz, S., Schneider, H.H., Stephens, D.N., and Weidmann, R. (1986). Tolerance to the anxiolytic action of diazepam in rats. *British Journal of Pharmacology*, **88**, 336P.

Gallager, D.W., Lakoski, J.M., Gonsalves, S.F., and Rauch, S.L. (1984). Chronic benzodiazepine treatment decreases postsynaptic GABA sensitivity. *Nature*, **308**, 74–7.

Gallager, D.W., Heninger, K., and Heninger, G. (1986). Periodic benzodiazepine administration prevents benzodiazepine withdrawal symptoms in primates. *European Journal of Pharmacology*, **132**, 31–8.

Gent, J.P., Feely, M.P., and Haigh, J.R.M. (1985). Differences between the tolerance characteristics of two anticonvulsant benzodiazepines. *Life Sciences*, **37**, 849–56.

Goldberg, M.E., Manian, A., and Efron, D. (1967). A comparative study of certain pharmacologic responses following acute and chronic administration of chlordiazepoxide. *Life Sciences*, **6**, 481–91.

Gonsalves, S.F. and Gallager, D.W. (1985). Spontaneous and Ro 15–1788 induced reversal of subsensitivity to GABA following chronic benzodiazepines. *European Journal of Pharmacology*, **110**, 163–70.

Gonsalves, S.F. and Gallager, W. (1986). Tolerance to anti-pentylenetetrazole effects following chronic diazepam. *European Journal of Pharmacology*, **121**, 281–4.

Gonsalves, S.F. and Gallager, D.W. (1988). Persistent reversal of tolerance to anticonvulsant effects and GABAergic subsensitivity by a single exposure to benzodiazepine antagonist during chronic benzodiazepine administration. *Journal of Pharmacology and Experimental Therapeutics*, **244**, 79–83.

Gonzales, J.P., McCulloch, A.J., Nicholls, P.J., Sewell, R.D.E., and Tekle, A. (1984). Subacute benzodiazepine treatment: observations on behavioural tolerance and withdrawal. *Alcohol and Alcoholism*, **19**, 325–32.

Goudie, A.J., and Leathley, M.J. (1990). Effects of the 5-HT$_3$ antagonist GR38032F (ondansetron) benzodiazepine withdrawal in rats. *European Journal of Pharmacology*, **185**, 179–86.

Goudie, A.J., And Leathley, M.J. (1991). An evaluation of the dependence potential of the selective 5-HT$_{1A}$ agonist ipsapirone in rats and of its effects on benzodiazepine withdrawal. *Psychopharmacology*, **103**, 529–37.

Greeley, J. and Cappell, H. (1985). Associative control of tolerance to the sedative and hypothermic effects of chlordiazepoxide. *Psychopharmacology* **86**, 487–93.

Griffiths, J.W. and Goudie, A.J. (1986). Analysis of the role of drug-predictive environmental stimuli in tolerance to the hypothermic effects of the benzodiazepine metabolism. *Psychopharmacology*, **90**, 513–21.

Grimm, V.E. and Hershkowitz, M. (1981). The effect of chronic diazepam treatment on discrimination performance and 3H-flunitrazepam binding in the brain of shocked and nonshocked rats. *Psychopharmacology*, **74**, 132–6.

Henauer, S.A., Gallaher E.J., and Hollister, L.E. (1984). Long-lasting single-dose tolerance to neurologic deficits induced by diazepam. *Psychopharmacology*, **82**, 161–3.

Heninger, C. and Gallager, D.W. (1988). Altered γ-aminobutyric acid/benzodiazepine interaction after chronic diazepam exposure. *Neuropharmacology*, **27**, 1073–6.

Heninger, C., Saito, N., Tallman, J.F., Garrett, K.M., Vitek, M.P., Duman, R.S., and Gallager, D.W. (1990). Effects of continuous diazepam administration on GABA$_A$ subunit mRNA in rat brain. *Journal of Molecular Neuroscience*, **2**, 101–7.

Herberg, L.J. and Montgomery, A.M.J. (1987). Learnt tolerance to sedative effect of chlordiazepoxide on self stimulation performance, but no tolerance to facilitatory effects after 80 days. *Psychopharmacology*, **93**, 214–17.

Hitchcott, P.K., File, S.E., Little, H.J., and Nutt, D.J. (1989). Diazepam withdrawal: decreased seizure threshold and increased anxiety reversed by FG 7142 and flumazenil. *Society of Neuroscience Abstracts*, **15**, 414.

Hitchcott, P.K., File, S.E., Ekwuru, M., and Neal, M.J. (1990). Chronic diazepam treatment in rats causes long-lasting changes in central [³H]-5-hydroxytryptamine and [¹⁴C]-γ-aminobutyric acid release. *British Journal of Pharmacology*, **99**, 11–12.

Hollister, L.E., Motzenbecker, F.P., and Degan, R.O. (1961). Withdrawal reaction from chlordiazepoxide (Librium). *Psychopharmacologia* **2** 63–8.

Hoogland, D.R., Miya, T.S., and Bousquet, W.F. (1966). Metabolism and tolerance studies with chlordiazepoxide in the rat. *Toxicology and Applied Pharmacology*, **9**, 116–23.

Jenner, P., Chadwick, D., Reynolds, E.H., and Marsden, C.D. (1975). Altered 5-HT metabolism with clonazepam, diazepam and diphenyl hydantoin. *Journal of Pharmacy and Pharmacology*, **27**, 707–10.

Jori, A., Prestini, P.E., and Pugliatti, C. (1969). Effect of diazepam and chlordiazepoxide on the metabolism of other drugs. *Journal of Pharmacy and Pharmacology*, **21**, 387–90.

Juhasz, L. and Dairman, W. (1977). Effect of subacute diazepam administration in mice on the subsequent ability of diazepam to protect against metrazole and bicuculline induced convulsions. *Federation Proceedings*, **36**, 377.

Kaplan, S.A., Jack, M.L., Alexander, K., and Winfeld, R.E. (1973). Pharmacokinetic profile of diazepam in man following single intravenous and oral and chronic oral administration. *Journal of Pharmacological Sciences*, **62**, 1789–96.

Killam, E.K., Matsuzaki, M., and Killam, K.F. (1973). Effects of chronic administration of benzodiazepines on epileptic seizures and brain electrical activity, in Papio papio. In *The benzodiazepines* (ed. S. Garattini, E. Mussini, and L.O. Randall), pp.443–60. Raven Press, New York.

King, D.A., Bouton, M.E., and Musty, R.E. (1987). Associative control of tolerance to the sedative effects of a short-acting benzodiazepine. *Behavioural Neuroscience*, **101**, 104–14.

Kunchandy, J. and Kulkarni, S.K. (1986). Reversal by alpha-2 agonists of diazepam withdrawal hyperactivity in rats. *Psychopharmacology*, **90**, 198–202.

Lader, M.H. and File, S.E. (1987). The biological basis of benzodiazepine dependence. *Psychological Medicine*, **17**, 539–47.

Lader, M.H. and Morton, S. (1991). Benzodiazepine withdrawal syndrome. *British Journal of Psychiatry*, **158**: 435.

Lewin, E., Peris, J., Bleck, V., Zahniser, N.R., and Harris, A.R. (1989). Diazepam sensitizes mice to FG 7142 and reduces muscimol-stimulated ³⁶Cl–flux– *Pharmacology, Biochemistry and Behavior*, **33**, 465–8.

Lippa, A.S. and Regan, B. (1977). Additional studies on the importance of glycine and GABA in mediating the actions of benzodiazepines. *Life Sciences*, **21**, 1779–84.

Lister, R.G. and File, S.E. (1983). Changes in regional concentrations in the rat brain of 5-hydroxytryptamine and 5-hydroxyindoleacetic acid during the development of tolerance to the sedative action of chlordiazepoxide *Journal of Pharmacy and Pharmacology*, **35**, 601–3.

Lister, R.G. and Nutt, D.J. (1986). Mice and rats are sensitized to the proconvulsant action of a benzodiazepine receptor inverse agonist (FG 7142) following a single doze of lorazepam. *Brain Research*, **379**, 364–6.

Lister, R.G., File, S.E., and Greenblatt, D.J. (1983a). The behavioural effects of lorazepam are poorly related to its concentration in the brain. *Life Sciences*, **32**, 2033–40.

Lister, R.G., File, S.E., and Greenblatt, D.J. (1983b). Functional tolerance to lorazepam in the rat. *Psychopharmacology*, **81**, 292–9.

Lopez, F., Miller, L.G., Greenblatt, D.J., Chesley, S., Schatzki, A., and Shader, R.I. (1990). Chronic administration of benzodiazepines—V. Rapid onset of behavioural and neurochemical alterations after discontinuation alprazolam. *Neuropharmacology*, **29**, (3), 237–41.

Mally, J., Connick, J.H., and Stone, T.W. (1990). Chronic benzodiazepine treatment and cortical responses to adenosine and GABA. *Brain Research*, **530**, 353–7.

Marangos, P.J. and Crawley, J.N. (1982). Chronic benzodiazepine treatment increases [³H] muscimol binding in mouse brain. *Neuropharmacology*, **21**, 81–4.

Margules, D.L. and Stein, L. (1968). Increase of anti-anxiety activity and tolerance of behavioural depression during chronic administration of oxazepam. *Psychopharmacologia*, **13**, 74–80.

McMillan, D.E. and Leander, J.D. (1978). Chronic chlordiazepoxide and pentobarbital interactions on punished and unpunished behavior. *Journal of Pharmacology and Experimental Therapeutics*, **207**, 515–20.

Mele, L., Sagratella, S., and Massotti, M. (1984). Chronic administration of diazepam to rats causes changes in EEG patterns and in coupling between GABA receptors and benzodiazepine binding sites in vitro. *Brain Research*, **323**, 93–102.

Miller, L.G., Greenblatt, D.J., Roy, R.B., Summer, W.R., and Shader, R.I. (1988). Chronic benzodiazepine administration. 11. Discontinuation syndrome is associated with upregulation of GABA$_A$ receptor complex binding and function. *Journal of Pharmacology and Experimental Therapeutics*, **246**, 177–82.

Mohler, H., Okada, T., and Enna, S.J. (1978). Benzodiazepine and neurotransmitter receptor binding in rat brain after chronic administration of diazepam or phenobarbital. *Brain Research*, **156**, 391–5.

Oakley, N.R., Jones, B.J., and Tyers, M.B. (1988). Tolerance and withdrawal studies with diazepam and GR38032F in the rat. *British Journal of Pharmacology*, **96**, 764P.

Orme, M., Breckenridge, A., and Brooks, R.V. (1972). Interactions of benzodiazepines with warfarin. *British Medical Journal*, **3**, 611–14.

Prezioso, P.J. and Neale, J.H. (1983). Benzodiazepine receptor binding by membranes from brain cell cultures following chronic treatment with diazepam. *Brain Research*, **288**, 354–8.

Randall, L.O., Heise, G.A., Schallek, W., Bagdon, R.E., Banziger, R., Boris, A., Moe, R.A., and Abrams, W.B. (1961). Pharmacological and clinical studies on valium, a new psychotherapeutic agent of the benzodiazepine class. *Current Therapy Research*, **3**, 405–25.

Rastogi, R.B., Lapierre, Y.D., and Singhal, R.L. (1976). Evidence for the role of brain norepinephrine and dopamine in 'rebound' phenomenon seen during withdrawal after repeated exposure to benzodiazepines. *Journal of Psychiatric Research*, **13**, 65–75.

Rastogi, R.B., Lapierre, Y.D., and Singhal, R.L. (1978). Some neurochemical correlates of rebound phenomenon observed during withdrawal after long-term exposure to 1,4-benzodiazepines. *Progress in Neuro-Psychopharmacology*, **2**, 43–54.

Rattray, M., Andrews, N., Wu, P-Y., Singhui, S., and File, S.E. (1993). Diazepam treatment modulates in RNA for GAD and CCK in several rat brain regions. *British Journal of Pharmacology*, (In press).

Rock, R.S. and Barrett, R.J. (1987). Tolerance and withdrawal to the anticonflict properties of diazepam following chronic administration in rats. *Society of Neuroscience Abstracts*, **13**, 452.

Rosenberg, H.C. and Chiu, T.H. (1979). Decreased 3H-diazepam binding is a specific response to chronic benzodiazepine treatment. *Life Sciences*, **24**, 803–8.

Rosenberg, H.C. and Chiu, T.H. (1981). Regional specificity of benzodiazepine receptor down-regulation during chronic treatment of rats with flurazepam. *Neuroscience Letters*, **24**, 49–52.

Rosenberg, H.C., Smith, S., and Chiu, T.H. (1983). Benzodiazepine specific and non-specific tolerance following chronic flurazepam treatment. *Life Sciences*, **32**, 279–85.

Sansone, M. (1979). Effects of repeated administration of chlordiazepoxide on spontaneous locomoter activity in mice. *Psychopharmacology*, **66**, 109–10.

Savic, I., Widen, L., and Stone-Elander, S. (1991). Feasibility of reversing benzodiazepine tolerance with flumazenil. *Lancet*, **337**, 133–7.

Scherkl, R., Kurudi, D., and Frey, H.-H. (1988). Tolerance to the anticonvulsant effect of clorazepate and clonazepam in mice. *Pharmacology and Toxicology*, **62**, 38–41.

Schiller, G.D. and Farb, D.H. (1986). Enhancement of benzodiazepine binding by GABA is reduced rapidly during chronic exposure to flurazepam. *Annals of the New York Academy of Sciences*, **463**, 221–3.

Shearman, G.T., Miksic, S., and Lal, H. (1979). Lack of tolerance development to benzodiazipine in antagonism of the pentylenetetrazole discriminative stimulus. *Pharmacology, Biochemistry and Behavior*, **10**, 795–7.

Sher, P.K. (1983). Reduced benzodiazepine receptor binding in cerebral cortical cultures chronically exposed to diazepam. *Epilepsia*, **24**, 313–20.

Sher, P.K. (1986). Long-term exposure of cortical cell cultures to clonazepam reduces benzodiazepine receptor binding. *Experimental Neurology*, **92**, 360–8.

Sher, P.K. Study, R.E., Mazzetta, J., Barker, J.L., and Nelson, P.G. (1983). Depression of benzodiazepine binding and diazepam potentiation of GABA-mediated inhibition after chronic exposure of spinal cord cultures to diazepam. *Brain Research*, **268**, 171–6.

Shibla, D.B., Gardell, M.A., and Neale, J.H. (1981). The insensitivity of developing benzodiazepine receptors to chronic treatment with diazepam, GABA, and muscimol in brain cell cultures. *Brain Research*, **210**, 361–9.

Soderpalm, B. (1987). Pharmacology of the benzodiazepines; with special emphasis on alprazolam. *Acta Psychiatrica Scandinavica*, **76**, 39–46.

Stein, L. and Berger, B.D. (1971). Psychopharmacology of 7-chloro 5-(0-chlorophenyl)-1,3-dihydroxy-2H-1,4-benzodiazepines-2-one (Lorazepam) in squirrel monkey and rat. *Arzneimittel Forschung*, **21**, 1073–8.

Stephens, D.N. and Schneider, H.H. (1985). Tolerance to the benzodiazepine diazepam in an animal model of anxiolytic activity. *Psychopharmacology*, **87**, 322–7.

Suzuki, T., Fukumori, R., Yoshii, T., Yanaura, S., Satoh, T. and Kitagawa, H. (1980). Effect of p-chlorophenylalanine on diazepam withdrawal signs in rats. *Psychopharmacology*, **71**, 91–3.

Treit, D. (1985). Evidence that tolerance develops to the anxiolytic effect of diazepam in rats. *Pharmacology, Biochemistry and Behavior*, **22**, 383–7.

Vellucci, S.V. and File, S.E. (1979). Chlordiazepoxide loses its anxiolytic action with long-term treatment. *Psychopharmacology*, **62**, 61–5.

Warner, R.S. (1965). Management of the office patient with anxiety and depression. *Psychosomatics*, **6**, 347–51.

Wilson, M.A. and Gallager, D.W. (1987). Effects of chronic diazepam exposure on GABA sensitivity and on benzodiazepine potentiation of GABA mediated response of substantia nigra pars reticulata neurons of rats. *European Journal of Pharmacology*, **136**, 333–43.

Wise, C.D., Berger, B.D., and Stein, L. (1972). Benzodiazepines: anxiety reducing activity by reduction of serotonin turnover in the brain. *Science* **177**, 180–3.

Woods, J.H., Katz, J.L., and Winger, G. (1987). Abuse liability of benzodiazepines. *Pharmacological Reviews*, **39**, 251–413.

Yanagita, T. and Takahashi, S. (1973). Dependence liability of several sedative hypnotic agents. *Journal of Pharmacology and Experimental Therapeutics*, **185**, 307–16.

Yanaura, S., Tagashira, E., and Suzuki, T. (1975). Physical dependence on morphine, phenobarbital and diazepam in rats by drug-admixed food ingestion. *Japanese Journal of Pharmacology*, **25**, 453–63.

Yoong, Y.L., Lee, H.S., Gwee, M.C.E., and Wong, P.T.-H. (1986). Acute tolerance to diazepam in mice: pharmacokinetic considerations. *Clinical and Experimental Pharmacology and Physiology*, **13**, 153–8.

8 Benzodiazepine/alcohol dependence and abuse

Stefan Borg, Sten Carlsson, and Pierre Lafolie

Although chemical dependence may be developed for many different type of drugs, the abuse often involves only one main drug. However, primary benzodiazepine abuse can be associated with alcohol abuse, but is perhaps less common than primary alcohol dependence and abuse followed by benzodiazepine dependence and abuse. Both benzodiazepines and alcohol show common effects on cellular levels, and both also produce similar neuropsychological changes.

Effects of benzodiazepines and alcohol on the GABA-receptor site

Chronic exposure to alcohol

A major site of action of alcohol may be the GABA–benzodiazepine receptor complex (Nutt *et al.* 1989). Chronic exposure to alcohol reduces coupling between benzodiazepine agonist sites and the chloride channel, and this action may be responsible for the development of cross-tolerance between alcohol and benzodiazepine receptor agonists (Buck and Harris 1990). Chronic treatment with alcohol also selectively alters the receptor sensitivity to RO 15–4513, an inverse benzodiazepine agonist (Metha and Ticku 1989), indicating common cellular effects between benzodiazepines and alcohol.

The chloride channel

Alcohol effects, such as motor incoordination, hypnosedation, anti-anxiety, and anticonvulsant properties, are reported to be mediated by GABA. Cl-influx studies support this theory and suggest that the chloride channel is influenced by modulation at the GABA–benzodiazepine receptor ionophore complex (Ticku and Kulkarni 1988). The alcohol withdrawal syndrome may reflect alterations in the GABA–benzodiazepine–chloride receptor complex, and also stimulation of noradrenergic activity and hypothalamic–pituitary–adrenal axis stimulation (Adinoff *et al.* 1988).

Pharmacological aspects of benzodiazepine abuse

Pharmacokinetic factors such as rapid absorption, rapid distribution to the central nervous system, and short half-life have been reported to increase the likelihood of abuse for different benzodiazepines (Jaffe *et al.* 1983; Griffiths *et al.* 1984; Busto and Sellers 1986; Ciraulo *et al.* 1988, 1989).

Pharmacodynamic properties, e.g. induction of euphoria (Busto and Sellers 1986) reinforcement of drug-taking behaviour, (Meyer 1986), or termination of anxiety (Khantzian 1985), have also been reported to increase abuse liability for different benzodiazepines.

Combined abuse of alcohol and benzodiazepines

A common problem?

It has been reported that, upon admission to a clinic for treatment of alcohol withdrawal, 33 per cent of patients were positive for benzodiazepines in urine, and 54 per cent of these were considered to abuse benzodiazepines (Busto *et al.* 1983). Similar results were reported by Wiseman and Spencer-Peet (1985). In another report, 24 of 50 patients suffering from the alcohol dependence syndrome consumed minor tranquillizers prior to admission to the hospital for detoxification (Thomas *et al.* 1989). An indication of a genetic or social influence is reported by Ciraulo *et al.* (1989) who found that sons with a parental history of alcoholism were at greater risk of abusing benzodiazepines. Also, Ciraulo *et al.* (1988) showed that alcoholic men have a greater abuse liability for alprazolam. Benzodiazepines tend to be secondary drugs to a preferred primary intoxicant, e.g. alcohol (Senay 1989). Kryspin-Exner and Demel (1975) reported that long-term treatment with sedatives or hypnotics among alcoholics resulted in the development of dependence. For diazepam this potential was estimated to be 2.3 per cent. Thus the treatment of alcohol withdrawal only is not sufficient if the patient is a benzodiazepine abuser.

Risk factors for benzodiazepine abuse

Women are at a higher risk for benzodiazepine addiction (Chan 1984). Female gender, mild-to-moderate alcohol use, and neuroticism were all found to be significant predictors of benzodiazepine withdrawal severity and clinical outcome (Schweizer *et al.* 1990). Alcohol abuse by itself increases anxiety and depression and impairs judgement and performance. It is found that benzodiazepine abuse is more likely to occur in individuals who abuse other drugs, such as alcohol (Roth 1989).

The use of benzodiazepines in alcohol withdrawal

Research in the combined abuse of benzodiazepines and alcohol does not seem to have received great attention internationally. The literature containes surprisingly few references on the subject. Other research areas, such as the treatment of alcohol withdrawal with benzodiazepines, have been studied much more extensively, for instance by McMicken (1990) and Guthrie (1989).

Laboratory services for diagnosis of benzodiazepine abuse, tapering, and abstinence

It must be held in mind that most analytical assays are performed with immunological or chromatographic methods. This means that for most low-dose benzodiazepines (e.g. flunitrazepam, triazolam, alprazolam, lorazepam) problems arise with their detectability, especially in therapeutic doses. The sensitivity of the analysis differs among different methodological systems and also depends on the type of drug to be tested, the dose, and the time between last dose and testing.

Immunological testing is based on the identification of common metabolites by an antigen–antibody reaction. Mostly these types of antibodies recognize oxazepam the metabolite of diazepam, chlordiazepoxide, and other benzodiazepines, with a cross-reactivity of the antibodies against the other benzodiazepines not producing oxazepam. These tests are mainly used for detection in urine. They are easily performed and inexpensive. They detect benzodiazepines in general and do not reveal the specific drug.

Chromatographic tests are based on separation by the chemical characteristics of the molecules. These tests are specific and quantitative. They are used for analysis in plasma or as a verification of immunological testing. They are expensive. The ideal technology is often gas chromatography–mass spectrometry (GC–MS), which is a highly specific and sensitive procedure but also very expensive.

Detection in urine

Detection of benzodiazepines in urine is easily performed in many laboratories with immunological techniques, and lately these techniques have been further developed to provide a higher degree of sensitivity and selectivity (Minder *et al.* 1989; Beck *et al.* 1990). Still there are difficulties with the detectability of low-dose benzodiazepines.

Measurements in plasma

In order to standardize the procedure, blood samples must be taken at steady state on each dose level and at the same time after the dose. A relationship between blood levels of benzodiazepines and clinical effect in terms of reducing anxiety is reported by Lapierre (1983). In patients on diazepam tapering, measurements of diazepam and desmethyl–diazepam concentrations in plasma showed that patients with withdrawal symptoms had a significantly higher elimination rate of desmethyl–diazepam than patients without withdrawal symptoms, indicating *interindividual variations* in the pharmacokinetics (Tyrer and Owen 1981). A smooth fall in blood benzodiazepine concentration instead of steep decreases during tapering of benzodiazepines was reported to reduce withdrawal symptoms (Tyrer *et al.* 1983). In patients who dropped out during withdrawal treatment, a significant inverse relationship between plasma benzodiazepine level and severity of withdrawal symptoms was found (Rickels *et al.* 1990). During benzodiazepine tapering it is therefore recommended that the decrease in plasma benzodiazepine levels be monitored (Rickels *et al.* 1988, 1990; Schweizer *et al.* 1990). The concentrations may be fluctuating in an individual during tapering, indicating an *intraindividual pharmacokinetic variation* in some patients. A raise in plasma benzodiazepine concentrations must therefore not be due to a side-intake of drugs! (See also Table 8.1.)

Clinical aspects of the patient with combined abuse of benzodiazepine and alcohol

Symptomatology of withdrawal

Abstinence from benzodiazepines includes anxiety, depression, insomnia, tremor, perceptual changes, and various other symptoms. Seizures have been reported by several authors (Fialip *et al.* 1987; Schneider *et al.* 1987). Thus the symptoms in part correspond to alcohol withdrawal, but persist for a prolonged period of time (Benzer and Cushman 1980). According to Fontaine *et al.* (1984), a more intensive period persists in many patients for 2–3 weeks, while minor symptoms may be present for 13–27 weeks (Ashton 1984).

Table 8.1. Guidelines for the use of laboratory tests in benzodiazepine abuse

---

Diagnosis. Analysis of benzodiazepine in *urine*. A positive analysis without recorded prescription requires further exploration of the drug history

Tapering. Analysis of *plasma* concentrations of prescribed benzodiazepine. Samples must be obtained at steady-rate on each dose level and at the same dose-sampling time interval. Decline in concentrations should be smooth. Steep reduction in concentrations increases the risk for relapse

Adherence to abstinence. A negative analysis of benzodiazepine in *urine* may confirm the compliance

NB.
1. Not all examinations are performed at all laboratories.

2. In both urine and plasma, analysis of low-dose benzodiaxepines, e.g. of flunitrazepam, may be difficult.

Check the 'menu' with the local laboratory!

Table 8.2. Basis for combined abuse diagnosis

1. Precise drug history
2. Laboratory tests:
   blood markers for high alcohol consumption (e.g. MCV, GT);
   detection of benzodiazepines in urine/plasma

Diagnosis

In a comparison of patient drug history with blood alcohol and benzodiazepine metabolites in urine in 198 patients admitted to the hospital for medical or surgical treatment, it was found that 71 per cent of alcohol intake, but only 33 per cent of benzodiazepine intake, was recorded in the drug history (Lilja et al. 1986). This indicates the necessity for a detailed drug history, especially in patients where risk factors are identified. Laboratory testing may also be helpful in the diagnosis (Table 8.2).

Prognostic factors

Aside from the social, physical, and psychiatric decline, abusers are at medical risk if not diagnosed correctly. The overall incidence of seizures during alcohol detoxification was 10 per cent. These seizures were found in two categories of patients: (1) abusers of benzodiazepines; (2) patients known to develop seizures during alcohol detoxification with an erratic use of prescribed phenytoin (Hillbom and Hjelm-Jäger 1984). In patients who abused benzodiazepines exclusively the mortality was insignificantly raised, but in patients who abused benzodiazepines together with alcohol the mortality was significantly raised (Piesiur-Strehlow et al. 1984). Deaths following benzodiazepine intoxication are rare but have been reported by some authors (Sunter et al. 1988; Höjer et al. 1989).

Treatment of the combined abuse patients

No clear-cut articles report on this matter. It seems appropriate to detoxify the patient from alcohol with continued prescription of the abused benzodiazepine. Good experiences are also reported when short-acting agents are replaced with long-acting ones like diazepam (Sellers 1988). After this period an individualized tapering of the benzodiazepine for a prolonged period of time should be tried.

Neuropsychological changes in relation to the intake of benzodiazepine and/or alcohol

Although brain computer tomography shows different pictures in benzodiazepine abusers and alcoholics, the type of neuropsychological deficit is similar in both these patient groups with decreased capacity in category-test and block-test, indicating a decreased ability in abstraction and problem-solving (Grant *et al.* 1979; Bergman *et al.* 1980, 1983).

Therapeutic doses of benzodiazepines and short-term treatment

Even short periods of treatment with conventional doses of benzodiazepines give measurable effects on a number of neuropsychological functions. Lader *et al.* (1982) were able to show that intake of 1 mg flunitrazepam in the evening for 8 consecutive days decreased performance in psychometric tests, such as finger-tapping, symbol-copying, and the digit-symbol-substitution test. These tests primarily measure psychomotor ability, capacity of attention, and endurance. Changes were also noted in the electroencephalogram (EEG) and in critical flicker fusion. Similar results were noted by Bond *et al.* (1983) who compared eight healthy controls using 5 mg diazepam for 1 week with a placebo group.

Therapeutic doses of benzodiazepines and long-term treatment

In patients with chronic pain, chronic benzodiazepine use in therapeutic doses decreased neuropsychological functions in comparison with patients in whom narcotic drugs (opiates) were used. In patients on long-term benzodiazepines, EEGs were changed and cognitive ability, as measured with the Wechsler Adult Intelligence scale and Bender Gestalt test, was lowered (Hendler *et al.* 1980) In a report from Pétursson *et al.* (1983), 22 patients on long-term therapeutic doses of benzodiazepines were compared to matched controls. These patients showed decreased digit–symbol substitution and symbol-copying.

Summary

1. Surprisingly few studies report on the combined abuse of benzodiazepines and alcohol.

2. Both benzodiazepines and alcohol act on the GABA–ionophore complex, thereby influencing the chloride-channel function.

3. The abuse of benzodiazepine among alcoholics is more common than generally believed but can be detected by means of toxicological screening.

4. Diagnosis of benzodiazepine abuse and adherence to abstinence after tapering may be performed by urine benzodiazepine tests, but these tests may fail to detect intake of low-dose benzodiazepines.

5. Compliance during tapering may by followed by plasma benzodiazepine measurements, if inter- and intraindividual variations in pharmacokinetics are taken into account.

6. Even short-term treatment with benzodiazepines in therapeutic doses gives rise to measurable effects in a number of neuropsychological functions.

7. Benzodiazepine abusers and alcoholics both show decreased capacity in abstraction and problem-solving abilities.

8. In patients abusing both benzodiazepines and alcohol in which only one diagnosis of the combined abuse is detected, the clinical outcome, with respect to the patients prognosis, may be uncertain.

9. In patients with combined abuse of benzodiazepines and alcohol the treatment should start with alcohol detoxification while maintaining a full dose of benzodiazepines. After this, gradual tapering of the benzodiazepine is needed.

10. The problem with combined abuse of benzodiazepine and alcohol deserves increased attention regarding diagnosis, treatment, and follow-up.

References

Adinoff, B., Bone, G., and Linnoila, M. (1988). Acute ethanol poisoning and the ethanol withdrawal syndrome. *Medical Toxicology and Adverse Drug Experience*, **3**, 172–96.

Ashton, H. (1984). Benzodiazepine withdrawal: an unfinished story. *British Medical Journal*, **288**, 1135–40.

Beck, O., Lafolie, P., Odelius, G., and Boréus, L. (1990). Immunological screening of benzodiazepines in urine: improved detection of oxazepam intake. *Toxicology Letters*, **52**, 7–14.

Benzer, D. and Cushman, Jr, P. (1980). Alcohol and benzodiazepines: withdrawal syndromes. *Alcoholism: Clinical and Experimental Research*, **4**, 243–7.

Bergman, H., Borg, S., and Holm, L. (1980). Neuropsychological impairment and exclusive abuse of sedative or hypnotics. *American Journal of Psychiatry*, **137**, 215–17.

Bergman, H., Axelsson, G., Ideström, C., Borg, S., Hindmarch, T., Makower, J., and Mützell, S. (1983). Alcohol consumption, neuropsychological status and computer tomographic findings in a random sample of men and women from the general population. *Pharmacology, Biochemistry and Behavior*, **18**, 501–5.

Bond, A., Lader, M., and Shrotriya, R. (1983). Comparative effects of a repeated dose regime of diazepam and buspione on subjective ratings, psychological tests and the EEG. *European Journal of Clinical Pharmacology*, **24**, 463–7.

Buck, K. and Harris, R. (1990). Benzodiazepine agonist and inverse agonist actions on GABA receptor-operated chloride channels. II. Chronic effects of ethanol. *Journal of Pharmacology and Experimental Therapeutics*, **253**, 713–19.

Busto, U. and Sellers, E. (1986). Pharmacokinetic determinants of drug abuse and dependence. A conceptual perspective. *Clinical Pharmacokinetics*, **11**, 144–53.

Busto, U., Simpkins, J., Sellers, E., Sisson, B., and Segal, R. (1983). Objective determinations of benzodiazepine use and abuse in alcoholics. *British Journal of Addiction*, **78**, 429–35.

Chan, A. (1984). Effects of combined alcohol and benzodiazepine: a review. *Drug and Alcohol Dependence*, **13**, 315–41.

Ciraulo, D., Barnhill, J., Greenblatt, D., Shader, R.I., Ciraulo, A.M., Tarmey, M.F., Molloy, M.A., and Foti, M.E. (1988). Abuse of alprazolam in alcoholic men. *Journal of Clinical Psychiatry*, **49**, 333–7.

Ciraulo, D., Barnhill, J., Ciraulo, A., Greenblatt, D.J., and Shader, P.I. (1989). Parental alcoholism as a risk factor in benzodiazepine abuse: a pilot study. *American Journal of Psychiatry*, **146**, 1333–5.

Fialip, J., Aumaitre, O., Eschalier, A., Maradeix, B., Dordain, G., and Lavarenne, J. (1987). Benzodiazepine withdrawal seizures: analysis of 48 case reports. *Clinical Neuropharmacology*, **10**, 538–44.

Fontaine, R., Chouinard, G., and Annable, L. (1984). Bromazepam and diazepam in generalized anxiety: a placebo-controlled study of efficacy and withdrawal. *Psychopharmacology Bulletin*, **20**, 126–7.

Grant, I., Reed, R., Adams, K., and Carlin, A. (1979). Neuropsychological function in young alcohol and polydrug abusers. *Journal of Clinical Neuropsychology*, **1**, 39–47.

Griffiths, R., McCleod, D., Bigelow, G., Liebson, I., Roache, J., and Nowowieski, P. (1984). Comparison of diazepam and oxazepam: preference, linking and extent of abuse. *Journal of Pharmacology and Experimental Therapeutics*, **229**, 501–8.

Guthrie, S. (1989). The treatment of alcohol withdrawal. *Pharmacotherapy*, **9**, 131–43.

Hendler, N., Cimini, C., Terenca, M., and Long, D. (1980). A comparison of cognitive impairment due to benzodiazepines and narcotics. *American Journal of Psychiatry*, **137**, 828–30.

Hillbom, M. and Hjelm-Jäger, M. (1984). Should alcohol withdrawal seizures be treated with anti-epileptic drugs? *Acta Neurologica Scandinavica*, **69**, 39–42.

Höjer, J., Baehrendtz, S., and Gustavsson, L. (1989). Benzodiazepine poisoning: experience of 702 admissions to an intensive care unit during a 14-year period. *Journal of Internal Medicine*, **226**, 117–22.

Jaffe, J., Ciraulo, D., Nies, A., Dixon, R., and Monroe, L. (1983). Abuse potential of halozepam and of diazepam in patients recently treated for acute alcohol withdrawal. *Clinical Pharmacology and Therapeutics*, **34**, 623–30.

Khantzian, E. (1985). The self-medication hypothesis of addictive disorders: focus on heroin and cocaine dependence. *American Journal of Psychiatry*, **142**, 1259–64.

Kryspin-Exner, K. and Demel, J. (1975). The use of tranquillisers in the treatment of mixed drug abuse. *International Journal of Clinical Pharmacology*, **12**, 13–18.

Lader, M., Melhuish, A., and Harris, P. (1982). Residual effects of repeated doses of 0.5 and 1 mg flunitrazepam. *European Journal of Clinical Pharmacology*, **23**, 135–40.

Lapierre, Y. (1983). Are all benzodiazepines equivalent? *Progress in Neuro-Psychopharmacology and Biological Psychiatry*, **7**, 641–6.

Lilja, M., Arvela, P., Klintrup, H., and Jounela, A. (1986). Intake of alcohol and benzodiazepines and reliability of drug history in patients admitted to hospital. *Human Toxicology*, **5**, 281–2.

McMicken, D. (1990). Alcohol withdrawal syndromes. *Emergency Medical Clinics of North America*, **4**, 805–19.

Metha, A. and Ticku, M. (1989). Chronic ethanol treatment alters the behavioral effects of Ro 15–4513, a partially negative ligand for benzodiazepine binding sites. *Brain Research*, **489**, 93–100.

Meyer, R. (1986). Anxiolytics and the alcoholic patient. *Journal of Studies on Alcohol*, **47**, 269–73.

Minder, E., Schaubhut, R., and Simmler, F. (1989). Toxicological screening for benzodiazepines in urine: EMIT™ versus high-performance liquid chromatography with photodiode array detection. *Toxicology Letters*, **45**, 93–9.

Nutt, D., Adinoff, B., and Linnoila, M. (1989). Benzodiazepines in the treatment of alcoholism. *Recent Developments in Alcoholism*, **7**, 283–313.

Pétursson, H., Gudjonsson, G., and Lader, M. (1983). Psychiatric performance during withdrawal from long-term benzodiazepine treatment. *Psychopharmacology*, **81**, 345–9.

Piesiur-Strehlow, B., Strehlow, U., and Poser, W. (1984). Increased mortality associated with dependence on legal drugs? *Drug and Alcohol Dependence*, **14**, 97–9.

Rickels, K., Fox, I., Greenblatt, D., Sandler, K., and Schless, A. (1988). Clorazepate and lorazepam: clinical improvement and rebound anxiety. *American Journal of Psychiatry*, **145**, 312–17.

Rickels, K., Schweizer, E., Case, W., and Greenblatt, D. (1990). Long-term therapeutic use of benzodiazepines. I. Effects of abrupt discontinuation. *Archives of General Psychiatry*, **47**, 899–907.

Roth, S. (1989). Anxiety disorders and the use and abuse of drugs. *Journal of Clinical Psychiatry*, **50**, 30–5.

Schneider, L.S., Syapin, P.J., and Pawluczyk, S. (1987). Seizures following triazolam withdrawal despite benzodiazepine treatment. *Journal of Clinical Psychiatry*, **48**, 418–19.

Schweizer, E., Rickels, K., Case, W., and Greenblatt, D. (1990). Long-term therapeutic use of benzodiazepines. II. Effects of gradual taper. *Archives of General Psychiatry*, **47**, 908–15.

Sellers, E.M. (1988). Alcohol, barbiturate and benzodiazepine withdrawal syndromes: clinical management. *Canadian Medical Association Journal*, **139**, 113–20.

Senay, E. (1989). Addictive behaviours and benzodiazepines. 1. Abuse liability and physical dependence. *Advances in Alcohol and Substance Abuse*, **8**, 107–24.

Sunter, J., Bal, T., and Cowan, W. (1988). Three cases of fatal triazolam poisoning. *British Medical Journal*, **297**, 717.

Thomas, C., Spurrell, M., Hackett, R., and Hore, B. (1989). Severity of withdrawal in subjects exposed to a combination of alcohol and minor tranquillisers. *British Journal of Psychiatry*, **154**, 83–5.

Ticku, M. and Kulkarni, S. (1988). Molecular interactions of ethanol with GABAergic system and potential of Ro 15–4513 as an ethanol antagonist. *Pharmacology, Biochemistry and Behavior*, **30**, 501–10.

Tyrer, P. and Owen, R. (1981). Gradual withdrawal of diazepam after long-term therapy. *Lancet*, **i**, 1402–6.

Tyrer, P., Rutherford, D., and Hugget, T. (1983). Benzodiazepine withdrawal symptoms and propanolol. *Lancet*, **i**, 520–2.

Wiseman, S. and Spencer-Peet, J. (1985). Prescription for alcoholics: a survey of drugs taken prior to admission to an alcoholism unit. *Practitioner*, **229**, 88–9.

9 Oral and intravenous abuse of benzodiazepines

John Strang, Nicholas Seivewright, and Michael Farrell

The story of benzodiazepines and their relationship with the drugs field is a story that cannot yet be fully told, for the relationship is still developing and the uses and abuses that will be found for benzodiazepines have not all been adequately explored by either drug users or treatment or research personnel. Nevertheless, the extent of their use (by those already identified as drug abusers) has increased greatly over the last decade or two, and, during the last few years, there has been an emergence of novel patterns of abuse such as the intravenous self-administration of various benzodiazepines (notably temazepam capsules).

Six separate relationships are explored within this chapter. First, an examination is made of the stand-alone position of benzodiazepines in the field of drug abuse—the extent to which they have been deliberately abused or taken for hedonistic purposes either alone or in combinations, such as with alcohol. Second, attention will be given to the extent to which oral benzodiazepines are a widely used supplementary drug amongst populations of addicts (in particular opiate addicts) who are attending treatment services. Third, consideration will be given to the possible psychopharmacological interactions between benzodiazepines and other drugs (for example, between benzodiazepines and the opiates). Fourth, the intravenous abuse of benzodiazepines will be described and considered alongside the strategies that have been employed to reduce the spread of this novel pattern of abuse. Fifth, reports of an associated increase in HIV risk behaviour amongst benzodiazepine abusers will be considered. Finally, consideration will be given to the possible adaptive use of benzodiazepines, either as a prescribed detoxification agent for opiate or cocaine addicts (as with the treatment of the alcohol withdrawal syndrome) or, alternatively, as a drug used by out-of-treatment populations of drug users who attempt a do-it-yourself detoxification.

Benzodiazepines as an independent drug of abuse

Little attention has so far been paid to the extent to which benzodiazepines are abused with deliberate pursuit of some hedonic tone from the drug themselves. This is surprising in view of the considerable body of evidence of such abuse for earlier sedative and tranquillizer drugs such as the barbiturates, related drugs such as methaqualone, and alcohol.

Barbiturates were extensively abused during the 1960s and 1970s—not only for reasons of attempted self-medication, but also in wilful pursuit of psychoactive effects perceived as positive (Mitcheson *et al.* 1970). Some of this use was in the context of polydrug abuse at a time of increasing interest by the young in a range of drugs of potential abuse across much of the Western world. This was certainly associated with considerable morbidity and mortality (see Ghodse 1977; Ghodse and Rawson 1978; Royal College of Psychiatrists 1987). However, not all of this drug use was without perceived purpose, and Burr (1984) has argued that the use of barbiturates by punks and skinheads (often in combination with alcohol) can be seen within the context of their position within society, the statements they wished to make, and their underlying 'ideology of despair'. Bravado and disregard for possible personal harm were striking features of the injecting barbiturate abuser in London during the 1970s (see later section on intravenous use) where their presentation was in some ways more similar to that of the alcohol-intoxicated street-fighting man than to that of their fellow injectors who were using opiates. Extensive deliberate abuse of sedatives was also seen in many other countries, with similar intravenous abuse of barbiturates occurring in Australia. Sedative abuse by drug users became more widespread in the USA, perhaps especially on the West Coast (Smith and Wesson 1973). Methaqualone, known variously as Mandrax (Mandies) or Quaaludes (Ludes) in Europe and the USA, respectively, also achieved considerable popularity. More recently, during the 1980s, Mandrax has been extensively abused in the subcontinent of India and would appear to have been a forerunner of the more recent heroin-smoking and injecting epidemic in this part of the world.

Large-scale epidemiological surveys of drug usage provide an assessment of the extent of non-medical use of benzodiazepines; the data is limited by the fact that the relevant drug class is usually grouped simply as 'tranquillizers'. In recent years the vast majority of such figures refer to benzodiazepines. In the USA such surveys are regularly conducted by the National Institute of Drug Abuse (NIDA). For example, in the mid-1970s, 17 per cent of high school seniors had been involved in the non-medical use of tranquillizers, of whom 4.6 per cent had used them in the last month: by the mid-1980s there had been a reduction in these figures to 12 and 2 per cent, respectively (thus representing a trend in the opposite direction to that seen with cocaine) (Johnston *et al.* 1986). It was notable that in both these surveys virtually all reported tranquillizer use was on a non-daily basis. In the separate National Household Survey on Drug Abuse conducted by the NIDA (Miller *et al.* 1983) non-prescription use of tranquillizers was reported by 15 per cent of respondents aged 18–25, 5 per cent of respondents aged 12–17, and 4 per cent of respondents aged 26 and older. In the 1985 version of the National Household Survey, 3.5 per cent of the sample, which translated to some seven million people, had used tranquillizers non-medically in the previous year, with such use predominantly reported by those under 35 years of age and by males more than females. The latter finding is usual in surveys of this nature, apparently indicating that the male preponderance in drug abuse overrides the female preponderance typical of therapeutic-dose benzodiazepine usage.

Other studies have shown similar extensive non-prescription use of tranquillizers, especially amongst the young. Smart *et al.* (1981) reported on a household survey conducted in three countries (India, Mexico, and Canada), in all of which non-prescription tranquillizers were found to be widely used to an extent only exceeded, among the psychoactive drugs, by cannabis and amphetamines. The extent of use was, however, slightly less than in the previously mentioned NIDA high school survey. A recent study of 13–18 year olds in Oslo by Pedersen and Lavik (1991) found a past-year prevalence of anxiolytic or hypnotic use, considered to be primarily benzodiazepines, of 10 per cent, with most of that use non-prescribed. Interestingly, there was a strong association between the non-prescribed use of benzodiazepines by young people and by their parents.

There are a number of features that delineate sedative abuse: two key features appear to be supratherapeutic dosage often to extraordinarily high levels (Farrell and Strang 1988; Ruben and Morrison 1992) and intermittent binge usage. It would appear that some substances lend themselves to abuse more than others and the science of abuse liability testing continues to expand (Evans *et al.* 1991). A novel aspect of the methodology of assessing abuse liability in humans is the use of standard double-blind placebo-controlled trials that compare new compounds with substances of known abuse liability. Particular attention is paid to the complete dose–response curve with an awareness that abuse liability may vary along the range of the curve and, in most cases, abuse liability doses will be two to four times the typical therapeutic dose. Such studies need to be carried out in subjects with a history of recreational sedative abuse because they represent the group at risk for illicit high-dose misuse of a new sedative drug with potential for abuse (de Wit and Griffiths 1991).

Benzodiazepines appear to be abused frequently on the illicit drug scene in combination with other drugs—indeed in much the same way as seen previously with the barbiturates. Specifically, Perera *et al.* (1987) made reference to the mixing of benzodiazepines with alcohol to obtain a combined effect (similar to the previous reports by others including Burr (1984)), and they also describe the use of a combination of benzodiazepines with cyclizine (an over-the-counter anti-emetic marketed under various names including 'Marzine').

Supplementary use of benzodiazepines

In the UK use of sedative drugs by heroin addicts was almost entirely centred on barbiturates during the late 1960s, with Mitcheson *et al.* (1970) reporting that 62 of 65 heroin addicts attending day centres reported abuse of barbiturates as well as of heroin, but it is interesting to note that there was no use of non-barbiturate tranquillizers. Ghodse (1977) had found that half of the drug-dependent individuals presenting to London casualty departments had been taking barbiturates compared with only 10 per cent of the comparative non-dependent cases. By the late 1970s in the same city, Jauhar (1981) found that 80 of 100 consecutive clinic attenders had been recently abusing non-opiate drugs and, whilst a quarter had been taking barbiturates, nearly half had been abusing benzodiazepines.

Diazepam became a popular drug of abuse both in addicts attending methadone treatment programmes in the USA and also in addicts new to treatment (Woody *et al.* 1975*a*,*b*; Budd *et al.* 1979) and has also been reported more recently in UK samples of addicts entering a therapeutic community (Perera *et al.* 1987). Higher levels of benzodiazepine use among opiate addicts in treatment (compared with their counterparts who are not in treatment) were seen in the USA reports and have also recently been reported from the UK (Seivewright *et al.* in press). Between the US Drug Abuse Reporting Programme (DARP) studies in the 1970s and the Treatment Outcome Prospective Study (TOPS) reports from the mid-1980s, the extent of tranquillizer use amongst opiate addicts in treatment had increased considerably, so that by the early 1980s a quarter of subjects in methadone maintenance programmes were taking minor tranquillizers weekly or more frequently (Hubbard *et al.* 1984).

A different approach was used by Budd *et al.* (1979). They examined more than 8000 urine specimens from seven methadone maintenance clinics in Los Angeles during 1977. In addition to identifying widespread diazepam use among patients receiving methadone maintenance, they also found substantial variation among clinics with from 5 to 50 per cent of specimens being positive, and also considerable variation within each clinic from one month to the next. More advanced radioimmunoassay techniques were used in another study (Kaul and Davidow 1981) who found that about one-eighth of all urine specimens from methadone maintenance programmes in New York City were also positive for benzodiazepines. Much higher levels of use have been reported from other studies including that of Stitzer *et al.* (1981) who found a positive benzodiazepine urinalysis rate of 65–70 per cent in two clinics. That group subsequently went on to investigate the malleability of this behaviour and reported on the considerable success of contingency contracting as an approach to bring about reductions in benzodiazepine use in drug abuse treatment populations (Stitzer *et al.* 1982).

A drug-using population may also judiciously or injudiciously titrate drugs of differing effects to achieve particular subjective effects. The combination of stimulants and sedatives are one such example where somebody after a cocaine binge lasting many hours may begin to experience anxiety symptoms and wish to experience a more sedated subjective state. It is very clear from general knowledge of reported patterns of drug use that cocaine and amphetamine users frequently take benzodiazepines towards the end of a binge to settle down and sometimes to induce sleep. It is possible that the affective disturbance after heavy stimulant use that is initially medicated with sedatives may then enter into a cycle of anxiety, and benzodiazepines may be used to ameliorate such symptoms. In the wide-ranging study by Seivewright *et al.* (in press) of the prevalence of benzodiazepine use by illicit drug users, 43 (13.5 per cent) of 318 subjects, whose main drug was either amphetamine or cocaine, were reported as additionally using benzodiazepines.

With the recent surge in the interest and use of MDMA (Ecstasy), a combined stimulant and hallucinogen, among young 'rave' party attenders, there are also reports of benzodiazepine use to terminate the period of stimulation produced by this drug. As with other stimulants there are indications of high levels of affective disturbance and anxiety symptoms in the intermediate post-drug use period and such symptoms may be medicated with tranquillizers.

Is there an interaction between benzodiazepines and opiates?

Opiate addicts (at least some of them) appear to have formed the view that benzodiazepines might be used to enhance the effect they receive from opiates. There appears to be considerable overlap of the populations, as demonstrated by Busto *et al.* (1986) who noted that 10 per cent of patients attending a health service with an identified benzodiazepine dependence were also simultaneously taking opiates.

What possible benefit could there be to the drug user from combining these two different types of drug? Before discarding the possibility of any hitherto unidentified interaction, it would be well to remember that drug users have previously discovered interactions before they were identified either by clinicians or the pharmaceutical industry—for example, the apparently paradoxical interaction between amphetamines and barbiturates.

Kleber and Gold (1978) reported an increased use of oral diazepam among patients in methadone maintenance programmes, and also reported that some of the patients claimed that 25–50 mg of diazepam could be used to 'boost the high' achieved from the oral methadone. Stitzer *et al.* (1981) also reported that their methadone maintenance patients were seeking the same effect, and were taking the oral diazepam shortly after the daily methadone dose in order to achieve this boost. It is unclear whether this may be the same effect from oral use of diazepam as that already described by Woody *et al.*

(1975*a,b*). Perera *et al.* (1987) similarly report that a few of their subjects reported that the benzodiazepines helped to intensify the opiate 'high'. Strang (1984) also described this reported enhancement of opiate effect after the self-administration of benzodiazepines—in this case the simultaneous intravenous self-administration of the benzodiazepine flurazepam (Dalmane) in a network of injecting opiate addicts in Manchester who believed that the addition of flurazepam not only enhanced the effect, but also extended the duration of opiate effect.

Laboratory study of this possible interaction provides inconclusive or conflicting data. Animal studies have provided some evidence of an apparent pharmacodynamic interaction between diazepam and opiates (Bradshaw *et al.* 1973; Wiechman and Spratto 1982). *In vitro* diazepam has been found to inhibit the degradation of methadone in dependent rats (Spaulding *et al.* 1974), and prior loading with diazepam increases the levels of methadone found in brain and liver after subsequent administration of methadone (Shah *et al.* 1979). Other investigators (e.g. Shannon *et al.* 1976; Pond *et al.* 1982), have not found evidence of any interaction between diazepam and methadone. Human studies from Preston and colleagues in Baltimore initially found evidence of an interaction between diazepam and methadone when the drugs were concurrently administered orally with these effects being measurable both physiologically as well as subjectively (Preston *et al.* 1984). However, the analyses of their later study found no evidence of any pharmacokinetic interaction between these two drugs (Preston *et al.* 1986).

The intravenous abuse of benzodiazepines

Perhaps the most surprising observation regarding this aspect is that decades elapsed after the widespread prescribing of benzodiazepines was established (the 'relentless march of the psychotropic juggernaut'; Trethowan 1975) before the intravenous abuse potential of the benzodiazepines was discovered and developed by the injecting drug user. In most parts of the world, this intravenous abuse has not yet developed, but it is sobering to observe the speed of spread of this novel pattern of abuse in affected cities where it appears to have become one of the most widespread drugs of intravenous abuse within a matter of a few years (e.g. Sakol *et al.* 1989; Hammersley *et al.* 1990).

The first reports in the literature of intravenous abuse of benzodiazepines appeared in 1984. There were single case reports from New Zealand and from Israel (Kaminer and Modia 1984) of subjects feigning clinical conditions in order to obtain intravenous diazepam from physicians, and in the same year, the first report of intravenous abuse of benzodiazepines among injecting opiate addicts also occurred, describing the spread of concurrent injecting of flurazepam and blackmarket heroin in the UK (Strang 1984). In the study by Perera *et al.* (1987) of benzodiazepine use among drug addicts in the

UK, they found that about one-third of their subjects included intravenous benzodiazepine use in their varied previous drug use. Half of these subjects were taking the benzodiazepinealong with their main drug (usually an opiate), although about a third would take the drug during times of shortage or as an alternative to the main drug. At the time of this study (1985) diazepam was the most widely used benzodiazepine, with temazepam being used much less frequently.

Over the course of the next few years the intravenous abuse of temazepam capsules became widespread among injecting drug users in some cities (*Druglink* 1987; Stark *et al.* 1987; Farrell and Strang 1988; Sakol *et al.* 1989; Hammersley *et al.* 1990). This novel intravenous abuse of benzodiazepines related almost exclusively to the liquid-filled temazepam capsules—so-called 'soft eggs'. The manufacturers moved to alter the formulation of the capsules to a hard gel consistency (like candle wax, and hence presumed to be un-injectable) so as to prevent any further intravenous abuse (Drake and Ballard 1988; Launchbury *et al.* 1989). However, the 'hard eggs' were themselves also abused, with some addicts heating the hard capsules in an oven or microwave until the contents were sufficiently soft to enable injection through a wide-bore needle. The 'soft eggs' had themselves required a wide-bore needle, and appeared to be associated with an increased frequency of complications, and the early reports suggest that these physical sequelae were even more pronounced with the injection of the liquefied 'hard eggs' (Griffiths and Rothwell 1990; Grahame-Smith 1991). Most recently, Seivewright *et al.* (in press) have looked at the extent of oral and intravenous use of benzodiazepines by illicit drug users by reference to the most established of the network of anonymized UK regional drug misuse databases (Department of Health 1989; Donmall 1990; Strang *et al.* 1991). The study, which identified 661 illicit drug users using benzodiazepines in a reporting period of the 2 years 1988 and 1989, demonstrated that the injected abuse of benzodiazepines within the north-west of England at that time was dominated by temazepam, with abuse of diazepam and nitrazepam accounting for the remaining 10 per cent of injecting cases. The reformulation of temazepam capsules did not occur until the end of 1989 so that study did not include a significant period of reports that followed that change.

Green *et al.* (1992) have recently reported from Glasgow on the recent extensive intravenous use of triazolam (Halcion) up until it was banned by the Committee on Safety of Medicines in the UK. They interviewed 503 current injecting drug users in 1990; 226 (45 per cent) had used triazolam, of whom a quarter had injected the drug. Seven subjects were injecting triazolam on a daily basis.

One of the key indicators of abuse liability of a drug is the reported subjective effect. Inadequate attention has been paid to this dimension of benzodiazepine abuse. Evans *et al.* (1991) report in detail on the methodology of asking subjects how much they like a drug's effects and report that drug-liking measurements have a face validity for assessing potential for abuse and are a sensitive measure of subjective drug effect. Such drug-liking ratings may be compared to those for a placebo or for other drugs used. One study in a clinical setting of injecting drug users asked about the likeability of injecting temazepam (Farrell, Herrod, and Strang, unpublished data). This study was conducted in 1990 prior to the widespread availability of new formulation temazepam. Using a questionnaire with a likert scale rating for likeability in 38 injecting drug users, a total of 19 had taken temazepam and 14 (37 per cent) had injected temazepam. When asked to rate likeability of injected temazepam, 21 per cent of the injecting cohort liked injecting, 14 per cent did not mind injecting, while 64 per cent said they did not like injecting despite having injected more than once. Thus only 8 per cent of the total sample questioned rated intravenous temazepam as an experience they would wish to repeat, indicating a much lower rating for liking for injecting temazepam than was originally believed to be the case.

The speed with which intravenous abuse of benzodiazepines has been taken up by populations of injecting drug users in some cities would suggest that this unwelcome development was a discovery waiting to be made. It is likely that efforts will be made to nip in the bud any such growths of the drug problem, but it may well be that the acquisition of the information and an available variety of benzodiazepines with such abuse potential may be more powerful influences promoting the spread of benzodiazepine injecting. The wider abuse potential of temazepam has now been discovered, and with it the extensive abuse potential of the benzodiazepines in general: it may now be too late to wish that Pandora's box had not been opened.

Finally, it may be interesting to consider the modification of the temazepam product from the point of view of benefits and harms to personal and public health. It seemed clear that some action was required to interrupt the spread of intravenous abuse of the 'soft eggs' of temazepam. On first examination, the move to the 'hard egg' formulation appears to have been paradoxically harm-increasing, thus placing it apparently out of step with the growing harm minimization movement within the UK (O'Hare *et al*. 1992; Strang and Farrell 1992; Stimson, in press; Strang, in press). However, whilst the change to the new formulation has been harm-increasing at a personal level for those injectors who have continued to inject temazepam capsules, it is still possible that the intervention might be neutral or even harm-minimizing at the public health level, if the overall extent of temazepam injecting has reduced. To comment on this possible therapeutic Benthamism, it would be necessary to examine data on the overall extent of injecting of temazepam capsules before and after the reformulation, and to have data on the extent of morbidity in the abuse of the two forms. Temazepam has also been reformulated as a tablet and there is a need for research to compare the relative abuse liability of both formulations (Strang *et al*. 1992).

Other routes of administration may also be exploited by tomorrow's abuser of benzodiazepines. Sheehan *et al.* (1991) have recently reported on the snorting of benzodiazepines in a manner similar to the long-established practice of snorting blackmarket amphetamines or cocaine. While there have not been any reports yet in the UK of this novel method of benzodiazepine abuse, the snorting of pharmaceutical drugs has recently been reported in relation to the prescribed analgesic buprenorphine (Strang 1991), and so the potential would seem to exist already for this new twist in the benzodiazepine abuse problem.

The full extent of potential abuse of intravenous benzodiazepines has probably not been explored fully by the drug-using entrepreneurs. We have recently encountered cases of intravenous self-administration of the rapid-onset, short-acting benzodiazepine midazolam in physicians, who at the present time are one of the few groups who would have access to this drug.

At the present time, it is far from clear what the future holds in store with regard to intravenous benzodiazepine abuse.

Benzodiazepines and HIV risk behaviour

The single most serious development within the field of drug misuse in recent years has been the emergence of drug misusers as one of the main high-risk groups in the international epidemic of HIV infection and AIDS. The most obvious way in which drug misusers are implicated in the transmission of infection is through sharing contaminated injecting equipment; thus those users who are injecting are clearly at the highest risk. However, sexual spread is also a possible method of transmission in this population, and it seems likely that both general and specific aspects of the disinhibiting effects of using drugs (including alcohol) probably act to encourage spread through sexual contact. As a mainly heterosexually active group, drug misusers risk vertical transmission of the disease to newborn children, while it has frequently been pointed out that drug misusers probably represent the main route of spread of HIV and AIDS from high-risk groups into the general heterosexual population. A further complication is posed by the close links between drug misuse and prostitution with particular concern being expressed recently over the possibility that drug-using prostitutes may be the most likely to agree to unprotected sex for higher payments.

Amidst the various data now emerging on all these aspects, some early but potentially very important work has suggested that abuse of the benzodiazepine temazepam by polydrug users in the UK may be particularly associated with a range of high HIV risk injecting and sexual practices. The findings are contained in a study by Klee *et al.* (1990) of 272 injecting polydrug users in the north-west of England. Twenty-eight per cent were using temazepam, which was in turn strongly associated with multiple drug use (for example four or more drugs). Use of temazepam specifically was strikingly associated with the practice of sharing injecting equipment, with casual sexual contacts, and with unprotected sexual activity. Detailed analyses showed that the relationships between temazepam and sharing and casual sexual contacts held only for those using temazepam but not other tranquillizers, suggesting that the high-risk behaviour was a feature of those individuals who were using temazepam for purposes other than sedation, such as enhancing an opiate 'high' or substituting for heroin. Temazepam use was also associated with high involvement in criminal activity and a history of drug overdosage.

The authors point out that their findings were to some extent serendipitous in that it became clear from additional rather than central study information that effects of this sort were occurring with temazepam. No detailed information was collected on temazepam usage unless it was a subject's main drug and the authors suggest that more detailed study is now indicated to assess the meaning of their findings. This is certainly so, but meanwhile it is clear that use of temazepam must be taken very seriously in the assessment of drug use in harm-reduction treatment programmes. As to the reasons why it might be that use of temazepam is related to the extent to which individuals indulge in high HIV risk behaviours, it is at this stage possible to speculate in two areas. First, it may be that the particular effects of temazepam appeal selectively to those drug users who tend anyway towards more chaotic drug use and associated risky behaviours. Second, it may be that some of the risky behaviours occur at the height of the disturbed behavioural effects, particularly characterized by amnesia, which high-dose temazepam appears to produce (Ruben and Morrison, 1992). It seems to us that there should be no surprise at the fact that the high-dose injected benzodiazepines produce amnesia, as this is one of the reasons for which intravenous benzodiazepines are used prior to various procedures in general medical practice. It may well prove to be the case that future research will demonstrate that there are particular aspects of the usage and effects of benzodiazepines that relate more closely and specifically to high HIV risk behaviours than can be accounted for in terms of the general, for instance disinhibiting, effects of any drug abuse.

Adaptive use of benzodiazepines?

Caution is definitely required in suggesting any adaptive use of benzodiazepines by illicit drug users especially if that might involve prescribing benzodiazepines, as, clearly, the whole widespread abuse situation with its sometimes severe associated problems originates with prescribed supplies. However it is also probably wrong to consider all use of benzodiazepines by illicit drug users to be definitely misuse, and brief consideration is given here to the possible circumstances in which use of benzodiazepines might be of some benefit rather than harmful. Two recent studies provide an insight into such situations, one relating to treatment with benzodiazepines in an in-patient setting, and the other to drug misusers' usage of benzodiazepines in their own attempts at self-detoxification.

Drummond *et al.* (1989) describe a conventional double-blind controlled trial of chlordiazepoxide and methadone in in-patient detoxification from opiates. Although on purely neuropharmacological grounds a benzodiazepine could not be expected to relieve the specific features of opiate withdrawal (Seivewright and Tyrer 1984) that study found only minor differences in the severity of withdrawal symptoms in the two treatment groups. The authors suggested that chlordiazepoxide could be popular with doctors wary of misuse of methadone or of the legal formalities involved in its prescription. While the results of the study need to be accepted as evidence for a possible useful treatment method with in-patients, for an out-patient detoxification the potential misuse of benzodiazepines is in its way just as problematic as that of methadone, and the climate of opinion now would probably be more in favour of providing methadone rather than a benzodiazepine in such circumstances (Department of Health 1991).

Although it is possible to be sceptical about the effectiveness of benzodiazepines in relieving opiate withdrawal symptoms, it is of interest that drug misusers do appear to use benzodiazepines in such circumstances. Gossop *et al.* (1991) asked attenders at a treatment service in some detail about the methods they had employed at times in the past when they had attempted to stop using opiates themselves. Benzodiazepines were found to be the most frequently used drug group for that purpose, and appeared to have had a similar efficacy in the short term to other approaches used by the study subjects.

In a review of large-scale epidemiological studies of non-medical use of tranquillizers, Cole and Chiarello (1990) observe that such terms can include an extremely wide range of behaviours, from one borrowed tablet on one occasion through to extensive polydrug abuse. It is certainly necessary to be aware that the harmfulness of such usage is very variable, and to counter the view that all use of benzodiazepines by illicit drug users constitutes abuse. Going a little further, we may observe that some behaviours that on the face of it seem to suggest abuse may have a beneficial side: thus the methadone patients referred to earlier who use a benzodiazepine to enhance the effect of their opiate may at least be managing on a smaller dose of methadone than might otherwise be the case! In such circumstances it is useful for a clinician to refer to the concept of harm reduction to examine the relative harm produced by alternative patterns of drug-taking, and to consider whether sometimes the use of benzodiazepines can be adaptive rather than purely disadvantageous.

Conclusion

In many countries of the world in recent years, information from treatment centres and elsewhere has shown that benzodiazepines have become firmly established in patterns of polydrug use by drug misusers. In addition, there is evidence of significant misuse of benzodiazepines by young people and by alcoholics. Although diverse behaviours are included in such statistics, and some of this usage may be of little serious significance, at the other end of the spectrum lies extremely harmful benzodiazepine abuse, including that by injection. The recent phenomenon in the UK of extensive high-dose injecting of temazepam has produced evidence of highly disturbing behavioural effects and severe physical complications, and may well be associated with behaviour that leads to HIV infection and AIDS. Unlike some forms of drug abuse, benzodiazepine abuse derives solely from pharmaceutical supplies. Major educational initiatives are required to reduce unwise prescribing of benzodiazepines. Indeed, it is possible that some changes may be required in the degree of controlled status of certain of this group of drugs.

Much is now known about the patterns of benzodiazepine misuse prevalent within specific groups such as treatment samples or in different geographical areas. While more documentation will be valuable, the focus of future research must also shift towards the management of benzodiazepine misuse. Virtually all such evidence relates solely to in-patient detoxification (e.g. Harrison *et al.* 1984) but as with opiates, although specific data are lacking, this is likely to be followed by a high rate of relapse amongst samples of drug misusers. Other measures that attempt to tackle benzodiazepine misuse, suitable for ambulatory care, urgently require investigation.

References

Bradshaw, E.G., Biswas, T.K., and Pleuvry, B.J. (1973). Some interactions between morphine and diazepam in the mouse and rabbit. *British Journal of Anaesthesia*, **45**, 1185–90.
Budd, R.D., Walkin, E., Jain, N.C., and Sneath, T.C. (1979). Frequency of use of diazepam in individuals on probation and in methadone maintenance programmes. *American Journal of Drug and Alcohol Abuse*, **6**, 511–14.
Burr, A. (1984). The ideologies of despair: a symbolic interpretation of punks and skinheads usage of barbuturates. *Social Science and Medicine*, **19**(9), 928–9.
Busto, U., Sellers, E.M., Naranjo, C.A., Kappell, H.D., Sanchez-Craig, M., and Simpkins, J. (1986). Patterns of benzodiazepine abuse and dependence. *British Journal of Addiction*, **81**, 87–94.
Cole, J.O. and Chiarello, R.J. (1990). The benzodiazepines as drugs of abuse. *Journal of Psychiatric Research*, **24**, 135–44.
de Wit, H. and Griffiths, R.R. (1991). Testing the abuse liability of anxiolytic and hypnotic drugs in humans. *Drug and Alcohol Dependence*, **28**, 83–111.
Department of Health (1989). *Health Services management. Services for drug misusers—regional databases* HC (89) 30. Department of Health, London.
Department of Health (1991). *Drug misuse and dependence: guidelines on clinical management*. Her Majesty's Stationery Office, London.
Donmall, M.C. (1990). Towards a national drug database. *Druglink*, **5**, 10–12.
Drake, J. and Ballard, R. (1988). Misuse of temazepam: reply from the manufacturer. *British Medical Journal*, **297**, 1402.
Druglink (1987). Temazepam creates new 'barb freaks'. *Druglink*, **2**(6), 5.
Drummond, D.C. Turkington, D., Rahman, M.Z., Mullin, P.J., and Jackson P.

(1989). Chlordiazepoxide versus methadone in opiate withdrawal: a preliminary double blind trial. *Drug and Alcohol Dependence*, **23**, 63–71.

Evans, S., Critchfield, T.S., and Griffiths, R.R. (1991). Abuse liability assessment of anxiolytics/hypnotics: rationale and laboratory lore. *British Journal of Addiction*, **86**, 1625–32.

Farrell, M. and Strang, J. (1988). Misuse of temazepam. *British Medical Journal*, **297**, 1402.

Ghodse, A.H. (1977). Drug dependent individuals dealt with by London casualty departments. *British Journal of Psychiatry*, **131**, 273–80.

Ghodse, A.H. and Rawson, N.S. (1978). Distribution of drug related problems among London casualty departments. *British Journal of Psychiatry*, **132**, 467–72.

Gossop, M., Battersby, M., and Strang, J. (1991). Self-detoxification by opiate addicts: a preliminary investigation. *British Journal of Psychiatry*, **159**, 208–12.

Grahame-Smith, D. (1991). Misuse of temazepam. *British Medical Journal*, **302**, 1210.

Green, S., Goldberg, D., Frischer, M., and McKeganey, N. (in press). Triazolam as a substance of abuse among injecting drug users. *British Journal of Addiction*, **87**, 940–1.

Griffiths, S.J. and Rothwell, J.G. (1990). Misuse of temazepam. *Pharmaceutical Journal*, 9th June, p.675.

Hammersley, R., Lavelle, T., and Forsythe, A. (1990). Buprenorphine and temazepam—abuse. *British Journal of Addiction*, **85**, 301–3.

Harrison, M., Busto, U., Naranjo, C.A., Kaplan, H.L., and Sellers, E.M. (1984). Diazepam tapering in detoxification for high-dose benzodiazepine abuse. *Clinical Pharmacology and Therapeutics*, October, 527–33.

Hubbard, R.L., Rachal, J.V., Craddock, S.G., and Cavanagh, E.R. (1984). Treatment Outcome Prospective Study (TOPS): Client characteristics and behaviours before, during, and after treatment. In *Drug abuse treatment evaluation: strategies, progress and prospects* (NIDA Research Monograph no. 51) (ed. F.M. Timms and J.P. Ludford). National Institute on Drug Abuse, Rockville, Maryland.

Jauhar, P. (1981). Non-opiate abuse amongst opiate addicts. In *The misuse of psychotropic drugs* (ed. R.Murray, H.Ghodse, C.Harris, D. Williams, and P. Williams), pp.71–3. Gaskell, London.

Johnston, L.D., O'Malley, P.M., and Bachman, J.G. (1986). *Drug use among American High School students, college students and other young adults: national trends through* 1985, DHHS publication (ADM) 86–1450. National Institute on Drug Abuse, Rockville, Maryland.

Kaminer, Y. and Modia, I. (1984). Parenteral abuse of diazepam: a case report. *Drug and Alcohol Dependence*, **14**, 63–5.

Kaul, B. and Davidow, B. (1981). Drug abuse patterns of patients on methadone treatment in New York City. *American Journal of Drug and Alcohol Abuse*, **8**, 17–25.

Kleber, H.D. and Gold, M.S. (1978). Use of psychotropic drugs in treatment of methadone maintained narcotic addicts. *Annals of the New York Academy of Sciences* **311**, 81–98.

Klee, H., Faugier, J., Hayes, C., Boulton, T., and Morris, J. (1990). AIDS-related risk behaviour, polydrug use and temazepam. *British Journal of Addiction*, **85**, 1125–32.

Launchbury, A.P., Morton, F.S.S., and Lacy, J.E. (1989). The developing of temazepam gelthix. *Manufacturing Chemist*, December, 38–40.

Miller, J.D., Cisin, I.H., Gardner, K.H., Harrell, A.V., Wirtz, P.W., Abelson, H.I., and Fishburne, P.M. (1983). *National survey on drug abuse: main findings* 1982. DHHS publication (ADM) 83–1263. National Institute on Drug Abuse, Rockville, Maryland.

Mitcheson, M., Davidson, J., Hawks, D., Hitchens, L., and Malone, S. (1970). Sedative abuse by heroin addicts. *Lancet*, **i** 606–7.

O'Hare, P.A., Newcombe, R., Matthews, A., Buning, E., and Drucker, E. (1992). *The reduction of drug related harm.* Routledge, London.

Pedersen, W. and Lavik, N.J. (1991). Adolescents and benzodiazepines: prescribed use, self-medication and intoxication. *Acta Psychiatrica Scandinavica*, **84**, 94–8.

Perera, K.M.H., Tulley, M., and Jenner, F.A. (1987). The use of benzodiazepines among drug addicts. *British Journal of Addiction*, **82**, 511–15.

Pond, S.M., Tong, T.G., Benowitz, N.L., *et al.* (1982). Lack of effect of diazepam on methadone metabolism in methadone maintained addicts. *Clinical Pharmacology and Therapeutics*, **31**, 139–43.

Preston, K.L., Griffiths, R.R., Stitzer, M.L., Bigelow, G.E., and Liebson, I.A. (1984). Diazepam and methadone interactions in methadone maintenance. *Clinical Pharmacology and Therapeutics*, **36**, 534–41.

Preston, K.L., Griffiths, R.R., Cone, E.J., Darwin, W.D., and Gorodetzky, C.W. (1986). Diazepam and methadone blood levels following concurrent administration of diazepam and methadone. *Drug and Alcohol Dependence*, **18**, 195–202.

Royal College of Psychiatrists (1987). *Drug scenes: a report on drugs and drug dependence by the Royal College of Psychiatrists.* Royal College of Psychiatrists, London.

Ruben, S.M. and Morrison, C.L. (1992). Temazepam misuse in a group of injecting drug users. *British Journal of Addiction*, **87**(10), 1387–92.

Sakol, M.S., Stark, C., and Sykes, R. (1989) Buprenorphine and temazepam abuse by drug takers in Glasgow: an increase. *British Journal of Addiction*, **84**, 439–41.

Seivewright, N., Donmall, M., and Daly, C. (in press). Benzodiazepines in the illicit drugs scene: the UK picture and some treatment dilemmas. *International Journal of Drug Policy*.

Seivewright, N. and Tyrer, P. (1984). Use of beta-blocking drugs in withdrawal states. *Postgraduate Medical Journal*, **60**, 47–50.

Shah, N.S., Patel, V.O., and Donald, A.G. (1979). Effects of diazepam, desmethylimipramine and SKF 525-A on the disposition of levo-methadone in mice after single or double injection. *Drug Metabolism and Disposition*, **7** 241–2.

Shannon, H.E., Holtzman, S.G., and Davis, D.C. (1976). Interactions between narcotic analgesics and benzodiazepine derivatives on behaviour in the mouse. *Journal of Pharmacology and Experimental Therapeutics*, **199**, 389–99.

Sheehan, M.F., Sheehan, D.V., Torres, A., Koppola, A., and Francis, E. (1991). Snorting benzodiazepines. *American Journal of Drug and Alcohol Abuse*, **17** 457–68.

Smart, R.G., Mora, M.E., Terroba, G., and Varma, V.K. (1981). Drug use among non-students in three countries. *Drug and Alcohol Dependence*, **7** 125–32.

Smith, D.E. and Wesson, D.R. (ed.) (1973). *Uppers and downers.* Prentice-Hall, Englewood Cliffs, New Jersey.

Spaulding, T.C., Minimum, L., Kotake, A.N., and Takemori, A.E. (1974). The effects of diazepam on the metabolism of methadone by the liver of methadone dependent rates. *Drug Metabolism and Disposition*, **2** 458–63.

Stark, C., Sykes, R., and Mullin, P. (1987). Temazepam abuse. *Lancet*, **ii**, 284–5.

Stimson, G.V. (in press). Harm minimisation for drug users. In *Responding to drug abuse: the 'British System'* (ed. J. Strang and M. Gossop). Oxford University Press, Oxford.

Stitzer, M.L., Griffiths, R.R., McLellan, A.T., Grabowski, J., and Hawthorne, J.W. (1981). Diazepam use among methadone maintenance patients: patterns and dosages. *Drug and Alcohol Dependence*, **8** 189–99.

Stitzer, M.L., Bigelow, G.E., Liebson, I.A., and Hawthorne, J.W. (1982) Contingent reinforcement for benzodiazepine-free urines: evaluation of a drug abuse treatment intervention. *Journal of Applied Behavioural Analysis*, **15**, 493–503.

Strang, J. (1984). Intravenous benzodiazepine abuse. *British Medical Journal*, **289**, 964.

Strang, J. (1991). Abuse of buprenorphine (Temgesic) by snorting. *British Medical Journal*, **302**, 969.

Strang, J. (in press). Harm reduction: responding to the challenge. In *Psychotropic drugs and harm reduction: from faith to science* (ed. N. Heather, A. Wodak, and P. O'Hare). Whurr Publishers, London.

Strang, J. and Farrell, M. (1992). Editorial: Harm minimisation for drug users: when second best may be best first. *British Medical Journal*, **304**, 1127–8.

Strang, J., Donmall, M., Webster, A., Abbey, J., and Tantam, D. (1991). *A bridge not far enough: community drug teams and doctors in the North Western Region 1982–1986*, ISDD Research Monograph, No. 3. Institute for the Study of Drug Dependence, London.

Strang, J., Seivewright, N., and Farrell, M. (1992). Intravenous and other novel abuses of benzodiazepines: the opening of Pandora's Box? *British Journal of Addiction*, **87**(10), 1373–5.

Trethowan, W. (1975). Pills for personal problems. *British Medical Journal*, **3**, 749–51.

Wiechman, B.E. and Spratto, G.R. (1982). Body temperature response to cocaine and diazepam in morphine-treated rats. *Pharmacology*, **25**, 308–19.

Woody, G.E., O'Brien, C.P., and Greenstein, R. (1975*a*). Misuse and abuse of diazepam: an increasingly common medical problem. *International Journal of the Addictions*, **10**, 843–4.

Woody, G.E., Mintz, J., O'Hare, K., et al. (1975*b*). Diazepam use by patients in a methadone program—how serious a problem? *Journal of Psyched Drugs*, **7**, 373–9.

10 The assessment of anxiety and benzodiazepine dependence

John Pecknold

Differences between normal and pathological anxiety

Evaluation of primate behaviour indicates that there are situations in which displays of fear or anxiety represent perfectly normal, developmentally appropriate reactions most likely shaped by natural selection (Suomi 1986). Bowlby (1973) recognizes that fear which is focused, as well as anxiety which is diffuse and anticipatory, evoke the same cluster of reactions. He suggests that alarm and anxiety are two variants of the overall emotion of fear. Alarm appears to be avoidance of the feared object, while anxiety arises from non-availability of an attachment figure; both serve the biological function of protection. Species-specific, biologically determined tendencies interact with universal learning experiences in the child to produce negative affect in infants to sudden stimuli change. Later in development, strange people and separation from the mother evoke distress (Campbell 1986). Anxiety plays a compensatory, adaptive, and protective role. It is the basis for caution, reconsideration, and comparison of objectives and capabilities and the regulation of drives and motivations.

In contrast to the normal anxiety seen in childhood and in adulthood, there is the question of pathological anxiety. The three-systems definition considers anxiety to be a constellation of three response channels : (1) verbal reports of the experience of anxiety, fear, dread, panic, worry, obsessions, guilt, inability to concentrate, lack of self-efficacy, and insecurity (cognitive self-report); (2) avoidance behaviour, e.g. escape, vigilance, dysfunctional immobility, compulsive mannerisms, and deficits in attention, performance, and control (behaviour motoric); (3) patterns of visceral and somatic activation, e.g. increase in heart rate, blood pressure, sweating, generalized muscle tension, and concomitant biochemical changes (psychophysiological) (Lang 1971). When these three systems, all reflections of anxiety, move at the same rate and pace they are said to be synchronous. When one or another of the patterns of verbal reports, behaviour, and somatic activation are out of alignment, they are desynchronous (Rachman and Hodgson 1974). Discrepancies in synchrony can be measured and may characterize particular personalities or syndromes.

Diagnosis and clinical aspects

The term neurosis was coined by Cullen in 1787 to encompass a whole range of non-inflammatory diseases of the central and peripheral nervous system. As organic ideologies were identified, neurosis as a diagnosis was restricted to diseases of an unknown origin (Berner and Walter 1986). Via Kraepelin (1896), the international classification of diseases (ICD-9) came to a phenomenological view of neurotic disorders, which included anxiety states, hysteria, phobic states, obsessive–compulsive disorder, neurotic depression, neurasthenia, depersonalization syndrome, and hypochondriasis. Klerman (1986, 1990), outlined the continuum model of anxiety states in which anxiety appears in a continuum of increasing severity, modified by biological, psychodynamic, and behavioural paradigms.

The development of research diagnostic criteria evolved into the DSM-III (*Diagnostic and statistical manual of mental disorders* (3rd edn); APA 1980). Neurosis as a modifying diagnostic category was abandoned and instead separate categories were created, including anxiety disorders, affective disorders, and eating disorders. The DSM-III formulations were particularly criticized by several British psychopathologists (Marks 1969; Boyd *et al.* 1984; Goldberg and Simpson 1985).

Assessment of anxiety

A review of the assessment of anxiety by Borkovec *et al.* (1977) contained 191 references to rating instruments. Many of the methods of assessing anxiety have been developed specifically in the psychological literature and focus on a global assessment of anxiety, especially as it relates to personality variables and utilize a continuum between normal and pathological anxiety. Finney (1985) reviewed the assessment of anxiety by objective personality tests, especially the Minnesota Multiphasic Personality Inventory (MMPI) and its derivatives, including the Taylor Manifest Anxiety Scale, the Welsh Anxiety Scale, and the Finney Anxiety Scale. He also assessed several questionnaires, including those of Cattell (the Sixteen Personality Factors, the Clinical Analysis Questionnaires, the Institute for Personality and Ability Testing (IPAT); Cattell and Scheier 1957) and the Spielberger State Trait Anxiety Inventory (STAI). Finney found that all these measures are highly interconnected, whether derived by including items that have face validity, factoring pooled items, or by selecting items that correlate with an external criterion. In commentary Uhlenhuth (1985) noted that these instruments are diagnostic; they detect anxiety and do not measure change, particularly in pharmacological trials. Another group of observer-related instruments was required to quantify pathological levels, e.g. the Hamilton Anxiety Scale (Hamilton 1959) and the Covi Anxiety Scale (Lipman 1982). There have been many modifications of the Hamilton Anxiety Scale, produced in order to measure anxiety more accurately.

At the present time there are two sets of instruments that are widely used in the evaluation of anxiety disorders both for psychopharmacological studies and for epidemiological and other studies. The first set is essentially diagnostic and includes the Schedule of Affective Disorders and Schizophrenia (Endicott and Spitzer 1978), the Diagnostic Interview Schedule (Robins *et al*. 1981), the Structured Clinical Interview for DSM-III and DSM-III (R) (SCID; Spitzer and Williams 1982), the DIS (Diagnostic Interview Schedule), and the ADIS (Anxiety Disorders Interview Schedule (diNardo *et al*. 1983)). In the second category are some of the newer check-lists and scales (clinician and patient-scored) that focus on more specific symptoms and syndromes (the Sheehan Patient-Rated Anxiety Scale (SPRAS) and its equivalent psychiatrist-scored scale). This category may contain self-monitoring procedures, self-rating questionnaires, and check-lists or clinical ratings of a general scale (Fyer *et al*. 1987). For example, Zung (1971) constructed an observer-rated Anxiety States Inventory (ASI) and a patient Self-rating Anxiety Scale (SAS).

The relationship between anxiety and the benzodiazepine withdrawal syndrome

Chronicity of the illness

Generalized anxiety disorder may begin before adolescence or in early adulthood and can persist for decades with a waxing and waning pattern (Raskin *et al*. 1982; Anderson *et al*. 1984; Barlow *et al*. 1986; Thyer *et al*. 1985).

Panic disorder, too, is a chronic illness with only some degree of spontaneous recovery. Coryell *et al*. (1983) found that, in a 5-year outcome study of 116 panic disorder patients, only 15.5 per cent of the patients recovered. In panic disorder and agoraphobia, the symptoms of panic attack, anxiety, and phobic avoidance are generally intermittent and variable (Errera and Coleman 1963; Roberts 1964; Marks 1970; Breier *et al*. 1986). Several long-term outcome studies have reported substantial psychopathology in follow-up in 50 to 95 per cent of patients with panic disorder and agoraphobia, and agoraphobia with panic attacks (Wheeler *et al*. 1953; Coryell *et al*. 1983), although it has been reported that symptom-free periods may occur (Marks 1970; Burns and Thorpe 1977; Thorpe and Burns 1983).

Phenomena of discontinuation

The phenomena associated with discontinuation of anxiolytic medication may be separated into symptoms due to relapse, rebound, and withdrawal. Unfortunately, there may be considerable overlap in these symptoms with resultant uncertainty as to which category of discontinuation the symptoms appertain.

Relapse is the recurrence of the original condition from which the panic patient suffered. In panic disorder and agoraphobia the symptoms of panic attack, anxiety, and phobic avoidance are generally intermittent and variable; thus discontinuation of effective medical treatment may be followed by relapse. The same is true in the other anxiety disorders. Rickels and Schweitzer (1986) observed an anxiety recurrence rate of 65 per cent within a 12-month follow-up period and showed in two controlled double-blind studies that, over a 6-month treatment period, patients suffering from chronic anxiety did not develop tolerance to the anxiolytic effects of their benzodiazepines (Rickels *et al.* 1985). It appears that the benzodiazepines retain their anxiolytic efficacy during more chronic use. Indeed, long-term treatment may be required for selected patients with severe generalized anxiety as well as for patients with panic disorder (Sheehan *et al.* 1984) or those suffering from non-psychiatric medical disorders (Hollister *et al.* 1981). Rickels and Schweitzer (1986) described a rather chronically anxious and depressed population of 119 long-term benzodiazepine users, more than 90 per cent of whom had been given a psychiatric diagnosis. While for many of the patients benzodiazepine therapy appeared appropriate, for many others it was not. A follow-up of 62 of the patients, 6 to 12 months after study participation, indicated that 24 per cent were without medication, 37 per cent had been treated with antidepressants, and 39 per cent were still taking benzodiazepines frequently on an as-needed or low daily dosage. Nonetheless, it is evident in these long-term follow-ups that generalized anxiety, being a somewhat chronic illness, recurs after discontinuation of medication. In obsessive–compulsive disorder, there have been very few long-term studies. Recently, Pato *et al.* (1988), in a discontinuation study of clomipramine, found a recurrence rate of almost 90 per cent among patients with obsessive–compulsive symptoms after almost a year's treatment. It is clear, therefore, that in these chronic illnesses relapse will occur after the discontinuation of an effective medicine.

Rebound is relapse characterized by greater symptom intensity than that present before treatment. With hypnotic benzodiazepines rebound insomnia involves an increased time of sleep onset, more periods of wakefulness, a temporary worsening of sleep compared with the period before the hypnotic agent was first taken, and changes in rapid eye movement (REM) and slow-wave sleep (Kales *et al.* 1978, 1979). In a review of rebound insomnia and anxiety Kales *et al.* (1983) specifically suggested criteria for rebound insomnia. Lapierre (1981) noted that abrupt cessation of benzodiazepine therapy may also be followed by a rebound anxiety (Marks 1978). This was confirmed in studies comparing clobazam, a short-acting benzodiazepine, and diazepam, a longer-acting compound (Lapierre *et al.* 1982). In a single-blind 72 placebo wash-out this group noticed pronounced return of anxiety after withdrawal of medication. Rastogi *et al.* (1976) noted in a series of studies of bromazepam and diazepam the existence of a type of rebound phenomena in rats. Locomotor activity 48 h after cessation of diazepam and bromazepam was greater than the pre-treatment level. Several other investigators (Allen and Oswald 1976; Hallström and Lader 1981; Pétursson and Lader 1981*a,b*; Pecknold *et al.* 1982; Lader 1983) have noticed an increase in anxiety as rated on the Hamilton Anxiety Scale, peaking during the withdrawal of anxiolytic benzodiazepines and subsiding in generalized anxiety. Using this anxiety scale it was found that 44 per cent of such patients suffered rebound anxiety of at least 10 per cent above baseline (Fontaine *et al.* 1984).

Pecknold and Swinson (1985) presented a preliminary report of the first placebo control discontinuation study in a well-defined population with panic disorder and a final definitive report was presented by Pecknold and colleagues in 1988. Subsequent reports of discontinuation of alprazolam in panic were reported by Mellman and Uhde (1986) and Fyer *et al.* (1987). Finally, Roy-Byrne *et al.* (1989) reported on a group of 40 patients who discontinued after 7 weeks of treatment with alprazolam, diazepam, or placebo. There was no significant difference in the anxiety scores and the frequency of panic attacks among the three groups at the end of the initial 2-week taper. One week after discontinuation those patients who had been on alprazolam and diazepam had a greater increase of anxiety but no more panic attacks than occurred in the patients on placebo.

Pecknold *et al.* (1988) examined the gradual discontinuation of an effective antipanic medication (alprazolam) in a placebo-controlled study in a well-defined population with panic disorder. They found that there was a rebound of panic attacks that occurred, despite this taper schedule, in 27 per cent of the alprazolam-treated group and not at all in the placebo-treated group. The phenomenon of rebound panic did not occur at all in the placebo-treated group and could not be attributed to pseudowithdrawal. It was speculated by the authors that alprazolam blocks operant pathways to the locus ceruleus or other noradrenergic centres (Fyer *et al.* 1987) and decreases noradrenergic function (Charney and Heninger 1985). Consistent with this speculation is the finding that alprazolam, in contrast to diazepam, acts as an α-adrenergic agonist in rats (Eriksson *et al.* 1986) so that alprazolam may prevent panic by interfering with α-adrenergic mechanisms (Eriksson 1987). Animal studies have shown that benzodiazepines decrease the release of noradrenaline (Rastogi *et al.* 1976, 1978*a*) and enhance levels of serotonin (Agarwal *et al.* 1977). Deafferentation may produce receptor hypersensitivity distal to the point of blockage (Brown 1982); hence discontinuation of benzodiazepines may result in the release of noradrenaline (Rastogi *et al.* 1978*a*; Cowen and Nutt 1982). Although Pétursson *et al.* (1983) did not find evidence of noradrenergic overactivity during diazepam withdrawal, alprazolam discontinuation may increase noradrenergic activity in the locus ceruleus due to its action on α-adrenoceptors. Charney *et al.* (1987) have found that administration of yohimbine, an α-adrenergic agonist, will produce panic attacks in 50 per cent of patients with panic disorder. The yohimbine-like activity resulting from alprazolam withdrawal coupled with hypersensitive noradrenergic receptors may result in rebound panic attacks. Recently Pecknold *et al.* (1991) reported on a multicentre discontinuation study in alprazolam comparing regular alprazolam, alprazolam SR (slow release), and placebo, and found that the Los Angeles site that replicated the fast taper of the active agents essentially had a similar rebound pattern to that recorded in the 1988 report of Pecknold *et al.* The Montreal site, which had a very slow taper over a period of 19 weeks, had no rebound whatever. The Rhode Island site, which was intermediate between the two groups in terms of the length of taper, had an intermediate rebound pattern, which, however, much more closely resembled that of the Montreal site.

The *benzodiazepine withdrawal syndrome* was defined by Lader (1983) as 'the emergence of a well-defined syndrome with predictable onset, duration and offset of action containing psychological and bodily symptoms not previously complained of by patients. It can be suppressed by the reinstitution of discontinued medication.' Owen and Tyrer (1983) divided the syndrome into minor forms, including symptoms such as tremor, diaphoresis, and tachycardia, and major forms, such as seizure, abnormal perceptions or hallucinations, or delirious confusion. Mellor and Jain (1982) noted the waxing and waning of such symptoms on discontinuation of diazepam. Physical dependency was recognized as early as 1961 (Hollister *et al.* 1961; Covi *et al.* 1973) following high doses of chlorodiazepoxide therapy and has been documented and extensively reviewed (Marks 1978; Browne and Hauge 1986; Swinson *et al.* 1987). Tyrer *et al.* (1983) have shown that, despite gradual discontinuation of diazepam in controlling pseudowithdrawal symptoms, 44 per cent of patients reported a withdrawal syndrome.

Comparison of buspirone and benzodiazepine in the discontinuation of medication in patients with generalized anxiety disorder

Murphy *et al.* (1984), in a study of buspirone and diazepam, found a significant increase in symptoms of anxiety after the cessation of diazepam but not after the cessation of buspirone. Rickels *et al.* (1988) provided convincing evidence of withdrawal symptoms after long-term maintenance treatment with benzodiazepines and the lack of such a syndrome with buspirone. Pecknold *et al.* (1991) carried out a prospective placebo-controlled discontinuation study after short-term treatment with diazepam and buspirone and found a significant increase in symptoms after the cessation of diazepam but not after that of placebo or buspirone. In addition, they found that patients previously treated with benzodiazepines and later placed on buspirone did not have the same improvement as those who did not have previous benzodiazepine treatment. In fact, the buspirone group with the previous benzodiazepines performed at the level of the placebo groups. Patients on diazepam who were previously treated with benzodiazepines had a more difficult discontinuation than other groups. Thus the use of a non-benzodiazepine anxiolytic can provide a description of the difference between the rebound and withdrawal syndrome and that of relapse due to a gradual return of symptoms of anxiety.

Development of specific assessment techniques in discontinuation studies carried out with benzodiazepines

Table 10.1 shows the development of assessment techniques based on controlled trials and Table 10.2 shows the new symptoms found by most authors in benzodiazepine withdrawal. The first group to assess benzodiazepine withdrawal was Hollister *et al.* (1961) who gave chlordiazepoxide 100–600 mg daily to 36 hospitalized psychotics for periods of 1–7 months. Eleven of these patients were abruptly changed to placebo on a single-blind basis and 10 developed subjective or objective signs interpreted as those of withdrawal.

Table 10.1. Assessment techniques used in benzodiazepine discontinuation trials

Author	Year	No. of patients	Assessment technique
Hollister *et al.*	1961	11	Clinical symptoms and signs
Covi *et al.*	1972	39	Symptom check-list
Hartelius *et al.*	1978	117	Sleep questionnaire
Winokur *et al.*	1980	1	HAM-A, HAM-D, Hopkins Check-list, check-list of symptoms
Hallström and Lader	1981	10	HAM-A, withdrawal symptoms
Tyrer *et al.*	1981		Covi's symptom check-list
Petursson and Lader	1981	16	HAM-A, Digit-Symbol Substitution Test, symptom check-list
Laughren *et al.*	1982	24	HAM-A, SCL, POMS
Mellor and Jain	1982	10	Alcohol Withdrawal Rating Scale (Gross)
Pecknold *et al.*	1982	29	HAM-A, BWCL
Tyrer *et al.*	1983	41	CPRS
Harrison *et al.*	1984	16	Spielberger STAI, sleep questionnaire, withdrawal check-list, vital signs
Fontaine *et al.*	1984	16	HAM-A, Self-Rating Scale (Guy 1976), New Symptom Check-list
Busto *et al.*	1986	40	Clinical Institute Withdrawal Assessment—Benzodiazepine
Fyer *et al.*	1987	17	Symptom check-list
Pecknold *et at.*	1988	119	Panic scale, HAM-A, CGI, BWCL, Merz, SSEC

Table 10.2 New symptoms characteristic of the benzodiazepine withdrawal syndrome reported in most studies

---

Minor symptoms

Apprehension, agitation, tenseness, headache, dizziness, difficulty in concentrating, dysphoria, irritability, fatigue, depersonalization

Nausea, vomiting, abdominal cramps, anorexia, difficulty with micturition, sweating, muscle weakness, tremor, muscle pain, muscle twitching, ataxia

Hypersensitivity to light, sound, taste, and sensation; tinnitus

Major symptoms

Hyperthermia, convulsions, psychosis

The symptoms appeared mainly between day 4 and day 8 and decreased by day 10. Covi *et al.* (1973) studied abrupt discontinuation of 45 mg per day of chlordiazepoxide given to anxious neurotic patients for 20 weeks.

Wikler (1968), on the basis of barbiturate dependence studies, divided the withdrawal symptoms into minor (apprehension, muscular weakness, tremors, postural hypertension, anorexia, and muscle twitching) and major (hyperthermia, convulsions, and psychosis). This analysis of symptoms was supported by Marks (1978) in a critical analysis of 118 publications in the medical literature between 1961 and 1977 in which abstinence symptomatology was reported. Hallström and Lader (1981*a*) studied a withdrawal syndrome with drug tapering in 10 patients on benzodiazepines. The same team (Pétursson and Lader 1981*b*) studied 16 patients under placebo-controlled conditions. The symptoms included sleep disturbances and anxiety, intolerance to bright light and loud noise, unsteady gait, numbness and tingling feelings, muscular pain, loss of appetite or nausea, pressure on the face, aggressive feelings, depression, weakness, sore eyes, hallucinations, delusions and paranoid ideas, and grand mal seizure. Tyrer *et al.* (1981), in a propranolol over placebo replacement study of chronic users of benzodiazepines, employed the criteria of the presence of two or more new symptoms during withdrawal period and an increase in self-rating of symptoms during withdrawal to greater than 50 per cent of baseline levels followed by a return to lower values. As a symptom check-list, they used the symptoms noted by Covi *et al.* (1973). Forty-five per cent of patients reported two or more of the following symptoms: epileptic seizures, muscle twitching and pain, extreme dysphoria, sensory changes to touch, noise, vision, smell, depersonalization and derealization, impaired perception of movement, difficulty in focusing, retching or vomiting, persistent headache, and/or head throbbing. On the Hamilton Anxiety Scale (HAM-A) there was a slight elevation after 4 weeks off diazepam and the 58-item Symptom Check-list (SCL; Derogatis *et al.*

1974), the POMS, and the 10 items from the SCL-58. Only the HAM-A was a relatively objective measure of anxiety and appeared to be more reliable on multiple administrations than the two self-report measures.

Mellor and Jain (1982) studied 10 patients and used the alcohol withdrawal rating scale developed by Gross *et al.* (1974). They found three major groups of symptoms and signs that clustered in different parts of the withdrawal cycles. Rebound symptoms (group A) were found throughout and included a characteristic benzodiazepine withdrawal—tremor, anorexia, sweating, anxiety, agitation, insomnia, and myoclonus. Group B occurred during the first 10 days and resembled alcohol and barbiturate withdrawal symptoms, and group C included the perceptual disorders: heightened perceptions, photophobia, hyperacusis, cutaneous and ataxic sensations, as well as subjective feeling of incoordination. Tyrer *et al.* (1983) studied 41 patients using the Comprehensive Psychopathological Rating Scale (CPRS) of Asberg *et al.* (1978). In a comparison between true withdrawal and pseudowithdrawal symptoms they also used the concept of new symptoms—for example, reduced sleep, depersonalization, apparent sadness, reduced appetite, derealization, and worrying over trifles. Harrison *et al.* (1984) studied 23 patients, tapered medication, and used four assessments, including the Spielberger STAI; a sleep questionnaire; a check-list of withdrawal symptoms, which included nervousness, fatigue, tenseness, irritability, fearfulness, concentration difficulties, loss of appetite, sensory disturbance, palpitations, stomach cramps, uncontrolled thoughts, and headaches; and four objective nursing assessments that included vital signs, blood pressure, pulse, respiration, and temperature, as well as observations of sleep, appetite, tremor, agitation, sweating, nausea, and sensory disturbance.

Fontaine *et al.* (1984) studied 16 patients with abrupt discontinuation of benzodiazepines and they compared these with 13 patients on placebo. Forty-four per cent of the benzodiazepine patients had rebound anxiety on the Hamilton Anxiety Scale. They also measured the emergence of new symptoms suggestive of a withdrawal syndrome.

Assessment of withdrawal in panic disorder patients treated with alprazolam

In the evaluation of the withdrawal syndrome in panic disorder treated with alprazolam (Pecknold and Swinson 1985; Pecknold and Suranji-Cadotte 1986; Pecknold *et al.* 1988), there were no previous studies to use as a model. Many of the symptoms of discontinuation, like depersonalization, are part of the panic syndrome. We used the definition of Lader for the benzodiazepine withdrawal syndrome, that is, 'the emergence of a well-defined syndrome with predictable onset, duration, and offset of action containing psychological and bodily symptoms not previously complained of by patients. It can be suppressed by the reinstitution of the discontinued medication.' We used three scales to assess the discontinuation. These were the Symptoms and Side Effect Check-list (SSEC), the Benzodiazepine Withdrawal Check-list, (BWCL), and the patient-scored (Merz) questionnaire. The three scales were scored at baseline, during active treatment, during taper, and post-discontinuation. The SSEC is essentially a check-list used by the patient and corroborated by the physician of all the physical and bodily symptoms that can occur, whether pertinent to the withdrawal syndrome or not. The BWCL is a 19-item list of questions about symptoms, rated from 0–3 in terms of severity, which are derived from those symptoms reported by Hallström and Lader (1981) and Pétursson and Lader (1981) and revised by Pecknold *et al.* (1982). The Merz Withdrawal Scale (Merz 1982; Merz and Ballmer 1982), consists of 14 questions of withdrawal symptom rated from 0–3 and was originally derived by Merz using questions taken from the Zung Anxiety Scale and related to alcohol sedative withdrawal symptoms. In evaluating the criteria for the withdrawal syndrome, we accepted the definition of Lader and empirically identified any new symptoms from all three check-lists, BWCL, Merz, and SSEC. Although an unequivocal separation of relapse and rebound from the withdrawal syndrome is not possible, we reasoned that, if the symptom were frequent before starting treatment, then that same symptom appearing as a discontinuation emergence symptom would most probably be due to relapse or rebound. Conversely, if a discontinuation emergence symptom were not found before treatment or if it were not a symptom of panic-related disorder, then it would most probably be due to a withdrawal syndrome. We used the baseline period as well as the active treatment period to screen for any evidence of new symptoms and, if these occurred during taper or post-taper, they were considered to be part of the withdrawal syndrome.

Once indicator symptoms were identified, individual patient data were examined to identify the patients who most probably experienced withdrawal syndrome. The presence of any four indicator symptoms was selected as a criterion for separating patients in the placebo-treated group from patients in the alprazolam-treated group with a withdrawal syndrome. The indicator symptoms were confusion (patients self-report feeling confused), clouded sensorium, clinically observed disorientation in time, place, or person, heightened sensory perception, dysosmia, abnormality in taste or smell, paraesthesiae, muscle cramps, muscle twitches, blurred vision, diarrhoea, decreased appetite, and weight loss. This list cannot comprehensively describe the symptoms of the benzodiazepine withdrawal syndrome; it gives frequent symptoms that, in our study, appear to indicate withdrawal and be least obscured by the returning symptoms of panic disorder. The 11 symptoms are not unique to benzodiazepine withdrawal. In fact, in this study, 71 per cent (35 of 49) of the placebo-treated patients had at least one of these indicator symptoms at some time during taper or post-taper, 24 per cent (12 of 49) had two or more of them in a single week, 12 percent (6 of 49) had three or more in 1 week, and 2 per cent (one patient) had four of these indicator symptoms once. To minimize falsely identifying too many placebo-treated patients as suffering from benzodiazepine withdrawal symptoms, a weekly cluster of four or more of the withdrawal indicator symptoms occurring in any week were selected as the criterion for designating a patient as having the syndrome. Twenty-one alprazolam-treated patients and one placebo-treated patient met this criterion at 1 or more taper or post-taper weeks. Only the benzodiazepine-treated patients had clusters of five or more symptoms: seven patients had five symptoms; three had six symptoms; three had seven symptoms; and two had eight symptoms. The symptoms of withdrawal occurred most often during taper and the first post-taper week. No patient had detectable withdrawal symptoms during the first week of taper. The withdrawal syndrome lasted for 1 week for about half the patients and for as long as 3 weeks in three patients. In this study 21 (35 per cent) of 60 patients solely in the alprazolam-treated group experienced a detectable withdrawal syndrome. In no case was this incapacitating or life-threatening. However, we noted that, in terms of patients who had a withdrawal syndrome, a number also met criteria of simultaneous rebound, for example, those who had a minimal withdrawal syndrome (13 per cent) met rebound criteria and experienced a mean number of 4.0 indicator symptoms. Those who had a mild abstinence syndrome included 12 per cent of the alprazolam-treated group: 57 per cent of them met rebound criteria and they experienced a mean number of 5.1 indicator symptoms. The alprazolam patients experiencing a moderate withdrawal syndrome included 1C per cent of the population. One hundred per cent of those patients met rebound criteria of either panic or anxiety and experienced a mean number of 6.3 indicator symptoms. It is of interest that there is this connection between rebound and the withdrawal syndrome. Dosage at the end of an 8-week treatment period of alprazolam did not appear to be a significant factor in the withdrawal syndrome, as it ranged from 2 to 10 mg per day in the 21 patients who experienced the abstinence syndrome. Fyer *et al.* (1987) in an uncontrolled taper discontinuation of alprazolam in a panic disorder patient reported symptoms of malaise, weakness, insomnia, tachycardia, dizziness, and lightheadedness.

In a further study, we (Pecknold *et al.* 1991) reported discontinuation of alprazolam and alprazolam SR versus placebo in patients with panic disorder and agoraphobia. It was a multicentre trial and each centre used a different taper protocol. The Los Angeles site used a mean of 3 weeks to taper, the Rhode Island site used a mean of 5 weeks to taper, and the Montreal site used a mean of 18 weeks to taper. In a comparison of these three sites the same protocol for the abstinence syndrome was followed as in our earlier work. We used the SSEC, which had been modified to include all symptoms found in the BWCL and in addition used the SPRAS (Sheehan) as a further patient-rated control on emergent new symptoms. We used the same 11 indicator symptoms and found a striking difference in discontinuation at the three sites. The Montreal site had essentially no withdrawal syndrome. Two patients, one each taking alprazolam and alprazolam SR, had both elected to have a rapid taper, similar to that of the Los Angeles site. Apart from these two patients, there was no evidence of a withdrawal syndrome. The most severe withdrawal syndrome occurred in the Los Angeles site and the Rhode Island site was somewhat intermediate.

Biological markers of the withdrawal syndrome

A biological marker may be defined as a structural and/or functional sign of a relatively specific disorder. The marker may be expressed symptomatically, subclinically, or as a latent factor carried in the gene pool. As there may be aetiological or pathogenetic implications, markers may indicate the presence or potential for a disorder (Tuma and Maser 1985). There are few markers of benzodiazepine withdrawal: these include sleep laboratory evaluations, EEG abnormalities, and some neurotransmitter studies.

Sleep laboratory evaluations provide an objective means to study the effect of drug withdrawal on the pattern of sleep as well as on the specific sleep architecture changes. Oswald and Priest (1965) first documented REM sleep rebound after the withdrawal of 400 mg of sodium amylobarbitone. Kales *et al.* (1974) defined drug withdrawal insomnia as an intense sleep disturbance associated with REM rebound upon abrupt withdrawal of large doses of non-benzodiazepine hypnotics for protracted periods. This was extended (Kales *et al.* 1978) to identify a sleep rebound insomnia syndrome following abrupt withdrawal of benzodiazepines with short and intermediate elimination half-lives. Kales *et al.* (1983) extensively reviewed their own studies and those of other sleep laboratories and redefined the criteria for rebound insomnia, i.e. 'a statistically significant increase as an increase of 40% or greater in the mean group value for total wake time for a single withdrawal night or the entire withdrawal condition as compared to baseline'. In the same review they observed that only benzodiazepines with long elimination half-lives (flurazepam and quazepam) do not produce an appreciable worsening of sleep following abrupt withdrawal. They presented findings from studies by multiple authors demonstrating rebound insomnia in a number of short to intermediate half-life benzodiazepines. Non-benzodiazepine hypnotics may perform differently. In one study of zopiclone (Pecknold *et al.* 1986), a short-acting cyclopyrrolone, we found no evidence of rebound (sleep or REM) in abrupt discontinuation after 2 months of administration.

Neurotransmitter changes on benzodiazepine withdrawal

Rastogi *et al.* (1976) first evaluated brain monoamine changes in rats following abrupt benzodiazepine withdrawal and attempted to explain the evidence of 'rebound' as a parallel phenomenon in human subjects. In chronically diazepam-treated rats, discontinuation of the drug produced significantly elevated synaptosomal catecholamine synthesis above the values of treated as well as of normal control animals. Despite increased synthesis, the synaptosomal levels of noradrenaline and dopamine in withdrawn groups were decreased. This appeared to be due to compensatory release of these monoamines as well as to altered re-uptake of noradrenaline which was diminished by 24 per cent. The levels of HVA (homovanillic acid) and MHPG (3-methoxy, 4-hydroxy phenylglycol) increased by more than 190 per ent. Further studies by this group (Agarwal *et al.* 1977; Rastogi *et al.* 1978*a*) documented serotonin (5-HT) changes as well. The rate of synthesis of 5-HT and the level in synaptosomes decreased. They suggested that enhanced release and decreased re-uptake of catecholomines and 5-HT were responsible for the hyperexcitability noted during rebound. Rastogi *et al.* (1978*b*) also noted rebound excretion of MOPEG; this finding was not confirmed by Pétursson *et al.* (1983) who noted that, upon discontinuation of benzodiazepines in human chronic users, a characteristic withdrawal reaction recurred with an increase toward normal values of the MOPEG excretion levels and increased excretion during withdrawal of 5-HIAA (5-hydroxyindoleacetic acid). They noted no change in 24-h urine cortisol or HMMA (3-methoxy-hydroxy-mandelic acid—another measure of noradrenaline catabolism). Thus Pétursson *et al.* (1983) confirmed withdrawal data in human chronic benzodiazepine users concordant with animal withdrawal data. The increase in 5-HIAA and the gradual and prolonged increase of MOPEG may represent neurochemical changes—peripheral but possibly also central—associated with a benzodiazepine withdrawal. Nutt and Molyneux (1987) confirmed an increase in MHPG during benzodiazepine withdrawal.

Hallström and Lader (1981) evaluated the EEG and evoked auditory responses during benzodiazepine withdrawal of patients abruptly discontinued from both high and low doses of diazepam. They noted a decrease in the proportion of fast-wave activity (13.5–26 Hz). The mean decrease for all patients was significantly different from the baseline measure between days 5 and 15 after discontinuation. The amplitude of the auditory evoked response increased by an average of 89 per cent during the withdrawal phase and was significant 10–15 days after discontinuation. These results were replicated by Pétursson and Lader (1981).

Comment

In this chapter on the assessment of anxiety and benzodiazepine dependence, I have attempted to review some of the salient and voluminous literature on the difference between normal and pathological anxiety, measurement of anxiety and the benzodiazepine withdrawal syndrome, and related aspects of the phenomena of discontinuation. Finally, I made a brief mention of the biological markers that have been used to assess discontinuation.

The discontinuation of benzodiazepines varies considerably from cases of

156   The assessment of anxiety and benzodiazepine dependence

use by chronic drug abusers to those of patients on short- and long-term medical prescription. The pattern of withdrawal appears to differ in patients with panic disorder. In the medically treated patient it may be difficult to differentiate relapse from the rebound and withdrawal syndrome. The comparison with a non-benzodiazepine anxiolytic such as buspirone is clinically instructive.

The use of biological markers or probes is of considerable interest in elucidating neurochemical or physiological events in the brain that are precipitated by the discontinuation syndrome and are revealing of the mechanism of action of these drugs.

A final comment must be made about discontinuation. There is evidence in some of the studies reviewed that taper reduces discontinuation symptomatology considerably and thus alleviates some of the clinical fears of dependency on benzodiazepines.

References

Agarwal, R.A., Lapierre, Y.D., Rastogi, R.B., and Sinhal, R.L. (1977). Alternatives in brain 5-hydroxytyptamine metabolism during the 'withdrawal' phase after chronic treatment with diazepam and bromazepam. *British Journal of Psychopharmacology*, **60**, 3–9.

Allen, S. and Oswald, I. (1976). Anxiety and sleep after fosazepam. *British Journal of Psychopharmacology*, **3**, 165–8.

APA (American Psychiatric Association) (1980). *Diagnostic and statistical manual of mental disorders* (3rd. edn). American Psychiatric Press, Washington, DC.

Anderson, D.J., Noyes, R., Jr, and Crowe, R.R. (1984). A comparison of panic disorder and generalized anxiety disorder. *American Journal of Psychiatry*, **141**, 572–5.

Asberg, M., Montgomery, S.A., Perris, C., Schalling, D., and Sedvall, G. (1978). A comprehensive psychopathological rating scale. *Acta Psychiatrica Scandinavica*, **271**, (Suppl.) 5–27.

Barlow, D.H., diNardo, P.A., Vermilyea, B.B., Vermilyea, J., and Blanchard, E.B. (1986). Co-morbidity and depression among the anxiety disorders: issues in diagnosis and classification. *Journal of Nervous and Mental Disorders*, **17**, 63–72.

Berner, P. and Walter, H. (1986). Diagnostic issues in neurotic disorders. In *Drug treatment of neurotic disorders* (ed. M.H. Lader and H.C. Davies), pp.61–79. Churchill Livingstone, Edinburgh.

Borkovec, T.D., Werts, T.C., and Bernstein, D.A. (1977). Assessment of anxiety. In *Handbook of behavioral assessment* (ed. A. Ciminero, K.Calhoun, and H. Adams), pp.367–428. Wiley, New York.

Bowby, J. (1973). *Separation: anxiety and anger*. Basic Books, New York.

Boyd, J., Burke, J., Gruenberg, E., Holzer, C.E., Ray, D.S., George, L.K., *et al.* (1984). Exclusion criteria of DSM-III. *Archives of General Psychiatry*, **41**, 983.

Breier, A., Charney, D.S., and Heninger, G.R. (1986). Agoraphobia with panic attacks: development diagnostic stability and course of illness. *Archives of General Psychiatry*, **43**, 1029–36.

Brown, I.R. (1982). *Molecular approaches to neurobiology*. Academic Press Inc, Orlando, Florida.

browneowne, J.L. and Hauge, K.J. (1986). A review of alprazolam withdrawal. *Drug Intelligence and Clinical Pharmacy*, **20**, 837–40.

Burns, L.E. and Thorpe, G.L. (1977). The epidemiology of fears and phobias. *Journal of International Medical Research*, **5**, 1–7.

Busto, U., Sellers, E.M., Naranjo, C.A., Cappell, H., Sancez-Craig, M., and Sykora, K. (1986). Withdrawal reaction after long-term therapeutic use of benzodiazepines. *New England Journal of Medicine*, **315**, 854–9.

Campbell, S.B. (1986). Developmental issues in childhood anxiety. In *Anxiety disorders of childhood* (ed. R. Gittleman), pp.24–57. Guilford Press, New York.

Cattell, R.B. and Scheier, I.H. (1957). *Handbook for the IPAT Anxiety Scale*. Institute for Personality and Ability Testing, Champaign, Illinois.

Charney, D.S. and Heninger, G.R. (1985). Noradrenergic function and the mechanism of action of antianxiety treatment. *Archives of General Psychiatry*, **42**, 473–81.

Charney, D.S., Woods, S.M., Goodman, W.K., and Heninger, G.R. (1987). Neurobiological mechanisms of panic anxiety: biochemical and behavioral correlates of yohimbine-induced panic attacks. *American Journal of Psychiatry*, **144**, 1030–6.

Coryell, W., Noyes, R., and Clancy, J. (1983). Panic disorder and primary unipolar depression: an outcome. *Journal of Affective Disorders*, **5**, 311–17.

Covi, L., Lipman, R.S., Pattison, J.H., Derogatis, L.R., and Uhlenhuth, E.H. (1973). Length of treatment with anxiolytic sedatives and response to their sudden withdrawal. *Acta Psychiatrica Scandinavica*, **49**, 51–64.

Cowen, P.J. and Nutt, D.J. (1982). Abstinence symptoms after withdrawal of tranquilizing drugs: is there a common neurochemical mechanism? *Lancet*, **ii**, 360–2.

Cullen, W. (1787). *First lines in the practice of physic*, 4 volumes, Elliot, Edinburgh.

Derogatis, L.R., Lipman, R.S., Riebels, K., Uhlenhuth, E.H., and Covi, L. (1974). The Hopkins Symptom Checklist (HSCL): a self-report system inventory. *Behavioral Science*, **19**, 1–5.

diNardo, P.A., O'Brien, G.T., Barlow, D.H., Waddell, M.T., and Blanchard, E.B. (1983). Reliability of DSM-III anxiety disorder categories using a new structured interview. *Archives of General Psychiatry*, **40**, 1070–4.

Endicott, J. and Spitzer, R.L. (1978). A diagnostic interview: the Schedule for Affective Disorders and Schizophrenia. *Archives of General Psychiatry*, **35**, 837–44.

Eriksson, E. (1987). Brain neurotransmission in panic disorder. *Acta Psychiatrica Scandinavica*, **76** (suppl. 335), 31–7.

Eriksson, E., Carlsson, H., Nisson, C., and Soderpach, B. (1986). Does alprazolam in contrast to diazepam, activate alpha-2-adrenoceptors involved in the regulation of rat growth hormone secretion? *Life Sciences*, **38**, 1491–8.

Errera, P. and Coleman, J.V. (1963). A long-term follow-up study of a phobic anxiety state. *Journal of Nervous and Mental Disorders*, **136**, 267–71.

Finney, V.C. (1985). Anxiety: its measurement by objective personality tests and self-report. In *Anxiety and the anxiety disorders* (ed. A.H. Tuma and J.D. Maser), pp.645–73. Lawrence Erlbaum Assoc. Inc, Hilldale, New Jersey.

Fontaine, R. Chouinard, G., and Annable, L. (1984). Rebound anxiety in anxious patients after abrupt withdrawal of benzodiazepine treatment. *American Journal of Psychiatry*, **141**, 848–52.

Fyer, A.J., Liebowitz, M.R., Gorman, J.M., Compeas, R., Levin, A., Davies, S., Goetz, D., and Klein, D. (1987). Discontinuation of alprazolam treatment in panic patients. *American Journal of Psychiatry*, **144**, 303–8.

Goldberg, D. and Simpson, N. (1985). The diagnosis of anxiety in primary care settings. In *Drug treatment of neurotic disorders: focus on alprazolam* (ed. M.H. Lader and H.C. Davies). Churchill Livingstone, Edinburgh.

Gross, M.M., Lewis, E., and Hastey, J. (1974). Acute alcohol withdrawal syndrome. In *Biology of alcoholism*, Vol. 3. *Clinical Pathology* (ed. B. Kissin and H. Begleiter), pp.191–263. Plenum, New York.

Guy, W. (1976). *ECDELI assessment manual for psychopharmacology*, (revised), Biometric Laboratory, The George Washington University, Kensington. US Department of Health, Education, and Welfare, Washington, DC.

Hallström, C. and Lader, M.H. (1981). Benzodiazepine withdrawal phenomena. *International Pharmacopsychiatry*, **16**, 235–44.

Hamilton, M. (1959). The assessment of anxiety states by rating. *British Journal of Medical Psychology*, **32**, 50–5.

Harrison, M., Busto, U., Naranjo, C.A., Kaplan, H.L., and Sellers, E.M. (1984). Diazepam tapering in detoxification for high-dose benzodiazepine abuse. *Clinical Pharmacology and Therapeutics*, **36**, 527–33.

Hartelius, H., Larsson, A.K., Lepp, M., Malm, U., Arvidsson, A., and Dahlstrom, H. (1978). A controlled long-term study of flunitrazepam, nitrazepam, and placebo, with special regard to withdrawal effects. *Acta Psychiatrica Scandinavica*, **58**, 1–15.

Hollister, L.E., Motzenbecker, F.P., and Degan, R.O. (1961). Withdrawal reactions from chlordiazepoxide (Librium). *Psychopharmacologia*, **2**, 63–8.

Hollister, L.E., Conley, F.K., Britt, R.H., and Suer, L. (1981). Long-term use of diazepam. *Journal of the American Medical Association*, **246**, 1568–70.

Kales, A., Bixler, E.O., Tou, T.L., Scarf, M.B., and Kales, J.D. (1974). Chronic hypnotic-drug use: ineffectiveness, drug-withdrawal insomnia, and dependence. *Journal of the American Medical Association*, **227**, 513–17.

Kales, A., Scharf, M.B., and Kales, J.D. (1978). Rebound insomnia: a new clinical syndrome. *Science*, **201**, 1039–41.

Kales, A., Scharf, M.B., Kales, J.D., and Soldatos, C.R. (1979). Rebound insomnia : A potential hazard following withdrawal of certain benzodiazepines. *Journal of the American Medical Association*, **241**, 1692–5.

Kales, A., Soldatos, C.R., Bixler, E.O., and Kales, J.D. (1983). Rebound insomnia and rebound anxiety : a review. *Pharmacology*, **26**, 121–37.

Klerman, G.L. (1986). Historical perspectives on contemporary schools of psychotherapy. In *Contemporary directions in psychopathology: towards the DSM-IV* (ed. T. Millon and G.L. Klerman), pp.3–28. Guilford Press, New York.

Klerman, G.L. (1990). Historical perspectives of modern concepts of anxiety and panic. In *Clinical aspects of panic disorder* (ed. J.C. Ballenger), pp.3–12. Wiley-Liss Inc, New York.

Kraepelin, E. (1896). *Psychiatrie*, (5th edn). Barth, Leipzig.

Lader, M. (1983). Benzodiazepine withdrawal states. In *Benzodiazepines divided* (ed. M.R. Trimble), pp.17–31. John Wiley, New York.

Lang, P.J. (1971). The application of psychophysiological methods to the study of psychotherapy and behaviour modification. In *Handbook of psychotherapy and behavior* (ed. A.E. Bergin and S.L. Garfield). John Wiley, New York.

Lapierre, Y.D. (1981). Benzodiazepine withdrawal. *Canadian Journal of Psychiatry*, **26**, 93–5.

Lapierre, Y.D., Tremblay, A., Gagnon, A., Montpremier, P., Berliss, H., and Oyewumi, L.K. (1982). A therapeutic and discontinuation study of clobazam and diazepam in anxiety neurosis. *Journal of Clinical Psychiatry*, **43**, 372–4.

Laughren, T.P., Bailey, Y., and Greenblatt, D.J. (1982). A controlled trial of diazepam withdrawal in chronically anxious outpatients. *Acta Psychiatrica Scandinavica*, **65**, 171–9.

Lipman, R.S. (1982). Differentiating anxiety and depression in anxiety disorders : use of rating scales. *Psychopharmacology Bulletin*, **18**, 69.

Marks, I.M. (1969). *Fears and phobias*. Academic Press, New York.

Marks, I.M. (1970). Agoraphobic syndrome (phobic anxiety state). *Archives of General Psychiatry*, **23**, 538–53.

Marks, J. (1978). The benzodiazepines : use, overuse, misuse, abuse. MTP Press Ltd, Lancaster, England.

Mellman, T.A. and Udhe, T.W. (1986). Withdrawal syndrome with gradual tapering of alprazolam. *American Journal of Psychiatry*, **143**, 1464–6.

Mellor, C.S. and Jain, V.K. (1982). Diazepam withdrawal syndrome : its prolonged and changing nature. *Canadian Medical Association Journal*, **127**, 1093–6.

Merz, W.A. (1982). Standardized assessment of the symptoms of the benzodiazepine withdrawal syndrome prior to, during and after treatment of anxiety with a benzodiazepine by means of a novel self-rating scale, abstracted. Abstracts of the Scientific Proceedings of the 13th Collegium Internationale Neuropsychopharmacologium Congress, Jerusalem, 20–5 June 1982.

Merz, W.A. and Ballmer, V. (1982). Symptoms of the barbiturate/benzodiazepine withdrawal syndrome in healthy volunteers, abstracted. Abstracts of the Scientific Proceedings of the 13th Collegium Internationale Neuropsychopharmacologium Congress, Jerusalem, 20–5 June 1982.

Murphy, S.M., Owen, R.T., and Tyrer, P.J. (1984). Withdrawal symptoms after 6 weeks treatment with diazepam. *Lancet*, **i**, 389.

Nutt, D.J. and Molyneux, S.G. (1987). Benzodiazepines, plasma MHPG and alpha-adrenoceptor function in man. *Institute of Clinical Psychopharmacology*, **2**, 151–7.

Oswald, I. and Priest, R.G. (1965). Five weeks to escape the sleeping-pill habit. *British Journal of Medicine*, **ii**, 1093–5.

Owen, R.T. and Tyrer, P. (1983). Benzodiazepine dependence : a review of the evidence. *Drugs*, **25**, 385–98.

Pato, M.T., Zohar-Kadouch, R., Zohar, J., and Murphy, D.L. (1988). Return of symptoms after discontinuation of clomipramine in patients with obsessive–compulsive disorder. *American Journal of Psychiatry*, **145**, 1521–5.

Pecknold, J.C. and Swinson, R.P. (1985). Taper withdrawal studies in patients with panic disorder and agoraphobia. Presented at the NCDEU meeting, Key Biscayne, May 1985.

Pecknold, J.C., McClure, D.J., Fleuri, D., and Chang, H. (1982). Benzodiazepine withdrawal effects. *Progress in Neuro-psychopharmacology and Biological Psychiatry*, **6**, 517–22.

Pecknold, J.C., Swinson, R.P., Kuch, K., and Lewis, C.P. (1988). Alprazolam in panic disorder and agoraphobia : results from a multicenter trial. III. Discontinuation effects. *Archives of General Psychiatry*, **45**, 429–36.

Pecknold, J.C., Munjack, D., Alexander, P., and Luthe, L. (1991). Alprazolam and alprazolam SR in panic disorder: three patterns of discontinuation. Presented at the NCDEU Meeting, Key Biscayne, Florida, 28–31 May 1991.

Pétursson, H. and Lader, M.H. (1981*a*). Benzodiazepine dependence. *British Journal of Addiction*, **76**, 143–5.

Pétursson, H. and Lader, M.H. (1981*b*). Withdrawal from long-term benzodiazepine treatment. *British Medical Journal*, **283**, 643–5.

Pétursson, H., Bond, P.A., Smith, B., and Lader, M.H. (1983). Monoamine metabolism during chronic benzodiazepine treatment and withdrawal. *Biological Psychiatry*, **18**, 207–13.

Rachman, S. and Hodgson, R.J. (1974). Synchrony and desynchrony in fear and avoidance. *Behavioral Research and Therapy*, **12**, 311–18.

Raskin, M., Peeke, H.V.S., Dickman, W., and Pinsker, H. (1982). Panic and generalized anxiety disorders: Developmental antecedents and precipitants. *Archives of General Psychiatry*, **39**, 687.

Rastogi, R.B., Lapierre, Y.D., and Singhal, R.L. (1976). Evidence for the role of norepinephrine and dopamine in rebound phenomenon seen during withdrawal after repeated exposure to benzodiazepines. *Journal of Psychiatric Research*, **13**, 65–75.

Rastogi, R.B., Lapierre, Y.D., and Singhal, R.L. (1978a). Synaptosomal uptake of norepinephrine and 5-hydroxytopamine and synthesis of catacholamines during benzodiazepine treatment. *Canadian Journal of Physical Pharmacology*, **56**, 777–84.

Rastogi, R.B., Lapierre, Y.D., and Singhal, R.L. (1978b). Some neurochemical correlates of 'rebound' phenomena observed during withdrawal after long-term exposure to 1, 4-benzodiazepines. *Progress in Neuropsychopharmacology*, **2**, 43–54.

Rickels, K. and Schweitzer, E.E. (1986). Benzodiazepines for the treatment of panic attacks: a new look. *Psychopharmacology Bulletin*, **22**, 93–9.

Rickels, K., Schweitzer, E., Csanalosi, I., Case, W.G., and Chung, H. (1988). Long-term treatment of anxiety and risk of withdrawal. Prospective comparison of clorazepate and buspirone. *Archives of General Psychiatry*, **45**, 444–50.

Roberts, A.H. (1964). Housebound housewives : a follow-up study of a phobic anxiety state. *British Journal of Psychiatry*, **110**, 191–7.

Robins, I.N., Helzer, J.E., Croughan, J., and Ratcliff, R.S. (1981). National Institute of Mental Health Diagnostic Interview Schedule. *Archives of General Psychiatry*, **38**, 381–9.

Roy-Byrne, P.P., Dager, S.R., Cowley, D.S., Vitaliano, P., and Dunner, D. (1989). Relapse and rebound following discontinuation of benzodiazepine treatment of panic attacks : alprazolam versus diazepam. *American Journal of Psychiatry*, **146**, 860–5.

Sheehan, D.V., Coleman, J.H., Greenblatt, D.J., Sheehan, D.V., Coleman, J.H., Greenblatt, D.J., et al. (1984). Some biochemical correlates of panic attacks with agoraphobia and their response to a new treatment. *Journal of Clinical Psychopharmacology*, **4**, 66–75.

Spitzer, R.L. and Williams, B.W. (1982). Structured clinical interview for DSM-III. Biometric Research Department, New York State Psychiatric Institute, New York.

Suomi, S.J. (1986). Anxiety-like disorders in young nonhuman primates. In *Anxiety disorders of childhood* (ed. R. Gittleman), pp.1–23. Guilford Press, New York.

Swinson, R.P., Pecknold, J.C., and Kirby, M.E. (1987). Benzodiazepine dependence. *Journal of Affective Disorders*, **13**, 109–18.

Thorpe, G.L. and Burns, L.E. (1983). *The agoraphobic syndrome*. John Wiley, New York.

Thyer, B.E., Parrish, R.T., Curtis, G.C., et al. (1985). Ages of onset of DSM-III anxiety disorder. *Comprehensive Psychiatry*, **26**, 113–22.

Tuma, A.H. and Maser J.P. (ed.) (1985). Introduction. In *Anxiety and the anxiety disorders*, p.1. Lawrence Erlbaum Assoc. Inc, Hilldale, New Jersey.

Tyrer, P., Rutherford, D.M., and Huggett, T. (1981). Benzodiazepine withdrawal symptoms and propanolol. *Lancet*, **i**, 520–2.

Tyrer, P., Owen, R., and Dawling, S. (1983). Gradual withdrawal of diazepam after long-term therapy. *Lancet*, **i**, 1402–6.

Uhlenhuth, E.H. (1985). The measurement of anxiety : reply to Finney. In *Anxiety and the anxiety disorders* (ed. A.H. Tuma and J.D. Maser), pp.675–9. Lawrence Erlbaum Assoc. Inc, Hillside, New Jersey.

Wheeler, E.O., White, P.D., Reed, E.W., and Cohen, M.E. (1953). Neurocirculatory asthenia: a 20 year follow-up study of 173 patients. *Journal of the American Medical Association*, **142**, 878–89.

Wikler, A. (1968). *American Journal of Psychiatry*, **125**, 758.

Winokur, A., Rickels, R., Greenblatt, D.J., Snyder, P.J., and Schatz, N.J. (1980). Withdrawal reaction from long-term low dosage administration of diazepam. A double-blind placebo controlled case study. *Archives of General Psychiatry* **37**(1), 101–5.

Zung, W.W.K. (1971). A rating instrument for anxiety disorders. *Psychosomatics*, **12**, 371–9.

11 The epidemiology of neurosis and benzodiazepine use and abuse

Hans-Ulrich Wittchen and Cecilia Ahmoi Essau

Traditionally, epidemiology is defined as the field of research that estimates the frequency of a disorder and studies its distribution in various populations (Lilienfeld and Lilienfeld 1980). The scope of epidemiology, however, is much wider and includes: (1) establishing the dimensions of morbidity and mortality; (2) quantifying the risks of developing a disorder; (3) identifying and defining syndromes; (4) describing the natural history of disorders; (5) identifying factors that influence or predict clinical course; (6) searching for causes of disorders and related disability; and (7) evaluating specific methods of disease prevention and control (Morris 1975; von Korff and Eaton 1989). During the last decade, a considerable progress has been achieved in all these areas, strongly influenced by three major developments: (1) greater specificity of diagnoses for the so-called neurotic disorders and substance use disorders (i.e. DSM-III-R; American Psychiatric Association 1987); (2) the development of reliable diagnostic assessment instruments such as the Diagnostic Interview Schedule (DIS; Robins *et al.* 1982) and the Composite International Diagnostic Interview (CIDI; WHO 1990; Wittchen *et al.* 1991*a*); (3) the use of complex research designs (Regier *et al.* 1984). Consequently, there is now remarkable consistency in the prevalence of mental disorders especially that of 'neurotic' and substance use disorders. In this chapter we will briefly review recent epidemiological studies on the prevalence of neurotic and substance use (e.g. benzodiazepine) disorders.

Definitions of 'neurotic' and substance use disorders

One difficulty in reviewing epidemiological findings is the many conceptual changes in the definition of specific mental disorders. Since DSM-III (*Diagnostic and statistical manual of mental disorders*; APA 1980) burst on the world in 1980 there has been a tremendous change in the traditional grouping and definition of what were previously called neurotic or substance use disorders. One general trend, as reflected in Table 11.1, is the more detailed subgrouping of ICD-9 disorders in DSM-III, DSM-III-R (APA 1987), and also in ICD-10 (WHO 1991). This is particularly evident for anxiety and affective disorders. What was called depressive neurosis will fall in a yet

Table 11.1. Classification of neurotic disorders according to ICD-10, DSM-III-R, and ICD-9

	ICD-10	DSM-III-R*	ICD-9
Diagnoses			
F13	*Disorders resulting from use of sedatives or hypnotics*	Dependence on sedative, hypnotic, or anxiolytic	304.1 Dependence on barbiturates
		Abuse of sedative, hypnotic, or anxiolytic	305.4 Abuse of barbiturates and tranquillizers
F13.0	Acute intoxication		
F13.1	Harmful use		
F13.2	Dependence syndrome		
F13.3	Withdrawal states		
F13.4–9	Other psychopathology		
F34	*Persistent affective disorder*		
F34.1	Dysthymia	Dysthymic disorder	300.4 Depressive neurosis
F34.8	Other	†	
F34.9	Not specified	†	
		Depressive disorder NOS	
F40	*Phobic disorders*		
F40.0	Agoraphobia	Agoraphobia without history of panic disorder	300.2 Phobia
F40.1	Social phobia	Social phobia	
F40.2	Specific (isolated) phobia	Simple phobia	
F40.8	Other		
F40.9	Not specified		

Diagnoses cont.

	ICD-10	DSM-III-R*	ICD-9	
F45	*Somatoform disorders*	Somatoform disorders		
F45.0	Somatization	Somatization disorder		
F45.1	Undifferentiated somatoform disorder	Undifferentiated somatoform disorder		
F45.2	Hypochondrical disorder	Hypochondriasis	300.7	Hypochondriacal neurosis
F45.3	Somatoform autonomic dysfunction	No equivalent	300.6	Physiological malfunction arising from mental factors
F45.4	Persistent pain disorder	Somatoform pain disorder		
F45.8	Other	Somatoform disorder NOS		
		Body dysmorphic disorder		
		Conversion disorder		
F46	*Other neurotic disorders* (e.g.neurasthenia, depersonalization– derealization syndrome)			

Table 11.1. cont.

	ICD-10	DSM-III-R*	ICD-9
F41	*Other anxiety disorders*		
F41.0	Panic disorder (episodic paroxysmal anxiety)	Panic disorder with or without agoraphobia	
F41.1	Generalized anxiety disorder	Generalized anxiety disorder	300.0 Anxiety neurosis
F41.2	Mixed anxiety and depressive disorder		
F41.3	Other mixed anxiety disorders		
F41.8	Other	Anxiety disorders NOS	
F41.9	Not specified	Anxiety disorders NOS	
F42	*Obsessive–compulsive disorder*	Obsessive–compulsive disorder	300.3 Obsessive–compulsive neurosis
F42.0	Predominantly obsessional thoughts or ruminations		
F42.1	Predominantly compulsive acts (obsessional rituals)		
F42.2	Mixed obsessional thoughts and acts		
F42.8	Other		
F42.9	Not specified		
F44	*Dissociative (conversion) disorders*	Dissociative disorders	300.1 Hysterical neurosis

Table 11.1. cont.

ICD-10	DSM-III-R*	ICD-9
Diagnostic instruments for assessing ICD-10, DSM-III-R, and ICD-9 disorders		
Schedules for Clincial Assessment in Neuropsychiatry (SCAN)	Schedules for Clinical Assessment in Neuropsychiatry (SCAN)	Present State Examination (PSE)
Composite International Diagnostic Instrument (CIDI)	Composite International Diagnostic Instrument (CIDI)	Standardized Psychiatric Examination Intercalated Interview (SPE)
	Diagnostic Interview Schedule (DIS)	Schedule for a Standardized Assessment of Depressive Disorders (SADD)
	Schedule for Affective Disorders and Schizophrenia—Lifetime version (SADS-L)	
	Structured Clinical Interview for DSM-III-R (SCID)	
	Anxiety Disorders Interview Schedule (ADIS)	
	Psychiatric Diagnostic Interview (PDI)	
	Structured Psychopathological Interview and Rating of the Social Consequences for Epidemiology (SPIKE)	

* NOS, Not otherwise specified   † Classified under depressive disorder NOS.

unclear manner into dysthymic disorder, major depressive episode without melancholic or psychotic features, and other subtypes. For anxiety disorders, specific criteria are now used for disorders where phobic avoidance is the main focus, as is the case for simple phobia, social phobia, and agoraphobia, and disorders with a predominance of autonomic symptoms such as panic disorder, generalized anxiety disorder, and less clearly defined mixed groups. Another major innovation is the concept of multiple diagnoses both on current as well as lifetime criteria. Whereas before 1980, we were more likely to subsume all clinical phenomena under one principal diagnosis such as neurosis, DSM-III-R and ICD-10 give more emphasis to multiple diagnoses in the same case (i.e. comorbidity).

With regard to substance use disorders—unlike the ICD-9—specific and rather strict diagnostic criteria have been proposed for each substance class in the new classification systems. Whereas there were no clearly defined criteria for abuse and dependence in ICD-9 where abuse and dependence were clinically frequently diagnosed on the basis of the amount of substance used, DSM-III-R (and ICD-10) have proposed a set of criteria that sometimes conflict with our clinical concepts. For example, the diagnostic criteria for benzodiazepine abuse in DSM-III-R require that not more than two phenomena be fulfilled in a defined time frame, of which at least one is a potentially harmful use or continued use of the substance in spite of clear negative social, physical consequences or health problems that are caused or exacerberated by its use (Table 11.2). The latter criteria may lead to some discrepancies with our clinical judgement because we are frequently prone to diagnose benzodiazepine abuse due to the development of tolerance and withdrawal symptoms.

All these changes have made it increasingly difficult to interpret and compare prevalence findings across epidemiological studies because there is no perfect match between diagnoses used in different diagnostic systems. But it also seems important to mention the fact that the advent of operational diagnoses have led to the development of diagnostic instruments that have produced remarkably consistent findings on the prevalence of mental disorders.

Prevalence of neurotic disorders

Prevalence of anxiety disorders

Recent epidemiological studies—using the DIS which generated DSM-III diagnoses—conducted in the USA (Epidemiological Catchment Area (ECA): Myers *et al.* 1984; Robins *et al.* 1984; Burnam *et al.* 1987; Karno *et al.* 1987; Regier *et al.* 1988; 1990a; Robins *et al.* 1984), Canada (Edmonton study: Bland *et al.* 1988a,b), Puerto Rico (Canino *et al.* 1987), Germany (Munich Follow-up Study (MFS): Wittchen 1988; Wittchen *et al.* 1991b, 1992), Taiwan (Hwu *et al.* 1989), Korea (Lee *et al.* 1990), and New Zealand (Wells *et al.* 1989)

Table 11.2. DSM-III-R diagnostic criteria for psychoactive substance abuse and dependence

DSM-III-R diagnostic criteria for psychoactive substance dependence

A. At least three of the following:

(1) substance often taken in larger amounts or over a longer period than the person intended;

(2) persistent desire or one or more unsuccessful efforts to cut down or control substance use;

(3) a great deal of time spent in activities necessary to get the substance (e.g. theft), taking the substance (e.g. chain smoking), or recovering from its effects;

(4) frequent intoxication or withdrawal symptoms when expected to fulfil major role obligations at work, school, or home (e.g. does not go to work because hung over, goes to school or work high, intoxicated while taking care of his or her children), or when substance use is physically hazardous (e.g. drives when intoxicated);

(5) important social, occupational or recreational activities given up or reduced because of substance use;

(6) continued substance use despite knowledge of having a persistent or recurrent social, psychological, or physical problem that is caused or exacerberated by the use of the substance (e.g. keeps using heroin despite family arguments about it, cocaine-induced depression, or having an ulcer made worse by drinking);

(7) marked tolerance: need for markedly increased amounts of the substance (i.e. at least a 50% increase) in order to achieve intoxication or desired effect, or markedly diminished effect with continued use of the same amount

Note: The following items may not apply to cannabis, hallucinogens, or phencyclidine (PCP):

(8) characteristic withdrawal symptoms (see specific withdrawal syndromes under Psychoactive substance-induced organic mental disorders);

(9) substance often taken to receive or avoid withdrawal symptoms.

B. Some symptoms of the disturbance have persisted for at least 1 month, or have occurred repeatedly over a longer period of time.

Table 11.2. cont.

DSM-III-R diagnostic criteria for psychoactive substance abuse

A. A maladaptive pattern of psychoactive substance use indicated by at least one of the following:

(1) continued use despite knowledge of having a persistent or recurrent social, occupational, psychological, or physical problem that is caused or exacerbated by use of the psychoactive substance;

(2) recurrent use in situations in which use is physically hazardous (e.g. driving while intoxicated).

B. Some symptoms of the disturbance have persisted for at least 1 month, or have occurred repeatedly over a longer period of time.

C. Never met the criteria for psychoactive substance dependence on this substance.

---

have shown phobias as the most common anxiety disorder, with lifetime prevalences of about 10 per cent and a 6-month prevalence of about 5 per cent (Table 11.3). The most frequent subtypes of phobic disorders are simple phobia (range 5.4–8.6 per cent), followed by agoraphobia (range 2.9–6.9 per cent). Social phobia (range 0.5–3.1 per cent), as well as obsessive–compulsive (range 1.9–3.2 per cent) and panic disorders (range 1–2.4 per cent) are less frequent, with lifetime prevalences of about 2 per cent. Although panic disorder is rare, panic attacks are relatively common, with a 6-month prevalence of about 3 per cent and a lifetime rate of about 9 per cent (range 7.6–11.6 per cent) (von Korff *et al.* 1983; Wittchen 1986; Weissman 1990).

Epidemiological data on anxiety disorders based on the older *Research Diagnostic Criteria* (RDC) or other clinical instruments (e.g. SADS, SPIKE for DSM-III) are available from three community studies. In the New Haven survey (Weissman and Myers 1980), the current prevalence for generalized anxiety was 2.5 per cent, 1.4 per cent for phobic disorder, and 0.4 per cent for panic disorder. Using data from the National Survey of Psychotherapeutic Drug Use, Uhlenhuth *et al.* (1983) reported that the 1-year prevalence of the agoraphobia-panic and 'other phobic' syndromes were 1.2 and 2.3 per cent, respectively. The rate for generalized anxiety was 6.4 per cent. In the Zurich Study (Angst and Dobler-Mikola 1985), the 1-year rates of various anxiety syndromes were: general anxiety, 5.2 per cent; panic, 3.1 per cent; simple phobia, 3.7 per cent; social phobia, 1.1 per cent; and agoraphobia, 2.5 per cent.

Based on the *Present State Examination* (PSE) aiming at a case-definition of ICD-8 compatible diagnostic classes, the 1-year prevalence for phobia among Canadian women in Edmonton was 19 per cent; for separation anxiety it was

0.13 per cent (Costello 1982). The 1-month prevalence of anxiety disorders among residents of Camberwell, London was 2.9 per cent (Bebbington, Contractor, Hurry, and Tennant 1982, unpublished data). Higher rates were found for general anxiety (7.6 per cent), agoraphobic (17.4 per cent), and obsessive–compulsive symptoms (10.8 per cent). Dean and colleagues (1983), in a study to compare various diagnostic systems in a group of women in Edinburgh, reported a 0.5 per cent prevalence for anxiety neurosis and 2.3 per cent for phobic neurosis (Catego/ICD-8). The rate for generalized anxiety disorder, based on the RDC, was 2.6 per cent and for panic disorder 0.7 per cent.

Prevalence of major depression and dysthymic disorder

As shown in Table 11.3, major depression has a lifetime prevalence of approximately 7 per cent (range 3.3–12.6 per cent). The lowest rates are reported in Korea and the highest in New Zealand. The 6-month rates (about 3 per cent) are remarkedly lower than that of the lifetime prevalence, with rates ranging from 2.2 per cent in Baltimore to 3.5 per cent in New Haven. Dysthymia has a lifetime rate of about 4 per cent, with rates ranging from 2.4 per cent in Baltimore to 6.4 per cent in New Zealand. Studies using the DIS generally do not report the 6-month prevalence of dysthymia because the DIS has no recency probes for this diagnosis.

The prevalence of major depression based on the DSM-III criteria or the RDC has also been reported by several authors. Murphy (1980), in a reanalysis of the Stirling Study data, found a prevalence of 4.1 per cent. The current prevalence of major depression in a group of Swedish females according to the DSM-III criteria was 6.9 per cent (Hallström 1983). In the Zurich Study (Angst *et al.* 1990), the 1-year prevalence for major depression at the 1981 interview was 6.8 per cent and, at the 1986 interview, it increased slightly to 7.8 per cent. Weissman *et al.* (1978), using the SADS and the RDC, found a current prevalence of 4.3 per cent for major depressive episode.

Prevalence of neurotic disorders according to ICD-8/9

Some studies have focused on the prevalence rates of neurotic disorders according to ICD-8/9 that are assigned by psychiatrists. Within the MFS (Wittchen *et al.* 1988), the lifetime prevalence for neurotic disorders is 15 per cent. The rates for the individual neurotic disorders are 2.5 per cent for anxiety neurosis, 6.4 per cent for phobia, 1.1 per cent for obsessive—compulsive, 6.1 per cent for neurotic depression, 0.8 per cent for other neurotic disorders, and 5.0 per cent for psychosomatic disorder. The 6-month rates for each of these disorders are much lower: neurotic disorders, 11.6 per cent; anxiety neurosis, 1.3 per cent; phobia, 4.8 per cent; obsessive—compulsive, 0.5 per cent; neurotic depression, 4.3 per cent; other neurotic disorders, 0.7 per cent; and psychosomatic disorder, 2.5 per cent. In Upper Bavaria, Germany (i.e. the Traunstein Study) the 6-month rates for anxiety neurosis/phobia are 2.1

Table 11.3. Lifetime and six-month prevalence rates of DIS/DSM-III disorders from recent epidemiological studies*

DIS/DSM-III DIAGNOSES†	MFS	ECA (Total)	ECA sites St. Louis	New Haven	Baltimore	Los Angeles	Puerto Rico	Edmonton, Canada	Seoul, Korea	Christchurch, New Zealand
	Life (6-mth)	Life (6-mth)	Life (6-mth)	Life (6-mth)	Life (6-mth)	Life (6)	Life (6-mth)	Life (6-mth)	Life	Life
Affective dis.	12.9 (6.9)	8.3 (5.8)	8.0 (6.2)	9.5 (6.5)	6.1 (4.6)	8.9 (6.2)	7.9 (2.9)	10.2 (5.7)	5.5	14.7
Major depression	9.0 (3.0)	5.9 (3.0)	5.5 (3.2)	6.7 (3.5)	3.7 (2.2)	6.4 (3.1)	4.6 (3.0)	8.6 (3.2)	3.3	12.6
Dysthymia‡	4.0	3.3	3.8	3.2	2.1	4.2	4.7	3.7	2.4	6.4
Anxiety dis.	13.9 (8.1)	14.6 (8.9)	11.1§ (6.6)	10.4§ (7.2)	25.1§ (14.9)	13.5 (7.2)	13.6 (7.5)§	11.2 (6.5)	9.2	10.5§
Panic disorder	2.4 (1.1)	1.6 (0.8)	1.5 (0.9)	1.4 (0.6)	1.4 (1.0)	1.5 (0.9)	1.7 (1.1)	1.2 (0.7)	1.1	2.2
Agoraphobia	5.7 (3.6)	5.2 (3.4)	– (2.7)	– (2.8)	– (5.8)	–	6.9 (3.9)	2.9 (–)	2.1	–
Simple phobia	8.0 (4.1)	10.0 (6.4)	– (4.5)	– (4.7)	– (11.8)	–	8.6 (4.4)	7.2 (–)	5.4	–
Social phobia	3.1 (–)	2.8 (1.5)	–	–	–	–	1.6 (1.1)	1.7 (–)	0.5	3.0
Obsess.-Comp.	2.0 (1.8)	2.5 (1.5)	1.9 (1.3)	2.6 (1.4)	3.0 (2.0)	2.1 (0.7)	3.2 (1.8)	3.0 (1.6)	2.3	2.2
Generalized anxiety	–	–	–	–	–	–	–	–	3.6	31.1
Somatization	0.8 (0.8)	0.1 (0.0)	0.1 (0.1)	0.1 (0.1)	0.1 (0.1)	0.0 (0.0)	0.7 (0.7)	0.0 (0.0)	0.0	< 0.1
Substance use dis.	(13.5) (1.6)¶	16.7 (6.1)	18.1 (5.8)	15.0 (6.1)	17.0 (7.2)	18.5 (6.5)	–	20.6 (6.3)	31.8	21.0
Alcohol ab/dep	(13.0) (1.2)¶	13.5 (4.8)	15.7 (4.5)	11.5 (4.8)	13.7 (5.7)	14.9 (4.9)	12.6 (4.9)	18.0 (5.4)	21.7	18.9
Drugs ab/dep	1.8 (0.6)	6.1 (2.0)	5.5 (2.0)	5.8 (1.8)	5.6 (2.2)	7.3 (2.4)	7.0 (2.7)	6.9 (1.7)	0.9	5.7
Barbiturates ab/dep	1.7	1.2 (0.1)	–	–	–	–	–	–		

Life, lifetime prevalence; 6-mth, 6-month prevalence; —, not reported.
* The Taiwanese study (Hwu et al. 1989) was not included in this table because their rates are broken down into three geographical areas: metropolitan Taipei, small towns, and rural villages.   † dis., Disorders; Obsess.–comp., obsessive–compulsive disorder; ab/dep, abuse/dependence.   ‡ There are no recency probes for dysthymia in the DIS.
§ Anxiety/somatoform disorders.   ¶ The alcohol abuse/dependence rating was modified from the original DIS (in the MFS).

per cent, for neurotic depression 12.8 per cent, for other neuroses 5.7 per cent, and for psychosomatic disorder 4.6 per cent (Dilling and Weyerer 1984; Fichter 1988). In the 'former' Stockholm County, the 1-year prevalence for neurotic disorders is 25.7 per cent (Halldin 1984). Among these subjects, 1.9 per cent have phobias, 0.2 per cent obsessions/compulsions, 0.8 per cent anxiety neurosis, 4.2 per cent depressive neurosis, and 18.5 per cent other neuroses. The rates for psychosomatic disorders are 16.1 per cent and for affective disorders 0.2 per cent. Based on the General Health Questionnaire (GHQ) in combination with PSE and ID-Catego, Henderson et al. (1979) found a current rate for depression in Canberra, Australia of 6.7 per cent in women and 2.6 per cent in men. The rates for anxiety states are 3 per cent for women and 4.1 per cent for men. The current prevalence for anxiety neurosis generally range from 0.5 to 1.8 per cent (Dean et al. 1983; Fichter 1988; Tress and Schepank 1990), for neurotic depression from 3.1 to 6.8 per cent (Fichter 1988; Tress and Schepank 1990), and for psychosomatic disorder from 2.5 to 11.6 per cent (Fichter 1988; Tress and Schepank 1990).

When comparing the prevalence of neurotic disorders based on the ICD-9-oriented approaches with recent DIS findings a relatively good concordance has been reported. However, there are some indications that DIS/DSM-III prevalences for anxiety disorders were higher than for depression (see Table 11.3), whereas on the ICD-9 higher rates were found for neurotic depression (Dean et al. 1983; Fichter 1988; Wittchen et al. 1988; Tress and Schepank 1990).

Risk factors for neurotic disorders

Rates for agoraphobia (female, 1.8–23.3 per cent; male, 3–5.2 per cent) and simple phobia (female, 8.5–25.9 per cent; male, 3.8–14.5 per cent) are remarkedly higher in females than in males (Robins et al. 1984; Wittchen 1986; Bourdon et al. 1988; Hwu et al. 1989; Eaton and Keyl 1990; Lee et al. 1990; Table 11.4). Similar but less pronounced female preponderance has been reported for panic disorder, social phobia, and obsessive–compulsive disorder (Robins et al. 1984; Wittchen 1986; Bland et al. 1988a; Hwu et al. 1989; Keyl and Eaton 1990; Wittchen et al. 1992). Lifetime rates for major depression are about two to three times higher in females than in males (Robins et al. 1984; Canino et al. 1987; Bland et al. 1988a; Wittchen 1988; Lee et al. 1990; Wittchen et al. 1992), with values ranging from 4.1 to 16.3 per cent for females, and from 2.3 to 8.8 per cent for males. Compared to major depression, the female preponderance for dysthymia is less pronounced (male, 1.3–3.8 per cent; female, 2.5–9.0 per cent).

The highest prevalence of panic disorder is found among subjects in the 25–44 year old age group, and the lowest among subjects 65 years and older (von Korff et al. 1983; Robins et al. 1984; Bland et al. 1988c; Lee et al. 1990; Regier et al. 1990a), while no consistent patterns emerged for agoraphobia and simple phobia. For major depression, the highest rate is found in the 25–44 years age group (Robins *et al.* 1984; Bland *et al.* 1988*c*; Wittchen 1988; Wells *et al.* 1989; Lee *et al.* 1990; Wittchen *et al.* 1992), and for dysthymia it is in the 45–64 year age group (Canino *et al.* 1987; Wittchen 1988; Wells *et al.* 1989; Lee *et al.* 1990; Wittchen *et al.* 1992).

Higher rates of panic disorder and agoraphobia have been reported in separated, divorced, or widowed than in married or never married subjects (von Korff *et al.* 1983; Bland *et al.* 1988*a*; Eaton and Keyl 1990; Regier *et al.* 1990*a*). The highest rates for major depression and dysthymia have also been reported in subjects who are separated, divorced, or widowed (Bland *et al.* 1988*a*; Wittchen *et al.* 1988).

Other factors such as education (von Korff *et al.* 1983; Robins *et al.* 1984; Canino *et al.* 1987), ethnic groups (Weissman and Myers 1980; Robins *et al.* 1984), urbanization (Robins *et al.* 1984; Blazer *et al.* 1985; Canino *et al.* 1987; Hwu *et al.* 1988; Lee *et al.* 1990), and employment status (Bland *et al.* 1988*d*; Robins *et al.* 1991) do not prove to be consistent and powerful risk factors for neurotic disorders.

Prevalence of substance use disorders

Substance use disorder has been reported in 13.5–31.8 per cent of the general populations studied (Table 11.3). Alcohol abuse/dependence has a lifetime prevalence ranging from 7 per cent in Puerto Rico to 21.7 per cent in Korea. The high rate of alcohol abuse/dependence in Korea was quite surprising given the past knowledge about Asian drinking norms (Lee *et al.* 1990). The 6-month rates of alcohol abuse/dependence were much lower, with values ranging from 1.2 to 5.4 per cent. Compared to alcohol abuse/dependence, the rates for drug abuse/dependence were considerably lower, the lifetime rates range from 0.9 per cent (in Korea) to 7.3 per cent (in the ECA: Los Angeles), and the 6-month rates vary from 0.6 per cent (in the MFS) to 2.4 per cent (in the ECA: Los Angeles). The lifetime prevalence for alcohol abuse/dependence based on the ICD-9 is 0.95 per cent and for drug abuse/dependence it is 1.78 per cent.

Unfortunately, only two of these recent epidemiological studies (ECA: Regier *et al.* 1990*a*; MFS: Wittchen *et al.* 1988) have reported the prevalence of psychotropic drug abuse/dependence. Using data from the ECA, Regier *et al.* (1990*a*) reported a 1.2 per cent lifetime rate for barbiturates abuse/dependence. In the MFS, a lifetime prevalence of drug abuse/dependence is 1.79 per cent; all of these are women with benzodiazepine abuse/dependence (Wittchen 1988).

In addition to these reports, a number of studies have assessed the extent of use of psychotropic drugs in the general population (Table 11.5). The largest study was that of Balter and colleagues (1984), which examined community samples from 10 Western European countries and the USA. According to this and several smaller community studies, between 7.4 and 31 per cent of

Table 11.4. Lifetime prevalence of DIS/DSM-III disorders by sex*

DIS/DSM III DIAGNOSES†	MFS	ECA sites						Christchurch New Zealand
		St Louis	New Haven	Baltimore	Puerto Rico	Edmonton, Canada	Seoul, Korea	
	M (F)	M (F)	M (F)	M (F)	M (F)	M (F)	M (F)	M (F)
Affective dis.	6.4 (18.7)	—	—	—	4.7 (10.9)	7.1 (13.2)	4.3 (6.6)	10.0 (19.4)
Major depression	4.0 (13.6)	2.5 (8.1)	4.4 (8.7)	2.3 (4.9)	3.5 (5.5)	5.9 (11.4)	2.4 (4.1)	8.8 (16.3)
Dysthymia	2.5 (5.4)	2.1 (5.4)	2.6 (3.7)	1.2 (2.9)	1.6 (7.6)	2.2 (5.2)	1.8 (3.0)	3.8 (9.0)
Anxiety dis.	9.1 (18.1)	—	—	—	11.2 (15.7)	8.7 (13.8)‡	5.3 (12.7)	4.4 (16.5)‡
Panic disorder	1.7 (2.9)	0.9 (2.0)	0.6 (2.1)	1.2 (1.6)	1.6 (1.9)	0.8 (1.7)	0.3 (1.8)	0.9 (3.4)
Agoraphobia	2.9 (8.3)	1.5 (6.4)	1.5 (5.3)	5.2 (12.5)	4.9 (8.7)	1.5 (4.3)	0.7 (3.3)	—
Simple phobia	5.5 (10.4)§	4.0 (9.4)	3.8 (8.5)	14.5 (25.9)	7.6 (9.6)	4.6 (9.8)	2.6 (7.9)	—
Social phobia	—	—	—	1.5 (1.6)	1.4 (2.0)	0.0 (1.0)	4.3 (3.5)	
Obsess.–comp.	1.8 (2.3)	1.1 (2.6)	2.0 (3.1)	2.6 (3.3)	3.3 (3.1)	2.8 (3.1)	2.2 (2.4)	1.0 (3.4)
Generalized anxiety	—	—	—	—	—	—	2.4 (4.3)	27.1 (35.1)
Substance use dis.	21.2 (6.1)	—	—	—		32.5 (8.6)	60.0 (5.2)‖¶	33.6 (8.7)
Alcohol ab/dep	21.0 (5.1)	28.9 (4.3)	19.1 (4.8)	24.9 (4.2)	24.6 (2.0)	29.3 (6.7)	=	32.0 (6.1)
Drug ab/dep	1.4 (2.0)	7.4 (3.8)	6.5 (5.1)	7.1 (4.4)	—	10.6 (3.2)	0.8 (0.9)	7.2 (4.1)

M, Male; F, Female; —, not reported.
* The Taiwanese study (Hwu et al. 1989) was not included in this table because their rates are broken down into three geographical areas: metropolitan Taipei, small towns, and rural villages.
† dis., Disorders; Obsess.–comp., obsessive–compulsive disorder; ab/dep, abuse/dependence.   ‡ Anxiety/somatoform disorders.
§ Rates for combined simple and social phobia.   ¶ Including tobacco dependence.
‖ In Seoul the rates for alcohol abuse were 25.6% for males and 1.6% for females; for alcohol dependence they were 17.2% for males and 1.0% for females.

the general population had consumed psychotropic drugs at some time in the year prior to the survey (Mellinger *et al.* 1971, 1974, 1984*a*; Parry *et al.* 1973; Balter *et al.* 1974; Uhlenhuth *et al.* 1983). Benzodiazepine accounted for approximately 70–85 per cent of all the psychotropic drugs used (Mellinger *et al.* 1984*b*; Siciliani *et al.* 1985). High rates in the use of benzodiazepine are not limited to adults, but are also found among adolescents. Pedersen and Lavik (1991) reported that about 10 per cent of the adolescents in Olso, Norway had taken benzodiazepine during the preceding year.

Among users of psychotropic drugs, chronic use (i.e. daily for at least 1 year) of psychotropic drug is estimated to range from 6.2 per cent (Sweden) to as high as 52.2 per cent (UK) (Balter *et al.* 1984; Dunbar *et al.* 1989); the rates of chronic use found in Belgium (33.2 per cent) and in France (31.5 per cent) are also relatively high. The prevalence of short-term use (i.e. daily for less than 1 month) generally vary from 21.8 per cent (Belgium) to 76.9 per cent (Sweden) (Balter *et al.* 1984).

Risk factors for substance use disorders

Males have almost four times higher rates of substance use disorders than females (Table 11.4). In the individual disorders, men show a clear predominance in alcohol abuse or dependence. Males also show higher rates of drug abuse/dependence than females; however, unlike alcohol abuse/dependence, this difference is less clear. Age differences in the rates of alcohol and drug abuse/dependence do not show any systematic patterns across studies.

The users of psychotropic drugs (e.g. benzodiazepines) are usually older—mostly over 50 years old (Murray *et al.* 1981; Uhlenhuth *et al.* 1983; Balter *et al.* 1984; Mellinger *et al.* 1984*a*; Dunbar *et al.* 1989; Fichter *et al.* 1989) tend to be women (Parry *et al.* 1973; Uhlenhuth *et al.* 1983; Balter *et al.* 1984; Mellinger *et al.* 1984*b*; Fichter *et al.* 1989; Vazquez-Barquero *et al.* 1989), have higher levels of psychological distress (Uhlenhuth *et al.* 1978; Murray *et al.* 1981; Mellinger *et al.* 1984*a*,*b*; Dunbar *et al.* 1989; Fichter *et al.* 1989; Vazquez-Barquero *et al.* 1989), have physical illness (Uhlenhuth *et al.* 1978; Mellinger *et al.* 1984*a*; Dunbar *et al.* 1989; Vazquez-Barquero *et al.* 1989), more frequent visits to the physicians (Murray *et al.* 1982; Mellinger *et al.* 1984*a*), have coexistent physical and mental illness (Vazquez-Barquero *et al.* 1989), and were separated, divorced, or widowed (Uhlenhuth *et al.* 1978). The relationships of psychotropic drugs use with other factors such as social class, education level, and occupation are less clear.

Co-occurrence of neurotic disorders and psychotropic drugs

Recent epidemiological studies conducted in different countries (Weissman *et al.* 1978, 1986; Angst and Dobler-Mikola 1985; Weissman and Merikangas 1986; Wittchen 1986, 1988; Wittchen and Essau 1989; Angst *et al.* 1990; Regier *et al.* 1990*b*; Robins *et al.* 1991; Wittchen *et al.* 1991*b*, 1992) have shown that

Table 11.5. Prevalence and patterns of psychotropic drug use in the community

References	Psychotropic drug classes included	Time frame	Countries	Prevalence (%)	Patterns of use
Mellinger et al. (1971)	Rx: stimulant, minor tranquillizer, hynotic, sedative, antispasmodic, major tranquillizer, antidepressant O-T-C: stimulant, sleeping pill, tranquillizer	1 year	USA	45* (F) 33* (M)	Rates of Rx drugs: 32% for female; 18% for male. Rates of O-T-C: 7% for female; 9% for male. Subjects aged 45 to 59 years used Rx drugs from medical sources, whereas O-T-C and Rx drugs from non-medical sources are most common among subjects 18 to 29 years old. Stimulant was most often used by 18–29 age group, and hypnotic by subjects 60 years and older. 17% of the female and 19% of the male psychotropic drug users consumed the medication for 6-months or longer
Parry et al. (1973); same database with Mellinger et al. (1974)	Rx: Major tranquillizers, minor tranquillizers (mostly benzodiazepine), antidepressants, sedatives, hypnotics O-T-C: stimulants, tranquillizer, sleeping pill	1 year	USA	31*	Rates for RX drugs: 19%; rates for Rx and O-T-C: 3%; for O-T-C: 9%. Higher rates in females (37%) than in males (22%). In males, the rates increased in the 30–44 year age group, and among those over 59 years old. In female, the rate increased in the 30–44 year age group and then remained constant. O-T-C drugs were mostly used by subjects in the 18–29 year age group
Balter et al. (1974)	Anti-anxiety/sedative agents daily for one month or more during the past year (chlordiazepoxide, diazepam, phenobarbital)	1 year	Belgium France Sweden Denmark UK Germany Netherlands Italy Spain	16.8 16.7 15.8 15.1 14.2 14.2 12.7 11.2 9.7	In every country, females have higher rates than males. Higher rates were generally found in age groups over 35 years. Among users, between 30% (in Italy) and 64% (in Netherlands) have used anti-anxiety/sedative agents daily for one or more during the past year

References	Psychotropic drug classes included	Time frame	Countries	Prevalence (%)	Patterns of use
Uhlenhuth et al. (1978)	Minor tranquillizer, sedative	1 year	USA	20	10% of the users consumed psychotropic drugs regularly for less than 2 weeks, 4% for at least 1 week, and 6% for at least 2 weeks. Female (27%) and older subjects had higher rates than male (12%) and younger subjects. Use of tranquillizer increased with more health problems. Male non-users consumed more alcohol than users, whereas female users consumed more alcohol and coffee/tea than non-users
Murray et al. (1981)	Major and minor tranquillizers, antidepressants, hypnotics, stimulants	2 weeks	UK	10.9	Women had two times higher rates than males. The use of hypnotics increased with age, but that of tranquillizers and antidepressants decreased
Balter et al. (1984)	Anti-anxiety/sedative drugs (e.g. diazepam, clorazepam, lorazepam, phenobarbital)	1 year	Belgium France Switzerland Spain USA Germany Denmark Italy UK Sweden Netherlands	17.6 15.9 14.6 14.2 12.9 12.0 11.9 11.5 11.2 8.6 7.4	In every country, over 60% of the psychotropic drug users were females. In most countries, high use of psychotropic drug was found in the middle and older age groups; in Switzerland and in USA, about equal percentages were found in the younger, middle, and older age groups

Table 11.5. cont.

References	Psychotropic drug classes included	Time frame	Countries	Prevalence (%)	Patterns of use
Mellinger *et al.* (1984a)	Anxiolytic	1 year	USA	11.0	Benzodiazepine accounted for 84% of the anxiolytics used. Persons with agoraphobia/panic syndrome used anxiolytics the most frequently, followed by those with 'other phobias' and generalized anxiety syndromes. Anxiolytic users were older, had high level of psychological distress and impairment, multiple health problems, and more visits to a physician than non-users. Agoraphobics (22%) were usually regular users of anxiolytics, and other phobics and those with generalized anxiety were mostly occasional users
Vazquez-Barquero *et al.* (1989)	Neuroleptic, antipsychotic, anxiolytic (mainly benzodiazepine), non-benzodiazepine, hypnotics, barbiturates, tricyclic antidepressants, MAO inhibitors, stimulants	2 weeks	Spain	6.9	High use of psychotropic drug was associated with female higher age and mental illness coexistent with physical and mental illness. The female predominance was enhanced among older and married subjects, as well as among the unemployed and housewives.
Dunbar *et al.* (1989)	Benzodiazepine	1 week	UK	7.7 3.6	Male: female ratio was 1:2, Anxiolytics were used more frequently than hypnotics by young subjects, and hypnotics by the elderly. Benzodiazepine users are older and have more physical illness than non-users. 48.5% of the benzodiazepine users have taken the medication for more than 12 months; 54.5% had used it on a regular basis. 61% of the users had difficulties in stopping the medication. These people were those who had consumed benzodiazepine for more than 12 months, and those who were older than 45 years

References	Psychotropic drug classes included	Time frame	Countries		Prevalence (%)	Patterns of use
Fichter et al. (1989)	(see next column)	4 weeks	Germany			Those with high use of psychotropic drug tend to be female, older in age, and tend to be found among those with high psychiatric morbidity, higher somatic morbidity, reduced work capacity, and higher neuroticism. No association was found with social class and and personality factor
				Benzodiazepines	6.9	
				Lithium	0.1	
				Neuroleptics	1.8	
				Carbamine-acid derivatives	0.8	
				Antidepressants	1.5	
				Barbiturates	3.6	
				Opioids	2.2%	
				Tranquillizers	8.3	
				Barbiturate-like hypnotics	4.3	
Pedersen & Lavik (1991)	Benzodiazepine	1 year	Norway		10.0	Only 1% of the subjects used benzodiazepine more than 10 times in the past year. Benzodiazepine was taken for sleeping disturbances, anxiety, life events. Mother is the most important supplier of benzodiazepine, followed by the physician and the fathers. Many of the benzodiazepine users had poor mental health. Subjects who obtained their benzodiazepine from the 'illegal market' consumed more alcohol and cannabis than other adolescents

F, Females; M, Males; Rx, prescribed psychotropic drug; O-T-C, over-the-counter drug; *, Rx or O-T-C.

individuals who fulfil criteria for one type of neurotic disorder tend to have other neurotic disorders as well. Based on these studies, between 30 and 80 per cent of persons with an anxiety disorder have at least one other anxiety disorder, and between 32 and 50 per cent of all the subjects with anxiety disorder also fulfil criteria for major depression (Lepine, Wittchen, and Essau, in preparation; Wittchen 1986; Markowitz *et al.* 1989; Vollrath and Angst 1989; see also reviews by Stavrakaki and Vargo 1986; Winokur 1988; Noyes 1990; Wittchen and Essau 1991).

Well-controlled epidemiological evidence on the comorbidity of psychotropic drug and neurotic and other substance use disorders is sparse, with the exception of an analysis of the ECA data by Regier *et al.* (1990*b*). In that report, about 23.7 per cent of the ECA subjects with anxiety disorder also have substance abuse/dependence. Among those with barbiturates abuse/dependence, 36.4 per cent also fulfil the criteria for affective disorder, 42.9 per cent for anxiety disorder, and 71.3 per cent for alcohol abuse/dependence. In the MFS, 14.7 per cent of the subjects with an alcohol use disorder have anxiety disorders, mostly agoraphobia and phobic disorder (Bronisch and Wittchen 1992; Wittchen and Bronisch 1992).

Conclusions

Based on recent epidemiological studies, according to the DSM-III, the lifetime prevalence of neurotic disorders can be estimated as 9–15 per cent of the adult population. Anxiety disorders (range, 9.2–25.1 per cent) are more common than affective disorders (range, 15.5 to 14.7 per cent), with a high degree of overlap between both. The most common type of anxiety disorder is phobia, mostly simple or social phobia (range 5.4–8.6 per cent) and agoraphobia (range 2.9–6.9 per cent). The cross-sectional prevalences are considerably lower. No clear findings are available on the poorly defined concept of generalized anxiety disorder. Major depression has a lifetime prevalence of about 7 per cent, and dysthymia about 4 per cent. Substance use disorder has been reported in 13.5–31.8 per cent of the general population. Psychotropic drugs have prevalence rates ranging from 6.9 to 31 per cent, and benzodiazepines made up about 70–85 per cent of all the psychotropic drugs consumed.

Being female, divorced, and separated is associated with a higher prevalence of anxiety and affective disorders. Alcohol and drug abuse/dependence is far more frequent in males, whereas medication drug use tends to be associated with higher age, being female, widowed, frequent visits to physicians, high levels of psychological distress and impairment, multiple somatic physical illness, as well as with coexistent physical and mental illness.

At this point, there is a lack of well-controlled epidemiological studies that look at the prospective interrelationship of psychopathology with medication and other substance use; rather consistent findings have been reported with regard to early onset of illegal drug use prior to the development of major psychopathology for medication abuse and dependence. Poorly recognized psychosomatic conditions and their inappropriate treatment with psychotropic medication have repeatedly been reported to play a major aetiological role in the development of medication use and abuse in neurotic conditions (Sartorius *et al.* 1990). However, clear epidemiological evidence for this is still lacking.

References

APA (American Psychiatric Association) (1980). *Diagnostic and statistical manual of mental* disorders (3rd edn). American Psychiatric Press, Washington, DC.

APA (American Psychiatric Association) (1987). *Diagnostic and statistical manual of mental disorders* (3rd edn, revised). American Psychiatric Press, Washington, DC.

Angst, J. and Dobler-Mikola, A. (1985). The Zurich study. V. Anxiety and phobia in young adults. *European Archives of Psychiatric Neurological Science*, **234**, 408–18.

Angst, J., Vollrath, M., Merikangas, K.R., and Ernst, C. (1990). Comorbidity of anxiety and depression in the Zurich Cohort Study of young adults. In *Comorbidity of mood and anxiety disorders* (ed. J.D. Maser and C.R. Cloninger), pp.123–53. American Psychiatric Press, Washington, DC.

Balter, M., Levine, J., and Manheimer, D.I. (1974). Cross-national study of the extent of anti-anxiety/sedative drug use. *New England Journal of Medicine*, **4**, 769–74.

Balter, M., Mannheimer, D.I., Mellinger, G.D., and Uhlenhuth, E.H. (1984). A cross national comparison of anti-anxiety/sedative drug use. *Current Medical Research and Opinion*, **8** (suppl. 4), 5–20.

Bland, R.C., Orn, H., and Newman, S.C. (1988*a*). Lifetime prevalence of psychiatric disorders in Edmonton. *Acta Psychiatrica Scandinavica*, **77** (suppl. 338), 24–32.

Bland, R.C., Newman, S.C., and Orn, H. (1988*b*). Period prevalence of psychiatric disorders in Edmonton. *Acta Psychiatrica Scandinavica*, **77** (suppl. 338), 33–42.

Bland, R.C., Newman, S.C., and Orn, H. (1988*c*). Age of onset of psychiatric disorders. *Acta Psychiatrica Scandinavica*, **77** (suppl. 338), 43–49.

Bland, R.C., Stebelsky, H., Orn, H., and Newman, S.C. (1988*d*). Psychiatric disorders and unemployment in Edmonton. *Acta Psychiatrica Scandinavica*, **77**, (suppl. 338), 72–80.

Blazer, D., George, L.K., Landerman, R., Pennybacker, M., Melville, M.L., Woodbury, M., *et al.* (1985). Psychiatric disorders: A rural/urban comparison. *Archives of General Psychiatry*, **42**, 651–6.

Bourdon, K.H., Boyd, J.H., Rae, D.S., Burns, B.J., Thompson, J.W., and Locke, B.Z. (1988). Gender differences in phobias: results of the ECA community survey. *Journal of Anxiety Disorders*, **2**(3), 227–41.

Burnam, M.A., Hough, R.L., Escobar, J.I., Karno, M., Timbers, D.M., Telles, C.A., *et al.* (1987). Six-month prevalence of specific psychiatric disorders among Mexican Americans and Non-Hispanic whites in Los Angeles. *Archives of General Psychiatry*, **44**, 687–94.

Bronisch, T. and Wittchen, H.-U. (1992). Lifetime and 6-month prevalence of abuse and dependence of alcohol in the Munich Follow-up study. *European Archives of Psychiatry and Clinical Neuroscience*, **241**, 273–82.

Canino, G.S., Bird, H.R., Shrout, P.E., Rubio-Stipec, M., Bravo, M., Martinez, R., et al. (1987). The prevalence of specific psychiatric disorders in Puerto Rico. *Archives of General Psychiatry*, **44**, 727–35.

Costello, C.G. (1982). Fears and phobias in women: A community study. *Journal of Abnormal Psychology*, **91**, 280–6.

Dean, C., Surtees, P.G., and Sashidharan, S.P. (1983). Comparison of research diagnostic systems in an Edinburgh community sample. *British Journal of Psychiatry*, **142**, 247–56.

Dilling, H. and Weyerer, S. (1984). Prevalence of mental disorders in the small-town–rural region of Traunstein (Upper Bavaria). *Acta Psychiatrica Scandinavica*, **69**, 60–79.

Dunbar, G.C., Perera, M.H., and Jenner, F.A. (1989). Patterns of benzodiazepine use in Great Britain. *British Journal of Psychiatry*, **155**, 836–41.

Eaton, W.W. and Keyl, P.M. (1990). Risk factors for the onset of Diagnostic Interview Schedule/DSM-III Agoraphobia in a prospective, population-based study. *Archives of General Psychiatry*, **47**, 819–24.

Fichter, M.M. (1988). *Die Oberbayerische Verlaufsuntersuchung: psychische Erkrankungen in der Bevölkerung*. Psychiatrische Universitätklinik, München.

Fichter, M.M., Witzke, W., Leibl, K., and Hippius, H. (1989). Psychotropic drug use in a representative community sample: the Upper Bavarian study. *Acta Psychiatrica Scandinavica*, **80**, 68–77.

Halldin, J. (1984). Prevalence of mental disorder in an urban population in central Sweden. *Acta Psychiatrica Scandinavica*, **69**, 503–18.

Hallström, T. (1983). Point prevalence of major depressive disorder in a Swedish urban female population. *Acta Psychiatrica Scandinavica*, **69**, 52–79.

Henderson, S., Duncan-Jones, P., Byrne, D.G., Scott, R., and Adcock, S. (1979). Psychiatric disorder in Canberra. A standardised study of prevalence. *Acta Psychiatrica Scandinavica*, **60**, 355–74.

Hwu, H.G., Yeh, E.K., and Chang, L.Y. (1989). Prevalence of psychiatric disorders in Taiwan defined by the Chinese Diagnostic Interview Schedule. *Acta Psychiatrica Scandinavica*, **79**, 136–47.

Karno, M., Hough, R.L., Burnam, M.A., Escobar, J.I., Timbers, D.M., Santana, F., et al. (1987). Lifetime prevalence of specific psychiatric disorders among Mexican Americans and Non-Hispanic whites in Los Angeles. *Archives of General Psychiatry*, **44**, 695–701.

Keyl, P.M. and Eaton, W.W. (1990). Risk factors for the onset of panic disorder and other panic attacks in a prospective, population-based study. *American Journal of Epidemiology*, **131**(2), 301–11.

Lee, C.K., Kwak, Y.S., Yamamoto, J., Rhee, H., Kim, Y.S., Han, J.H., et al. (1990). Psychiatric epidemiology in Korea. Part II: Urban and rural differences. *Journal of Nervous and Mental Disorders*, **178**(4), 247–252.

Lilienfeld, A.M. and Lilienfeld, D.E. (1980). *Foundations of epidemiology* (2nd edn). Oxford University Press, New York.

Markowitz, J.S., Weissman, M.M., Quellette, R., Lish, J., and Klerman, G.L. (1989). Quality of life in panic disorder. *Archives of General Psychiatry*, **46**, 984–92.

Mellinger, G.D., Balter, M.B., and Manheimer, D.I. (1971). Patterns of psychotherapeutic drug use among adults in San Francisco. *Archives of General Psychiatry*, **25**, 385–94.

Mellinger, G.D., Balter, M.B., Parry, H.J., Manheimer, D.I., and Cisin, I.H. (1974). An overview of psychotherapeutic drug use in the United States. In *Drug use:*

epidemiological and sociological approaches (ed. E. Josephson and E.E. Carroll), p.333. Wiley, New York.

Mellinger, G.D., Balter, M.B., and Uhlenhuth, E.H. (1984*a*). Prevalence and correlates of the long term regular use of anxiolytics. *Journal of the American Medical Association*, **251**, 375–9.

Mellinger, G.D., Balter, M.B., and Uhlenhuth, E.H. (1984*b*). Anti-anxiety agents: duration of use and characteristics of users in the USA. *Current Medical Research and Opinion*, **8**, (suppl. 4), 21–36.

Morris, J.N. (1975). *Uses of epidemiology* (3rd edn). Churchill Livingstone, London.

Murphy, J.M. (1980). Continuities in community-based psychiatric epidemiology. *Archives of General Psychiatry*, **37**, 1215–23.

Murray, J., Dunn, P., Williams, P., and Tarnopolsky, A. (1981). Factors affecting the consumption of psychotropic drugs. *Psychological Medicine*, **11**, 551–60.

Murray, J., Williams, P., and Clare, A. (1982). Health and social characteristic of long-term psychotropic drug takers. *Social Science and Medicine*, **16**, 1595–8.

Myers, J.K., Weissman, M.M., Tischler, G.L., Holzer, C.E., Leaf, P.J., Orvaschel, H., *et al.* (1984). Six-month prevalence of psychiatric disorders in three communities. *Archives of General Psychiatry*, **41**, 959–67.

Noyes, R. (1990). The comorbidity and mortality of panic disorder. *Psychiatric Medicine*, **8**, 41–66.

Parry, H.J., Balter, M.B., Mellinger, G.D., Cisin, I.H., and Manheimer, D.I. (1973). National patterns of psychotherapeutic drug use. *Archives of General Psychiatry*, **28**, 769–83.

Pedersen, W. and Lavik, N.J. (1991). Adolescents and benzodiazepines: prescribed use, self-medication and intoxication. *Acta Psychiatrica Scandinavica*, **84**, 94–8.

Regier, D.A., Meyer, J.K., Kramer, M., Robins, L.N., Blazer, D.G., Hough, R.L., *et al.* (1984). The NIMH Epidemiologic Catchment Area (ECA) Program: historical context, major objective, and study population characteristics. *Archives of General Psychiatry*, **41**, 934–41.

Regier, D.A., Boyd, J.H., Burke, J.D., Rae, D.S., Myers, J. K., Kramer, M., *et al.* (1988). One-month prevalence of mental disorders in the United States: Based on five Epidemiological Catchment Area sites. *Archives of General Psychiatry*, **45**, 977–86.

Regier, D.A., Narrow, W.E., and Rae, D.S. (1990*a*). The epidemiology of anxiety disorders: The Epidemiologic Catchment Area (ECA) experience. *Journal of Psychiatric Research*, **24**, (suppl. 2), 3–14.

Regier, D.A., Farmer, M.E., Rae, D.S., Locke, B.Z., Keith, S.J., Judd, L.L. *et al.* (1990*b*). Comorbidity of mental disorders with alcohol and other drug abuse. Results from the Epidemiologic Catchment Area (ECA) Study. *Journal of the American Medical Association*, **264**, (19), 2511–18.

Robins, L.N., Helzer, J.E., Weissman, M.M., Orvaschel, H., Gruenberg, E., Burke, J.D.Jr., *et al.* (1984). Lifetime prevalence of psychiatric disorders at three sites. *Archives of General Psychiatry*, **41**, 949–59.

Robins, L.N., Helzer, J.E., Ratcliff, K.S., and Seyfried, W. (1982). Validity of the Diagnostic Interview Schedule, version II: DSM-III diagnoses. *Psychological Medicine*, **12**, 855–70.

Robins, L.N., Locke, B.Z., and Regier, D.A. (1991). An overview of psychiatric disorders in America. In *Psychiatric disorders in America. The Epidemiologic Catchment Area Study* (ed. L.N. Robins and D.A. Regier), pp.328–66. The Free Press, New York.

184   The epidemiology of neurosis

Sartorius, N., Goldberg, D., De Girolamo, G., Costa de Silva, J.A., Lecrubier, Y., and Wittchen, H.-U. (ed.) (1990). *Psychological disorders in general medical settings*. Hogrefe and Huber, Toronto.

Siciliani, O., Bellantuono, C., Williams, P., and Tansella, M. (1985). Self reported use of psychotropic drugs and alcohol abuse in South Verona. *Psychological Medicine*, **15**, 821–6.

Stavrakaki, C. and Vargo, B. (1986). The relationship of anxiety and depression: a review of the literature. *British Journal of Psychiatry*, **149**, 7–16.

Tress, W. and Schepank, H. (1990). Zur Epidemiologie psychogener Erkrankungen in der Stadtbevölkerung. In *Fortschritte in der Psychiatrischen Epidemiologie* (ed. M.H. Schmidt), pp.75–86. VCH Verlagsgesellschaft, Germany.

Uhlenhuth, E.H., Balter, M.B., and Lipman, R.s. (1978). Minor tranquilizers: clinical correlates of use in an urban population. *Archives of General Psychiatry*, **35**, 350.

Uhlenhuth, E.H., Balter, M.B., Mellinger, G.G., Cisin, I.H., and Clinthorpe, J. (1983). Symptom checklist syndromes in the general population: correlations with psychotherapeutic drug use. *Archives of General Psychiatry*, **40**, 1167–73.

Vazquez-Barquero, J.L., Diez Manrique, J.F., Pena, C., Arenal Gonzalez, A., Cuesta, M.J., and Artal, J.A. (1989). Patterns of psychotropic drug use in a Spanish rural community. *British Journal of Psychiatry*, **155**, 633–41.

Vollrath, M. and Angst, J. (1989). Outcome of panic disorder and depression in a seven-year follow-up: results of the Zurich study. *Acta Psychiatrica Scandinavica*, **80**, 591–6.

von Korff, M. and Eaton, W.W. (1989). Epidemiologic findings on panic. In *Panic disorder: theory, research and therapy* (ed. R. Baker), pp.35–50. John Wiley, New York.

von Korff, M., Eaton, W., and Keyl, P. (1983). The epidemiology of panic attacks and panic disorder: results of three community surveys. *American Journal of Epidemiology*, **122**, 970–81.

Wells, J.E., Bushnell, J.A., Hornblow, A.R., Joyce, P.R., and Oakley-Browne, M.A. (1989). Christchurch psychiatric epidemiology study. Part I: Methodology and lifetime prevalence for specific psychiatric disorders. *Australian and New Zealand Journal of Psychiatry*, **23**, 315–26.

Weissman, M.M. (1990). The hidden patient: unrecognized panic disorder. *Journal of Clinical Psychiatry*, **51**, (suppl), 5–8.

Weissman, M.M. and Merikangas, K.R. (1986). The epidemiology of anxiety and panic disorders: an update. *Journal of Clinical Psychiatry*, **47**, 11–17.

Weissman, M.M. and Myers, J.K. (1980). Psychiatric disorders in a U.S. community: The application of Research Diagnostic Criteria to a resurveyed community sample. *Acta Psychiatrica Scandinavica*, **62**, 99–111.

Weissman, M.M., Myers, J.K., and Harding, P.S. (1978). Psychiatric disorders in a US urban community. *American Journal of Psychiatry*, **135**, 459–462.

Weissman, M.M., Leaf, P.J., Blazer, D.G., Boyd, J.H., and Florio, L.P. (1986). Panic disorder: clinical characteristics, epidemiology, and treatment. *Psychopharmacology Bulletin*, **22**, 787–91.

Winokur, G. (1988). Anxiety disorders: relationships to other psychiatric illness. *Psychiatric Clinics of North America*, **11**, 287–93.

WHO (World Health Organization) (1990). *Composite International Diagnostic Interview*. World Health Organization, Division of Mental Health, Geneva.

WHO (World Health Organization) (1991). *ICD*-10, Chapter V, Mental and behavioral disorders (including disorders of psychological development)—diagnostic criteria for research, draft for field trails. World Health Organization, Division of Mental Health, Geneva.

Wittchen, H.-U. (1986). Epidemiology of panic attacks and panic disorders. In *Panic and phobias* (ed. I. Hand and H.-U. Wittchen), pp.18–28. Springer, Heidelberg.

Wittchen, H.-U. (1988). Natural course and spontaneous remissions of untreated anxiety disorders: results of the Munich Follow-up study (MFS). In *Panic and phobias* 2 (ed. I. Hand and H.-U. Wittchen), pp.3–17. Springer, Heidelberg.

Wittchen, H.-U. and Bronisch, T. (1992). Use, abuse, and dependence of alcohol in West Germany—lifetime and 6-month prevalence in the Munich Follow-up study. In *Comparison of rates of alcoholism* (ed. J. Helzer and G. Canino) p.161–81. Oxford University Press, New York.

Wittchen, H.-U. and Essau, C.A. (1989). Comorbidity of anxiety disorders and depression: does it affect course and outcome? *Journal of Psychiatry and Psychobiology*, **4**, 315–23.

Wittchen, H.-U. and Essau, C.A. (1991). Epidemiology of panic attacks, panic disorder, and agoraphobia. In *Panic disorder and agoraphobia: a comprehensive guide for the practitioner* (ed. J.R. Walker, R. Norton, and C. Ross), pp.103–49. Brooks/Cole Publishing Co, California.

Wittchen, H.-U., Hecht, H., Zaudig, M., Vogl, G., Semler, G., Pfister, H. (1988). Häufigkeiten und Schwere psychischer Störungen in der Bevölkerung—Eine epidemiologische Feldstudie. *Verläufe behandelter und unbehandelter Depressionen und Angststörungen in der Bevölkerungen*, (ed. H.-U. Wittchen and D. von Zerssen), pp.232–51. Springer, Heidelberg.

Wittchen, H.-U., Robins, L.N., Cottler, L., Sartorius, N., Burke, J., Regier, D., & Participants of the field trials (1991*a*). Cross-cultural feasibility, reliability and sources of variance of the Composite International Diagnostic Interview (CIDI)—Results of the multicenter WHO/ADAMHA field trials (Wave 1). *British Journal of Psychiatry*, **159**, 645–53.

Wittchen, H.-U. Essau, C.A., and Krieg, C. (1991*b*). Comorbidity: similarities and differences in treated and untreated groups. *British Journal of Psychiatry*, **159** (suppl. 12), 23–33.

Wittchen, H.-U., Essau, C.A., von Zerssen, D., Krieg, C.J., and Zaudig, M. (1992). Lifetime and six-month prevalence of mental disorders in the Munich Follow-up Study. *European Archives of Psychiatry and Clinical Neuroscience*, **241**, 247–58.

12 An international perspective on benzodiazepine abuse

Hannes Pétursson

Following their introduction in the 1960s, the use of benzodiazepines increased rapidly and, during the next 2 decades, they virtually replaced earlier drugs in the treatment of anxiety disorders and insomnia. In most areas of the world, the use of benzodiazepines peaked during the late 1970s, when critical questions were being asked about their extensive use. Subsequently, a sharp decline in benzodiazepine prescriptions was seen in many countries. However, within the last decade this downward trend has been reversed, perhaps as a result of the introduction of newer benzodiazepines as well as of a clearer understanding of their indications and the high incidence of anxiety and sleep disorders.

The current concerns about benzodiazepines relate to their use in medical as well as non-medical practice. In the first category, concerns are being expressed about the appropriateness of benzodiazepine usage, possible mis-use, and the occurrence of physiological dependence with long-term use of therapeutic doses, leading to difficult withdrawal problems (Pétursson and Lader 1984). The second area of concern is the abuse or non-medical use of these drugs. This includes illegal use as well as the use of prescribed benzodiazepines for purposes, durations, or at dosage levels not intended by the prescribing physician and outside appropriate medical guidelines. The present chapter focuses mainly on the latter category, i.e. abuse of benzodiazepines. This approach attempts to clarify a problem that is often characterized by confusion and lack of reliable information. It is in this respect important to draw a sharp distinction between, on the one hand, benzodiazepine dependence occurring within the clinical context, and on the other hand non-medical problems of abuse.

The substantial research literature on benzodiazepine abuse tends to focus on the various details of the context within which abuse of these drugs takes place. However, in order to assess the significance of abuse in relation to the extensive, worldwide clinical use of benzodiazepines, it is essential to examine these problems and potential solutions to them in the broader, international perspective. The present chapter will thus weigh the extent and nature of the actual use and abuse of benzodiazepines followed by a discussion of national and international measures and recommendations to minimize the abuse of these important medications.

Worldwide use of benzodiazepines

The extent of benzodiazepine use has been of much interest in recent years. Several methods have been used to try and assess the true level of benzodiazepine use, including investigation of sales figures, prescription audits, and population surveys. However, statistics on the extent of benzodiazepine use must be interpreted cautiously in view of the many factors that influence the utilization of drug consumption in general. The overall use of benzodiazepines may co-vary with factors such as marketing practices and regulation policies as well as with the cultural and economic characteristics of different populations.

In spite of large-scale multinational studies and efforts by international bodies such as the World Health Organization (WHO), there is still a wide geographical variation in the amount of epidemiological data available on the use of benzodiazepines. Traditionally, most of the information relates to use in the USA and Western and Northern European nations. In many areas, in particular in some developing countries, the information is still anecdotal with few published studies and inadequate record-keeping. A further problem is presented by the fact that information on the use of different benzodiazepines also varies markedly. Data on actual use are often limited to substances that have been available for relatively long periods of time in various countries. The WHO has adopted a method that expresses drug use in terms of 'defined daily doses' (DDD) per day per 1000 population (Bergman 1981). This method has proven helpful in comparing levels of benzodiazepine use from one country to another.

Sales figures

Sales data provide only indirect information about benzodiazepine consumption and can be quite inaccurate nationally and internationally, since prices can vary enormously. However, wholesale data can provide certain information regarding the supply, distribution, and availability in various countries at a given point in time. National studies of retail prescription sales in the USA and some European countries as well as in Australia, generally revealed increases in sales of these drugs from the mid- and late 1960s to at least the early 1970s. From then on sales decreased generally until the late 1970s when a second gradual increase was observed in some countries, in particular in relation to the use of benzodiazepines as hypnotics.

The Nordic countries have traditionally reported benzodiazepine use in terms of defined daily doses (DDD)/1000/day (Nordic Council on Medicines 1979, 1982). In terms of this measure sales of benzodiazepines increased in most of the Nordic countries from the mid-1960s through the next decade or so. Sales of benzodiazepines decreased in Sweden from about 1970 and sales of benzodiazepine hypnotics decreased in Finland and Sweden between 1966 and 1977. The sales of benzodiazepine tranquillizers were generally comparable for the Nordic countries during this period of time, but somewhat higher figures were reported for Iceland and Denmark. Worldwide retail sales indicated that in 1985 nine of the leading tranquillizers were benzodiazepines which together accounted for three-quarters of the world market (Woods *et al.* 1987). Some members of the benzodiazepine group, for example, diazepam and lorazepam, have traditionally accounted for a substantial proportion of the world market, but the introduction of newer benzodiazepines has resulted in changes in the sales and market shares of individual benzodiazepines.

Prescription audits

Compiling the number of prescriptions written by physicians at a given point in time in different countries is a frequently used technique to assess benzodiazepine usage. However, caution is necessary when comparing data from different areas (Marks 1983). In general, the available information indicates that tranquillizer prescriptions peaked in the USA around 1975 (Rickels 1983), and the same applies to most Western European countries (Boethius and Westerholm 1976).

In addition to providing an estimate of overall usage, surveys of prescriptions can also provide details about the prescriptions themselves as well as about the patients for whom the drugs are prescribed. Thus, survey data indicate that benzodiazepine anxiolytics and hypnotics tend to be used for chronic or recurrent conditions in a substantial majority of instances. Most patients receiving prescriptions for benzodiazepines are suffering from psychiatric disorders, but a substantial proportion are suffering from a wide variety of somatic complaints. It is also found that benzodiazepine use increases sharply with age and that middle-aged women receive almost twice as many prescriptions for these drugs as men do. Older patients also tend to have prescriptions for longer periods of time than do younger patients. Prescription survey data indicate that medical use of benzodiazepines is on the whole consistent with the clinical utility of these medications and that there appears to be little or no evidence for frequent, inappropriate prescribing, at least from these types of data (Woods *et al.* 1987).

Transforming benzodiazepine use into defined daily doses (DDD) has improved comparability of international data, but even this method may not be totally reliable due to the variation in average dose in different countries (Marks 1985*a*). In agreement with the previously mentioned data, this method indicates that the consumption of benzodiazepines was reasonably uniform from one country to another during the 1970s, followed by decreasing levels of use in most countries and a subsequent increase over the last few years. Audits of prescriptions for psychotropic drugs in Reykjavik and total sales (in DDD units) of psychotropic drugs in Iceland were conducted in 1974, 1984, and 1989. A substantial reduction in the use of tranquillizers and hypnotics was observed between 1974 and 1984 and sales figures show a similar trend through 1989. However, although the number of prescriptions for tranquillizers continued to decline somewhat between 1984 and 1989, the reverse was observed for hypnotics. The latter is probably due to changes in prescription regulations (Zoëga *et al.* 1992). But even the DDD method is not infallible when comparing data internationally. Countries with close socio-cultural ties and a common background such as the Nordic countries can have varied patterns of benzodiazepines being used either as anxiolytics or hypnotics. Finally, this method, like other techniques based solely on sales figures or prescription numbers does not take into account the fact that patients may actually consume far less tranquillizers than are prescribed (Marks 1981).

Population surveys

The type of information that is of direct relevance to the assessment of benzodiazepine abuse liability relates to the extent and appropriateness of actual usage of the drugs. Data on the extent and characteristics of long-term regular use is of particular importance in this respect. Population surveys may measure the proportion of individuals who have used the medication over a defined period of time, usually 1 year, or the usage at a point in time.

Studies reported in the early 1970s indicated that approximately one in six individuals had used a tranquillizer during the previous year (Balter *et al.* 1974; Parry *et al.* 1973). These studies found that a uniform 10–17 per cent of the populations of several European countries had used tranquillizers during the previous 12 months and that regular use was reported by 3–8 per cent. Cross-national interview data collected in 1981 in several Western European countries and the USA reported that an average of 12.5 per cent of adults had used prescribed anxiolytics or sedative medication in the previous 12 months (Woods *et al.* 1987). Thus, these data confirm the decline in the level of use over a 10-year period. In 1985–86, Ashton and Golding (1989) found that 3 per cent of respondents in a large-scale UK survey were using a tranquillizer or a hypnotic at the time of the study. Currently, it has been estimated that about one in 10 of the adult population in most industrialized countries receives a prescription for a tranquillizer during the course of 12 months and that the point prevalence may be about 2–3 per cent (Marks 1985*a*; Ashton and Golding 1989). As with other types of studies of benzodiazepine consumption, population surveys have indicated that tranquillizers are used most frequently by people in late middle age or the elderly and twice as often by women compared to men in most age categories. Although the various studies indicate that the benzodiazepines are generally used for relatively short periods of time, an average of one in five users in the USA reported having used tranquillizers regularly during the previous 12 months, and the same applied to one in 10 of those who had used prescription hypnotics in the previous year (Woods *et al.* 1987). Although clinical evidence would suggest that prevalence of long-term use may naturally be substantially less than suggested by the interview studies, the finding of a relatively high level of regular, long-term use of benzodiazepines is the source of serious concern regarding the dependence and abuse potential of these medications. On the other hand, the data indicate that long-term use of benzodiazepines is most likely to develop in elderly patients, perhaps with recurrent psychiatric problems of long duration or multiple somatic disorders, and therefore presents a very different problem from that of the non-medical abuse of benzodiazepines.

Extent of benzodiazepine abuse

Assessment of the abuse liability of drugs usually rests on investigations of physiological and psychological dependence, development of tolerance, and the reinforcing properties of the particular substance. These issues are then set in the context of possible adverse health effects and the appropriate social context.

As indicated before, it is important to make a clear distinction between benzodiazepine dependence within the clinical context on the one hand, and the non-medical abuse of benzodiazepines on the other. There is little evidence of dosage escalation within the clinical setting, even among patients who have used therapeutic doses of benzodiazepines for long periods of time. Nevertheless, experimental studies have revealed that significant levels of tolerance may develop within the clinical context (Pétursson and Lader 1984). The few reports of some patients developing tolerance and escalating their dosage to high levels are not characteristic for the clinical situation, in contrast to benzodiazepine abusers who commonly report a progressive need to increase their drug intake. Physiological dependence to high doses of benzodiazepines was demonstrated soon after their introduction in the early 1960s (Hollister *et al* 1961), and withdrawal effects have been demonstrated repeatedly following termination of normal-dose, long-term benzodiazepine therapy (Pétursson and Lader 1981; Hallström and Lader 1981).

A number of investigations have demonstrated the capacity of benzo-diazepines for reinforcement, i.e. their ability to maintain a drug-seeking behaviour. Studies in animals have indicated that, although benzodiazepines are self-administered, they are less powerful reinforcers than other drugs of abuse, for example barbiturates and stimulants. Most of the human studies have been conducted in drug abusers and alcoholic subjects who have shown a moderate liking for the benzodiazepines. Benzodiazepines are rarely pre-ferred by normal human subjects or even individuals with anxiety. Preference is demonstrated, however, by selected subjects such as heavier drinkers of alcohol (Griffiths and Sannerud 1987; de Wit and Johanson 1991). The apparent differences in relative abuse liability of individual benzodiazepines have been pointed out by Griffiths and Wolf (1990).

It is obvious from numerous reports and surveys of the non-medical use of benzodiazepines that these drugs are abused worldwide and frequently turn up in the illicit drug traffic. The distinction between drug abusers and normal subjects in respect of the reinforcing effects of benzodiazepines seems to be supported by epidemiologial surveys of benzodiazepine abuse. Therefore, and in view of the extensive worldwide use of benzodiazepines, it is essential to have a reasonably accurate estimate of the extent of the non-medical use of benzodiazepines in order to understand the magnitude of and trends in benzodiazepine abuse.

Primary benzodiazepine abuse

Although primary benzodiazepine abuse is probably rare (Smith and Marks 1985), there are a number of reports, notably from some European countries, of patients who appear to be abusing benzodiazepines exclusively. Marks (1978, 1983) has pointed out the fairly small number of cases of primary benzodiazepine abuse within the UK. Reports from other European countries, however, suggest primary benzodiazepine abuse among several hundred patients, although in many instances it is difficult to distinguish primary from secondary benzodiazepine abuse. An important survey of all Swiss physicians was carried out by Ladewig *et al.* (1981) and revealed a surprisingly high proportion of primary benzodiazepine abusers although the problem may well be a minor one taking into account the extensive appropriate medical use of benzodiazepines. Within the illicit drug scene the amount of primary benzodiazepine abuse appears minimal, although in recent years there has been a growing problem with frequently abused drugs such as methaqualon being counterfeited using diazepam (Smith and Marks 1985).

Benzodiazepines and multiple drug abuse

As previously noted, patients who are not drug abusers or alcoholics and who receive benzodiazepines for appropriate medical indications rarely escalate their doses or go on to abuse alcohol or other drugs of abuse. In contrast, the opposite is often seen, i.e. alcoholics or other drug abusers may start to abuse benzodiazepines as a secondary substance of abuse. This is the current situation with benzodiazepine abuse, i.e. the problem is a part of polydrug abuse, presently found in many countries. This applies to alcoholics and abusers of other drugs, the exact pattern of substances depending upon a variety of socio-cultural factors. Benzodiazepines are in this respect not used for euphoric effects, but rather as the sedative component of the polydrug mixture. Smith and Marks (1985) have pointed out that at present the benzodiazepines are accepted as the most commonly used sedatives. Furthermore, although this type of secondary abuse usually rises within the recreational drug scene, some may be due to unwise prescribing of benzodiazepines during drug and alcohol withdrawals.

Surveys of benzodiazepine abuse

Surveys of drug abuse have generally found that benzodiazepine abuse is associated with the abuse of other drugs including alcohol. As previously pointed out, it is uncommon for drug abusers to prefer benzodiazepines initially, but they are typically selected as substances of secondary abuse. Within this context, benzodiazepine abuse probably occurs at modest levels, at least compared to their extensive medical use. However, a number of surveys and investigations have shown that the level of abuse is significant.

In 1981 Mellinger and Balter (1983) discovered that 2.3 per cent of USA women and 2 per cent of men within the age range of 18–79 years reported that they had used prescription anxiolytics during the previous 12 months without appropriate prescriptions. However, in the vast majority of instances this abuse had only occurred infrequently. Woods *et al.* (1987) quote two types of surveys in the USA that have provided information on the non-medical use of drugs among young people. One survey has annually assessed non-medical use of drugs among adolescent students and another is a national household survey that has been conducted every few years during the last two decades. Ten years ago the two surveys showed that 14–15 per cent of school students and other young adults had admitted to non-medical use of anxiolytics, whereas 15–19 per cent reported previous non-medical use of sedatives in general. In 1985 a similar survey indicated that approximately 6.5 million Americans used benzodiazepines non-medically that year. However, as previously, the benzodiazepine abuse was sporadic, i.e. 10 times or less in a lifetime for more than half of those who had reported non-medical use of benzodiazepines. The majority of benzodiazepine abusers were male and three-quarters were under the age of 35 years. Most of the benzodiazepine abusers also reported substantial non-medical use of other drugs and substances of abuse. The regular, ongoing survey of adolescent students found that non-medical use of anxiolytics peaked in 1977 and has since substantially declined. Thus, in 1985, 5.5 per cent of young adults reported non-medical use of tranquillizers in the previous year; less than 2 per cent reported such a use in the previous month. Students who had been to college for 1 to 4 years reported a 3.5 per cent use of tranquillizers in the previous year as opposed to almost 7 per cent in 1980 (Johnston *et al.* 1986; Woods *et al.* 1987).

Although most of the large-scale community surveys of benzodiazepine abuse have originated in the USA, important epidemiological data have also been collected in other countries. Boethius and Westerholm (1977) investigated purchases of benzodiazepines over 5-year periods in a county of Sweden. Although most individuals significantly reduced such purchases over time, 0.6 per cent developed a regular purchasing pattern and a minute proportion demonstrated overuse or abuse of benzodiazepines. Studies reviewed by Woods *et al.* (1987) revealed that 20 years ago between 6 and 9.5 per cent of teenage school students in Halifax, Nova Scotia and in Toronto had experimented with tranquillizers during the previous 6 months. Similar studies of young adults and school students in Asia, Africa, South America, and New Zealand have been reported over the years. The lifetime prevalence of non-medical use of tranquillizers has varied considerably, i.e. from 1 to 20 per cent. In 1984 a survey of 0.7 per cent of all Icelanders in the age range 16–36 years found that approximately 25 per cent of respondents had experimented with illegal substances of abuse, primarily the cannabinoids (Kristmundsson 1985). Only 2.2 per cent admitted to having abused medicines in order to get 'high', and the pattern was exclusively of the polydrug type.

From the available survey data of the general population it appears that benzodiazepines are infrequently abused. Young adults and school students do abuse benzodiazepines, but the data indicate the experimental nature and the relative infrequency of benzodiazepine abuse, even among this age group. Another indicator for decreasing levels of benzodiazepine abuse stems from data collected by the Dawn system in the USA. This system involves structured emergency room reports of non-medical drug use and, although its reliability has been questioned, it provides supplementary information to national survey data. In 1985 it was evident that the 5-year trend data for the mentioning of anxiolytics in emergency room reports was decreasing (Woods et al. 1987). The Dawn data are thus generally consistent with national surveys that suggest that the incidence of benzodiazepine abuse, at least in the USA, has been decreasing in recent years. Similar data has been collected regularly on cases of self-poisoning admitted to the Reykjavík City Hospital casualty ward. In 1976–81 benzodiazepines were involved in 58 per cent of instances, compared to 52 per cent and 47 per cent for the periods 1983–84 and 1987–88, respectively (Hardarson et al. 1986; Oddsson et al. 1989; Sigurbergsson et al. 1991). Similarly, we found that benzodiazepines were involved in 42.6 per cent of suicide attempts in 1983–85 (Pálsson et al. 1990).

Drug abuse and alcoholism

Little data is currently available on benzodiazepine abuse patterns within the illicit drug scene, but a number of reports are available of studies of drug clinic populations. As previously stated, the benzodiazepines are most frequently used by multidrug abusers, usually in combination with other drugs, rather than as a primary drug of abuse. A review (Woods et al. 1987) of studies from the USA and a few European centres indicates that opiate abusers, in particular methadone maintenance patients, are frequently found to abuse benzodiazepines, in particular diazepam. Such individuals report using rather high doses of diazepam in order to increase the effects they obtain from the methadone. Although benzodiazepine abuse may thus represent a significant problem in some methadone maintenance clinics, there is significant variability across clinics. Currently, the magnitude of benzodiazepine abuse among methadone maintenance patients is unknown, and it is also not clear whether this type of drug abuse is characteristic for opiate abusers in general.

Studies of patients who attend alcohol treatment services suggest that problems with benzodiazepine abuse are quite frequent. A study of an alcohol detoxification unit in the USA in 1976 found that 29 per cent had abused hypnotics or anxiolytics (Schuckit and Morrissey 1979). In Canada Busto *et al.* (1982) detected benzodiazepines in the urine of 33 per cent of out-patients with chronic alcoholism compared to none in a control group of medical patients and 4–6 per cent of the general population. In the UK 41 per cent of more than a 100 patients admitted to an alcohol treatment service were using benzodiazepines at the time of admission (Wiseman and Spencer-Peet, 1985). We found that 31 per cent of attenders at a psychiatric emergency clinic had a previous history of benzodiazepine abuse, primarily in combination with abuse of alcohol, and in a few instances with abuse of illicit substances (Pálsson *et al.* 1990). Preliminary data from alcohol treatment services in Iceland indicate that as many as 30–40 per cent of patients admitted to such units may also abuse benzodiazepines (Bergsveinsson and Tyrfingsson, personal communication). Primary benzodiazepine abuse, however, is rarely detected, although as stated before, reports of such nature have occurred from a number of other European countries.

Current situation

Epidemiological studies have shown that the medical use of benzodiazepines reached its highest point in most countries in the mid-1970s followed by a significant decline until the early 1980s. In the last decade or so a slight increase in benzodiazepine use has been observed in many countries, but the overall levels are still substantially below those of the 1970s. The extensive long-term use of benzodiazepines and the occurrence of dependence within the clinical context are a source of major concern, but are not dealt with in this chapter.

Primary benzodiazepine abuse occurs rarely, and there is also very little evidence that patients who are not alcoholics or drug abusers go on to escalate their dose or to abuse alcohol or other drugs. The main problem with benzodiazepine abuse is within the multidrug abuse scene. Survey data have repeatedly demonstrated benzodiazepine abuse in association with use of other drugs and/or alcohol. Although benzodiazepine abuse appears to occur at relatively modest levels compared to their extensive medical use, abuse of benzodiazepines outside of medical practice is by no means trivial. Benzodiazepines are frequently abused along with other drugs or alcohol, and this problem seems to be particularly apparent in some groups of patients, such as opiate addicts during methadone maintenance treatment.

Epidemiological surveys among the general population as well as studies of casualty department attendances support the view that abuse of benzo-diazepines usually occurs in the context of polydrug abuse. In line with the overall reduction in the medical use of benzodiazepines, investigations of non-medical abuse of benzodiazepines suggest that the problem has declined in recent years. However, it is far from clear whether or to what extent clinical use of benzodiazepines may be causally related to their abuse.

On the contrary, most of the data indicate that the latter is a separate problem from problems of dependence within the clinical context. Misuse of benzodiazepines within medical practice may, however, be partly responsible for some instances of abuse, for example, by uncritical use of benzodiazepines among alcoholic patients.

Minimizing benzodiazepine abuse

Policies intended to reduce abuse of benzodiazepines must be based on two main considerations. First, patients for whom benzodiazepines are appropriately prescribed must be ensured continued access to their medication. Second, benzodiazepine abuse is not a unique phenomenon, but forms an intrinsic part of alcohol and multidrug abuse. However, it is clear that benzodiazepine abuse is a significant problem that must be addressed by appropriate regulatory measures and educational efforts at national and international levels. Health authorities concerned with the various forms of drug abuse often resort to use of legislation to try and curb the problem. Drug abuse frequently becomes a problem in several countries and may thus require the intervention of international organizations and control systems. Minimizing problems of drug abuse, however, requires other measures, such as educational efforts, and, on their own, international and national control measures may be inadequate and problematic in practice. (Committee of the Institute for Behaviour and Health 1988).

International control of benzodiazepines

The medical use of benzodiazepines is currently regulated by national laws in the majority of countries. In most places, benzodiazepines are available by prescription only, but certain differences exist between countries regarding details and additional controls attached to the prescription requirements. A further problem is presented by the fact that in some countries socio-economic circumstances may hinder effective implementation of the appropriate legislation and regulation.

International conventions

Throughout this century a number of international conventions and treaties have been negotiated in order to establish international co-operation in the control of drugs of abuse. In 1961 these systems were re-organized and consolidated under a single treaty, the Single Convention of Narcotic Drugs (WHO 1961). However, with the development of synthetic drugs, it became necessary to set up a new international convention for the control of drug abuse, the United Nations' Convention on Psychotropic Substances (1971). The 1971 convention imposes international control on drugs if they are liable to lead to abuse and to produce ill effects similar to those of drugs already scheduled under the conventions. In addition, there are alternative criteria regarding dependence liability and central nervous system effects. This means that new types of drugs, pharmacologically unrelated to presently controlled drugs, can be controlled under the 1971 convention. Evidence must also be demonstrated that 'the substance is being or is likely to be abused' to such an extent that it causes 'a public health and social problem warranting the placing of the substance under international control'. Finally, the risk of abuse of a drug must be weighed against its legitimate medical use.

WHO review process

The Secretary General of the United Nations is formally notified by the World Health Organization or any national government if information has come to light that a substance should be internationally controlled. The notification is then forwarded to the WHO which, with the advice of an expert committee, considers the appropriate scientific and medical evidence that an abuse problem may exist. The review process also includes assessment of therapeutic usefulness of the substance as well as the extent of the problem and international implications. Having considered the WHO report, the final decision whether a substance should be controlled under the 1971 convention rests with the United Nations and its Commission on Narcotic Drugs (CND).

Scheduling of benzodiazepines

The benzodiazepines were first considered for inclusion in schedule IV at the time when the 1971 convention was established. Schedule IV is the least stringent control of the convention and requires that distribution of substances shall be under licence only. Furthermore, drugs can only be dispensed on the basis of medical prescription and there are also reporting requirements on importation and exportation.

The WHO continued to review the status of the benzodiazepines, and recommendations were made during the next few years for the scheduling of benzodiazepines. However, it was not until 1984 that the United Nations' CND decided, upon the recommendation of a WHO expert committee (WHO 1983), to place 33 benzodiazepines in schedule IV of the 1971 Convention on Psychotropic Substances. Although the decision was taken on a substance-by-substance basis, it was pointed out that there are differences among the benzodiazepines and that further studies were needed to determine whether those differences were of sufficient magnitude to warrant differences in scheduling. In 1989, the expert committee reviewed a further four benzodiazepines and recommended that one of them should be included in schedule IV but recommendations on the other three were deferred (WHO 1989).

In 1990 the expert committee on drug dependence examined the available data on the 34 currently controlled benzodiazepines with the aim of determining whether or not they were appropriately scheduled under the 1971 convention. The committee conducted a review according to recently revised guidelines and paid particular attention to trends in abuse pattern and reports of illicit traffic that might reflect adverse effects for public health as well as social problems. Nineteen benzodiazepines were found to be appropriately controlled in their present level in schedule IV. For another 13 benzodiazepines which have been controlled since 1984, the committee found few reports of abuse or illicit activity and recommended that the WHO continue to monitor these substances in order to determine whether they should be placed again under critical review to consider possible descheduling. The committee found that diazepam and flunitrazepam showed higher incidence of abuse and association with illicit activity than other benzodiazepines and recommended that the WHO continue to keep these two substances under surveillance in order to determine the appropriateness of their level of scheduling. Based upon the available information on three additional benzodiazepines, the committee did not recommend scheduling of those substances (WHO 1991).

Consequences of scheduling

Review groups and expert committees of the WHO have repeatedly noted that little data is so far available on the consequences of controlling a substance under the international convention. There are inherent difficulties in studying the consequences of international control due to a number of complex issues. First, and most importantly, patients for whom the drugs are therapeutically indicated must be ensured continued and unhindered access to their medication. It is important to try and determine whether scheduling of a drug has an effect upon the extent and seriousness of abuse of that substance. As has been pointed out previously in this chapter, epidemiological studies are difficult in this field and information may not always be reliable or fully representative. However, such an ongoing assessment is essential and the WHO has recently made additional efforts to implement further evaluation to assist the review process.

Other control measures

The development of abuse of a particular drug depends on a number of factors acting concurrently. These include the pharmacological characteristics of the substance, the personality of the user, and the socio-cultural context within which the abuse takes place. Thus, it is obvious that drug abuse cannot be effectively controlled by regulating the supply of drugs alone. Efforts to reduce demand are even more important, but equally difficult to achieve.

Continued emphasis on the rational prescribing of benzodiazepines is needed. This approach has become increasingly important during the last 10–15 years in view of the development of benzodiazepines with different pharmacological profiles. The physician must also be particularly careful about monitoring the patients' use of alcohol and must inform patients about potential warning signs that benzodiazepine dependence and/or abuse may be developing. Drug and alcohol abusers represent a group of individuals who are particularly at risk for benzodiazepine abuse. Medical staff in alcohol and drug abuse treatment services need to be made more aware of the special vulnerability of their patients in this respect.

As previously noted, the total use of psychotropic medicines has been monitored in the Nordic countries for several years. This may have helped to reduce the overall use of benzodiazepines over the years but more data is required in this area. Some of the control measures applied by health authorities include the reduction in the size of single doses, the number of tablets prescribed at one time, and feeding back information to physicians on the extent and nature of repeat prescriptions. Such prescription surveys could possibly be used even more effectively, for example, to identify smaller populations of polydrug abusers or community areas where special problems may occur.

Further studies and recommendations

In order to identify the various approaches and effective methods to minimize benzodiazepine abuse, further studies are needed of the true extent, nature, and consequences of the problem. In particular, additional research is required to learn more about the role of benzodiazepine abuse in the multidrug abuse scene. Further research is required on the characteristics of the individuals who abuse benzodiazepines and the reasons for their abuse; studies within the field of alcoholism are particularly important. The problem of misuse of benzodiazepines within the medical context requires more attention and appropriate corrective measures. The following is a brief discussion of some of the important issues involved.

Rational use of benzodiazepines

To reduce benzodiazepine abuse, misuse, and dependence it is necessary that medical practitioners and their patients are fully and accurately informed about the rational use of benzodiazepines. Making proper information available to the media and the public in general can also help to avoid some of the stigmatizing effects on patients caused by sensationalism in the press. The WHO Expert Committee on Drug Dependence has urged continued support and expansion of national and international training programmes in the processing and assessment of public health and social problem data as well as the rational use of psychoactive substances. It is important to encourage universities and other institutions to expand their training curriculae with the psychoactive substances in general (WHO 1991). It is important that the effort to minimize benzodiazepine abuse should be undertaken both by government institutions and private sector concerns such as the pharmaceutical industry.

Improved treatment of multidrug abuse

Improved treatment of drug abuse is essential to the reduction of the problem and the research and development of medications to treat abuse disorders appear promising. However, additional basic research is required to clarify further the different patterns of polydrug abuse, the role played by benzodiazepine abuse, and the effects of socio-cultural factors and the relevant pharmacological characteristics of abused substances.

Further investigations are needed regarding the proper and thorough treatment of anxiety and insomnia as well as the treatment of alcohol and drug withdrawal states. In view of the particular vulnerability of drug and alcohol abusers, studies of the non-pharmacological treatment of anxiety and other psychiatric disorders among such individuals are needed. Within the treatment of alcoholism medical practitioners need to be reliably informed that benzodiazepines should normally be limited to short-term detoxification purposes and that every effort must be made to detect and reduce the non-medical use of any drugs in this abuse-prone population of patients.

Role of international organizations

As previously noted, most of the data evaluating overdose or abuse of benzodiazepines originate in the USA or Europe. There is a lack of systematic information-gathering in many parts of the world, and it has been recommended that international agencies, such as the WHO, should liaise with selected countries or institutions to facilitate assessment of benzodiazepine abuse problems in different regions of the world. Furthermore, a setting up of surveillance programmes as early monitoring systems for detecting abuse of drugs in medical use would be advantageous to future deliberations of national authorities and international organizations such as the WHO (WHO 1991).

Last but not least, the various WHO expert committees and working groups have repeatedly emphasized the importance of the studying of the consequences of scheduling of psychoactive substances. The WHO has initiated limited investigations of the impact of scheduling in a small number of countries. It goes without saying that control methods currently in use should be carefully monitored, the aim being to achieve the best level of control over benzodiazepine abuse, with minimum negative impact upon patients and legitimate medical practice.

Assessment of abuse liability

The benzodiazepines have served us well as safe and effective anxiolytics and hypnotics during the past 30 years or so. However, their use is not without problems of dependence and abuse, and thus safer alternatives are now being actively sought. Extensive research efforts are being expended in order to address the issue of abuse liability. Regulatory authorities are constantly pressing for more information in this area and at a recent conference on anxiolytic trial methodology, the need for early and effective screening of abuse liability of any new anxiolytic was emphasized (Pétursson, 1991).

Griffiths and Wolf (1990) have pointed out the apparent differences in abuse liability of different benzodiazepines. Compared to conventional agonist benzodiazepines, the newer drugs such as partial benzodiazepine agonists may have lesser reinforcing activity and lower abuse liability (Sellers *et al.* 1991). While retaining the desired effects of conventional benzodiazepines, partial benzodiazepine agonists appear to have a selective profile, i.e. reduced central nervous system depression and possibly less development of tolerance, physiological dependence, and reinforcement (Haefely 1991). Non-benzodiazepine anxiolytics are being extensively investigated, and some appear to have low dependence potential during initial clinical studies (Lader and Morton 1991; Garreau *et al.* 1991). While pre-clinical and clinical studies are helpful predictors of abuse and dependence, the relative problems of dependence and abuse of the newer anxiolytics as compared to benzodiazepines will only become known after extensive and long-term usage of the new medications.

References

Ashton, H. and Golding, J.F. (1989). Tranquillisers: prevalence, predictors and possible consequences. Data from a large United Kingdom survey. *British Journal of Addiction*, **84**, 541–6.

Balter, M.B., Levine, J., and Manheimer, D.I. (1974). Cross-national study of the extent of anti-anxiety/sedative drug use. *New England Journal of Medicine* **290**, 769–74.

Bergman, U. (1981). Studies on patterns and prevalence of psychiatric drug use—data from the Nordic countries. In *Epidemiological impact of psychotropic drugs* (ed. G. Tognoni, C. Bellantuono, and M. Lader), pp.183–7. Elsevier Science Publishers, Amsterdam.

Boethius, G. and Westerholm, B. (1976). Is the use of hypnotics, sedatives and minor tranquillisers really a major health problem? *Acta Medica Scandinavica*, **199**, 507–12.

Boethius, G. and Westerholm, B (1977). Purchases of hypnotics, sedatives and minor tranquillisers among 2566 individuals in the county of Jämtland, Sweden: a six year follow-up. *Acta Psychiatrica Scandinavica*, **156**, 147–59.

Busto, U., Sellers, E.M., Sisson, B., and Segal, R. (1982). Benzodiazepine use and abuse in alcoholics. *Clinical Pharmacology and Therapeutics*, **31**, 207–8.

Committee of the Institute for Behaviour and Health (1988). Abuse of benzodiazepines: the problems and solutions (ed. R.L. DuPoint). *American Journal of Drug and Alcohol Abuse*, **14** (suppl. 1), 1–69.

de Wit, H. and Johanson, C.E. (1991). Benzodiazepine abuse potential in normal and anxious individuals. In *Biological psychiatry* (ed. G. Racagni, N. Brunello, T. Fukuda), pp.771–4. Elsevier Science Publishers, Amsterdam.

Garreau, M., de Wilde, J., Frattola, L., L'Heritier, C., Boval, P., and Morselli, P.L. (1991). Anxiolytics and dependence. Two double-blind studies of alpidem versus benzodiazepines. In *Biological psychiatry* (ed. G. Racagni, N. Brunello, T. Fukuda), pp.696–8. Elsevier Science Publishers, Amsterdam.

Griffiths, R.R. and Sannerud, C.A. (1987) Abuse of and dependence on benzo-diazepines and other anxiolytics/sedative drugs. In *Psychparmacology: the third generation of progress* (ed. H.Y., Meltzer), pp.1535–4. Raven Press, New York.

Griffiths, R.R. and Wolf, B. (1990). Relative abuse liability of different benzo-diazepines in drug abusers. *Journal of Clinical Psychopharmacology*, **10** (4), 237–43.

Haefely, W. (1991). Pharmacology of partial agonists at the benzodiazepine receptor. In *Biological psychiatry* (ed. G. Racagni, N. Brunello, and T. Fukuda), pp.705–8. Elsevier Science Publishers, Amsterdam.

Hardarson, Th.H., Oddsson, G., Jonsson, B., and Sigurdsson, G. (1986). Lyfjaei-tranir á lyflaekningadeild Borgarspítalans árin 1976–1981. *Laeknabladid (Icelandic Medical Journal)*, **72**, 89–92.

Hallström, C. and Lader, M.H. (1981). Benzodiazepine withdrawal phenomena. *International Pharmacopsychiatry*, **16**, 235–44.

Hollister, L.E. Motzenbecker, F.P., and Degan, R.O. (1961). Withdrawal reactions from chlordiazepoxide ('Librium'). *Psychopharmacologia*, **2**, 63–8.

Johnston, L.D., O'Malley, P.M., and Bachman, J.G. (1986). *Drug use among American high school students, college students and other young adults: national trends through* 1985, DHHS Publication (ADM) no. 86–1450. US Public Health Service, Rockville, Maryland.

Kristmundsson, Ó.H. (1985). *Ólögleg ávana–og fíkniefni á Íslandi.* Dóms- og kirkjumálaráduneytid, Reykjavík.

Lader, M. and Morton, S. (1991) Anxiolytics and withdrawal signs: comparative studies of alpidem and benzodiazepines. In *Biological psychiatry* (ed. G. Racagni, N. Brunello, and T. Fukuda), pp.693–5. Elsevier Science Publishers, Amsterdam.

Ladewig, D., Banziger, W., and Lowenheck, M. (1981). Tranquilliser abuse—results of a nationwide Swiss survey. *Journal of Drug Research*, **6**, 1132–7.

Marks, J. (1978). The benzodiazepines: use, overuse, misuse, abuse. MTP Press, Lancaster.

Marks, J. (1981). Diazepam—the question of long-term therapy and withdrawal reactions. *Drug Therapy*, (special suppl.).

Marks, J. (1983). Benzodiazepines—for good or evil. *Neuropsychobiology*, **10**, 115–26.

Marks, J. (1985*a*). An international overview. *In the benzodiazepines, current standards for medical practice* (ed. D.E. Smith and D.R. Wesson), pp.67–86. MTP Press, Lancaster.

Marks, J. (1985*b*). Benzodiazepines: international legislation and relation to the Convention on Psychotropic Substances 1971. In *The benzodiazepines, current standards for medical practice* (ed. D.E. Smith and D.R. Wesson), pp.267–85. MTP Press, Lancaster.

Mellinger, G.D. and Balter, M.B. (1983). Psychotropic drugs: a current assessment of prevalence and pattern of use. In *Society and medication: Conflicting signals for prescribers and patients* (ed. J.P. Morgan and D.V. Kagan), pp.137–44. D.C. Heath and Co., Lexington, KY.

Prevalence and patterns of use of psychotherapeutic drugs: results from a 1979 national survey of American adults. In *Epidemiological impact of psychotropic drugs* (ed. G. Tognoni, C. Bellantuono, and M. Lader), pp.117–35. Elsevier/North Holland, Amsterdam.

Nordiska läkemedelsnämnden (Nordic Council on Medicines) (1979). *Nordisk Läkemedelsstatistik* 1978–1980. NLN publication no. 8, Uppsala.

Oddsson, G., Kristinsson, J., Hardarson, Th. H., and Jakobsson, F. (1989).

Lyfjaeitranir á brádamóttöku Borgarspítalans á sex mánada tímabili 1983– 1984. *Laeknabladid (Icelandic Medical Journal)*, **75**, 5–9.

Pálsson, S.P. Jónsdóttir, G. & Pétursson, H. (1990) Emergency psychiatry in a general hospital *Nordisk Psykiatrisk. Tidsskrift*, **44**, 345–52.

Parry, H.J., Balter, M.B., Mellinger, G.D., Cisin, I.H., and Manheimer, D.I. (1973). National patterns of psychotherapeutic drug use. *Archives of General Psychiatry*, **7** (28), 769–83.

Pétursson, H. (1991). Dependency risk as a target for clinical trials of anxiolytic drugs. In *Abstracts of the Fourth Consensus Conference: Methodology of Clinical Trials of Anxiolytic Drugs*, Münich, 27th-29th October 1991.

Pétursson, H. and Lader, M.H. (1981). Withdrawal from long-term benzodiazepine treatment. *British Medical Journal*, **283**, 643–5.

Pétursson, H. and Lader, M. (1984). *Dependence on tranquillisers*, Maudsley Monograph, no. 28. Oxford University Press, Oxford.

Rickels, K. (1983). Benzodiazepines in the treatment of anxiety: North-American experience. In *The benzodiazepines: from molecular biology to clinical practice* (ed. E. Costa), pp.295–310. Raven Press, New York.

Schuckit, M.A. and Morrissey, E.R. (1979). Drug abuse among alcoholic women. *Journal of Psychiatry*, **136**, 607–11.

Sellers, E.M., Busto, U., and Kaplan, H.L. (1991). Clinical abuse liability of partial and full agonist benzodiazepines: A comparison of bretazenil, diazepam and alprazolam. In *Biological psychiatry* (ed. G., Racagni, N. Brunello, and T., Fukuda), pp.709–12. Elsevier Science Publishers, Amsterdam.

Sigurbergsson F., Oddsson, G., and Kristinsson, J. (1991). Rannsóknir á lyfjaeitrunum á Borgarspítala 1987–1988. Tháttur ólöglegra ávana–og fíkniefna í lyfjaeitrunum. *Laeknabladid (Icelandic Medical Journal)*, **77**, 384–90.

Smith, D.E. and Marks, J. (1985). Abuse and dependency: an international perspective. In *The benzodiazepines: current standards for medical practice*, (ed. D.E. Smith and D.R. Wesson), pp.179–99. MTP Press, Lancaster.

Wiseman, S.M. and Spencer-Peet, J. (1985). Prescribing for alcoholics: a survey of drugs taken prior to admission to an alcoholism unit. *Practitioner*, **229**, 88–9.

WHO (World Health Organization) (1961). Convention on psychotropic substances, Publication E/CONF.58/6. United Nations, New York.

WHO (World Health Organization) (1983) *Eighth review of psychoactive substances for international control*, Document MNH/83.28. WHO, Geneva.

WHO (World Health Organization Expert Committee on Drug Dependence) (1989). *Twenty-sixth report*. WHO technical report series, no. 787. WHO, Geneva.

WHO (World Health Organization Expert Committee on Drug Dependence) (1991). *Twenty-seventh report*. WHO technical report series, no. 808. WHO, Geneva.

Woods, J.H., Katz, J.L., and Winger, G. (1987). Abuse liability of benzodiazepines. *Pharmacology Reviews*, **39** (4), 251–419.

Zoëga, T., Björnsson, J., and Helgason, T. (1992). Samanburdur á gedlyfjaávísunum utan sjúkrahúsa í Reykjavík í mars 1989 og í mars 1984. *Laeknabladid (Icelandic Medical Journal)*, **78**, 23–31.

13 Dependence on hypnotics

Anthony Clift

What is the point of concerning ourselves with dependence on prescribed drugs when all that doctors are doing is attempting to alleviate symptoms? The matter has recently been brought into perspective by the litigation against manufacturers and prescribers of benzodiazepine drugs. Many of the plaintiffs consider that they suffered unacceptable side-effects, especially on withdrawal from the drug, and, indeed, believe that they developed adverse effects while actually on the drug.

I must say I have some sympathy for the busy general practitioner who only wants to give relief and has neither the time nor the skills for lengthy psychotherapy applied to the numerous people who attend his surgery with complaints of anxiety, minor depression, and insomnia, which he may well feel should be dealt with in a non-medical setting.

As insomnia is a fairly well understood condition, at least in the sense that we all have had experience of inadequate sleep, the use of drugs for its relief lends itself to more precise study than other complaints requiring tranquillizers.

The general practitioner needs to know the following.

1. Which drugs can cause dependence?

2. Does dependence matter?

3. How can I prevent it occurring if I do prescribe a drug?

4. If I do suspect dependence what do I do?

Drug dependence—a confusion of definition

The WHO definition of drug dependence (WHO 1969) is generally accepted but as Seevers (1968) has pointed out, 'it has long been known that the phenomenon of physical dependence would never play a role in drug seeking behaviour with the depressants if the individual NEVER AT ANY TIME during his life suffered withdrawal from the drug. This fact in itself assigns the major role in drug-seeking behaviour with the depressant drugs to primary psychological dependence based upon reward . . .'

This aspect of primary psychological dependence, especially dependence on prescribed dosage without necessarily escalating the dose, will be familiar to general practitioners who may have patients on hypnotics for many years

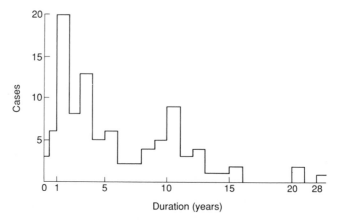

Fig. 13.1. Number of patients on regular sleeping medication in a British general practice. Taken with permission from Johnson and Clift (1968).

(Fig. 13.1). The reward is simply a good night's sleep or, at least, the temporary oblivion that the hypnotic drug obtains. Again, as Seevers points out, 'another parameter, secondary psychological dependence, is initiated and maintained as negative reinforcement from actual or contemplated drug withdrawal.' This may be a dominant factor especially as tolerance development diminishes the intensity of drug reward.

I think many general practitioners will recognize the strength of Seever's argument about the psychological component of dependence. Patients start with the request for a good night's sleep (for insomnia of whatever cause) and continue to take the drug as they enjoy the effect. The effect lessens and the patient possibly increases the dose. Finally, there is a continual further demand for the drug for fear of the possible insomnia that may follow withdrawal.

The problem of physical or psychological dependence is merely a matter of semantics for most general practitioners who may well not have observed, or had it reported to them that there was tolerance or escalation. It is hardly surprising that many patients will never report increased dose, side-effects such as morning drowsiness, or, especially, withdrawal effects as they fear that the general practition might well withdraw the crutch that has become an apparent necessity. In the author's experience of investigating patients who had apparently become dependent on tranquillizers and, indeed, recognized the fact themselves, many avoided bringing up the subject of side-effects in case the drug would be withdrawn by the prescriber.

Where was the drug prescribed?

As virtually all hypnotics require a medical prescription it follows, at least in the UK, that they must first be prescribed in hospital or general practice.

It is an ever-surprising source of amazement that hospitals still do not seem to have learned the lesson that much hypnotic prescribing starts when the patient is admitted for something unrelated to insomnia. A new environment and the worry of an operation and of leaving things unattended at home are just some of the myriad possible causes of insomnia in hospital patients. At least 20 per cent of chronic hypnotic prescribing starts in hospital (Johnson and Clift 1968) yet the practice of prescribing hypnotics is still very common, the initiative for the drug, after the initial doctor's prn prescription, being left with the ward sister. I suspect that most junior doctors prefer to sign the patient up for a hypnotic on admission rather than be called out at at night to prescribe for a restless patient.

The recent changes in the UK National Health Service (NHS) associated with indicative prescribing targets for general practitioners, many of whom will be managing their own budget, will undoubtedly lead to general practitioners demanding certain standards from hospitals who wish to have their contract. One such standard could certainly be that of not discharging patients with the expectation of their receiving continuing prescriptions for hypnotics. It may be that the only way to ensure this is to decline to prescribe them in hospital except in exceptional circumstances.

Which drugs are used?

In 1989, the last year for which figures are available, the UK Department of Health and Social Security (DHSS) listed no fewer than 66 different hypnotic drugs, although a few are duplicated by reason of physical state, e.g. tablets and capsules of temazepam, and also by reason of different dose tablets or capsules. The 'top 10' drugs are given in Table 13.1. Barbiturates are still used with the following number of prescriptions in the UK in 1989.

Drug	Prescriptions
Tuinal, 100 mg	73 800
Soneryl, 100 mg	69 100
Sodium amytal, 200 mg	50 200

This is despite the introduction of the controlled drug classification and the more irksome method of writing prescriptions associated with this.

The latest non-benzodiazepine drug, zopicolone (Zimovane), was prescribed 600 times as a generic drug and 9400 times under its trade name Zimovane despite its huge cost and (recently) doubts about its dependence capacity (Merec 1991).

Although, strictly speaking, we are not concerned about cost in this book, it must be of interest to both the NHS and the manufacturers and it is worth reminding ourselves of some differences in the price of drugs.

Table 13.1. The top 10 drugs

Drug	From	Dose	No. of prescriptions in 1989 ($\times 10^3$)
Temazepam	Capsule	10 mg	4684.2
Nitrazepam	Tablet	5 mg	4185.5
Temazepam	Capsule	20 mg	2275.5
Triazolam	Tablet	250 mcg	1423.2
Triazolam	Tablet	125 mcg	720.0
Heminevrin	Capsule		284.3
Welldorm	Tablet		182.4
Loprazolam	Tablet	1 mg	174.1
Lormetazepam	Tablet	1 mg	152.3
Temazepam	Tablet	10 mg	106.7

Obviously, a drug-dependent patient is a ready source of income to the pharmaceutical company concerned. The following figures are taken from the November 1990 copy of *MIMS*: Normison (temazepam), 10 mg, UK £6.66/100 tablets; Mogadon (nitrazepam), 5 mg, UK £4.80/100 capsules; Tuinat (barbiturate), 100 mg, UK £2.68/100 capsules; Zimovane (Zopiclone), 7.5 mg, UK £98.00/100 tablets (MIMS 1990).

No doubt zopiclone will come down in price in due course as has happened to other drugs before, but meanwhile we do not know its potential to give rise to dependence. It has a fairly short half-life of 5–6, the adverse effects reported have had a proportion of psychiatric reactions similar to those of the benzodiazepines (zopiclone is not a benzodiazepine), and some volunteers have reported anxiety and lighter sleep following withdrawal of the drug (Merec 1991).

In general, the literature does not distinguish different benzodiazepine drugs as more or less likely to give rise to drug dependence, but there is little doubt that, in recent years, it has become apparent that the short-acting drugs such as temazepam, lorazepam, and triazolam are more likely to give rise to adverse effects on sudden cessation (Tyrer *et al.* 1983). It is also clear that, despite promotional statements, all benzodiazepine drugs can be used as sleeping tablets.

What changes have occurred over the years?

The obvious change over the last 20 years has been the gradual substitution of benzodiazepines for barbiturates (Table 13.2). From Table 13.2 we can see that the total number of prescriptions for hypnotics has dropped somewhat and that drugs prescribed are predominantly in the non-barbiturate, mainly benzodiazepine group. This is not entirely accurate as, with the rise in prescription charges and possibly for other reasons, many doctors prescribe for more than a month at a time, and prescriptions may be for larger quantities than hitherto.

There is little doubt that the principal changes in hypnotic prescribing have arisen because of the dangers of overdose associated with the barbiturates and illustrated by the death of many prominent people often in show business.

Unfortunately, it is often forgotten that, although the benzodiazepines are relatively safe in overdose, they are still frequently used, often together with alcohol, for suicide attempts, and this combination can be successful. Moreover, the dangerous side-effects of barbiturate withdrawal, especially grand mal convulsions, *have* been reported with benzodiazepines (Hollister *et al.* 1961).

As far as hypnotics are concerned the principal changes over the years have been from bromides to barbiturates and then to benzodiazepines. There has long been a fashion for chloral hydrate and also for heminevrin in recent years but these have a comparatively small share of the market. One of the problems over the years has been confusion over the following two points.

1. Does sleep disturbance cause mental illness or is the reverse true?

2. Is a patient drug-dependent if he is only taking prescribed drugs and apparently not abusing them.

As to the first point, most commentators nowadays would regard insomnia as the result of some kind of mental disturbance rather than the cause of it. Numerous experiments on sleep deprivation have shown that it has little effect on normal volunteers except after marked deprivation over 200 hours when irritability and misperceptions can occur (Davis and Horne 1975).

As regards the second point, the concept of drug dependence on prescribed drugs has been difficult for general practitioners to accept—who would want to think they were responsible for creating a drug addict? Many general practitioners also find it difficult to prescribe a small quantity, say, 10 tablets knowing that the patient has to pay a prescription charge. It will be shown

Table 13.2. Barbiturates to benzodiazepines in 2 decades

| Year | No of prescription ($\times 10^6$) in given year | |
	Barbiturates	Non-barbiturates*
1971	11.7	7.7
1989	0.25	14.8

* Mainly benzodiazepines.

later, however, that it is generally the general practitioner who has allowed a significant number of patients to become dependent.

Certainly Marks (1978) considers that dependence cannot be considered present unless there has been a formal attempt to discontinue the drug, and that this attempt has been found impossible because of withdrawal symptoms. The matter was put to the test by Giblin and Clift (1983) in a group of patients taking hypnotics for at least 6 months with the following results.

1. All patients withdrawn from hypnotics suffered withdrawal effects.

2. Any withdrawal effects largely vanished over 10–14 days.

3. Without some kind of help people who try to stop taking sleeping pills tend to surrender to withdrawal effects within the first few days.

Historical aspects

The barbiturates held centre stage for over 60 years and during that time (Veronal was introduced in 1903) there was a long-standing dispute between those who maintained they were reasonably safe if not abused (represented by Maurice Craig) and those who were concerned about numerous cases of drug dependence and possible toxic sequelae (as represented by William Wilcox 1927. Wilcox certainly recognized the dangers

There can be no doubt that the very large group of barbituric acid derivatives occupies the foremost place amongst the drugs of addiction. The actual danger to the public in this country at present from addiction to these drugs is greater than that from any other group of drugs, even including the dangerous drugs, which are controlled by special Acts and Regulations . . . the risk of suicide from accidental or purposeful overdosage is very real and the medical profession should exercise great care in the prescription of these drugs.

The development of the benzodiazepines in the 1960s (nitrazepam was intro-duced in 1965 as 'the successor to the hypnotics' and with the claim that it had a unique mode of action . . . on the limbic rather than the reticular system of the brain as distinct from the barbiturates) led to controversy as to the dependence potential, which in some sense mirrored the previous controversy of the 1920s and 1930s relating to barbiturates. The fact that it was difficult to kill oneself with benzodiazepine overdosage made many doctors much less circumspect about their use but it was soon clear in a prospective longitudinal study (Clift 1972) that prescription of benzodiazepine hypnotics was as likely to lead to long-term use as prescription of barbiturates. The extensive monograph by Marks (1978) came to the conclusion that, 'although it is difficult to assess dependence risk in absolute terms because of its multifactorial nature, the risk for benzodiazepines is very low in relation to their wide availability over a period of almost 20 years, and extremely low in the therapeutic situation.'

Marks made it clear (at least in reference to hypnotics) that he was only prepared to accept that a patient was dependent if an attempt had been made by the physician to persuade the patient to give up taking the tablets. Thus he excluded the huge number of patients who continued to take the tablets simply because they felt they needed them even if they had been asked at the initial prescription to come off the drug as soon as they felt it possible. He did not recognize that this group (about 8 per cent of those prescribed hypnotics) were clearly different from those capable of taking hypnotics over a short period only in order to deal with a specific problem—usually one of situational anxiety. This situation was already well known with the barbiturates as most of those taking them long term were in fact on therapeutic dosage and rarely escalated the dose even if they declined to come off their 'steady state' of drugs (Johnson and Clift 1968).

It was the inadvertent cessation of such therapeutic drug usage that led researchers in Scandinavia to discover the danger of withdrawal convulsions in a number of patients who had been admitted to hospital for other reasons (Wulff 1955).

It would be foolish to consider only the dangers of convulsions, which must surely be an end-point for neurological damage. The fact that these can occur after certain doses of benzodiazepines (Hollister *et al.* 1961) should alert the doctor to the possibilities of more subtle changes that may not produce overt symptoms. I am indebted to Dr Paul Firth of Sale (personal communication) for a list of withdrawal symptoms (Table 13.3) that have been observed by doctors from time to time in patients prescribed benzodiazepine drugs. All

Table 13.3. Benzodiazepine withdrawal symptoms

Psychiatric	Central nervous system	Photophobia
		Hyperosmis
Anxiety	Tremor headache	Metallic taste
Agitation	Incoordination	
Irritability	Vertigo	**Miscellaneous**
Aversion	Convulsions	
Insomnia	Paraesthesia	Profuse perspiration
Depersonalization	Formication	Severe weight loss
Derealization	Hypersensitivity to touch	Palpitations
Disorientation	and pain	Anorexia
Dysphoria	Perioral numbness	Nausea
Depression	Increased reflexes	Weakness
Memory loss		Lack of energy
Confusion	**Special senses**	Constipation
Lack of concentration		Difficulties with micturition
Hallucinosis	Tinnitus	Muscular pains
Psychosis	Hyperacusis	Cramps
Paranoia	Blurred vision	Abdominal pains

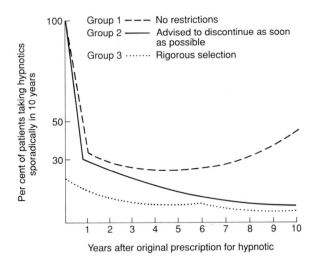

Fig. 13.2. Decrease in the use of hypnotics in groups given differing advice (Clift 1982).

the symptoms in Table 13.3 are equally likely to occur after benzodiazepine hypnotics are withdrawn and, as Firth points out in a useful review of the literature, long-term use at normal dosage is as likely to cause problems as is short-term treatment at high dosage.

Drug dependence as a longitudinal study

A long-term follow-up of three groups of patients who had been treated differently at the outset was reported by Clift (1975).

Group 1. This group had no restrictions on prescribing of hypnotics over the first year. A hypnotic was prescribed on request even if other treatment was given. As can be seen in Fig. 13.2, a large number of these patients continued hypnotic use for years. Such research at the time (1970) mirrored common practice. It would not now be ethical.

Group 2. This group were advised to discontinue hypnotics as soon as possible but prescriptions were given if requested. Otherwise they were treated as the first group.

Group 3. This group underwent rigorous selection before a hypnotic drug was prescribed as the only possible way of relieving insomnia, all other means having been exhausted. They were advised to discontinue the drug as soon as possible.

These groups were followed up over a 10-year period although some were lost to the practice because they left the area or for other reasons. The results (Fig. 13.2) show that there is a small number of patients who will take hypnotics on a long-term basis. There is, however, a large number of patients who will discontinue the drug within a few weeks. What is the difference between those patients and those who take hypnotics on a long-term basis? An analysis from the author's practice (Clift 1975) suggested that those prone to dependence tend to have the characteristics shown in Table 13.4.

In the general practice context, long-term use of a hypnosedative drug can be considered to be the same as dependence inasmuch as the patient continues to take the drug for fear of the consequences of not doing so. In practical terms it matters little if this is because of withdrawal effects such as muscle tremor, nausea, or heightened anxiety, or if it is because of fear of insomnia—the result is the same, namely continual use of the drug, taken not to manage a disease process such as cardiac disease or depressive illness but for the alleviation of inconvenient symptomatology, in this case insomnia.

Table 13.4. Characteristics of the dependence-prone patient

High personal disturbance (greater then 6 on the personal disturbance scale of Foulds)

A psychiatric cause for insomnia

Previous use of hypnotics in earlier life

Mixed or lacunary type insomnia

Vivid dreams

A tendency to increase the hypnotic dose from one to two tablets within the first 2 weeks of treatment.

Was the drug prescribed correctly?

Dependence cannot occur unless the drug is prescribed in the first instance.

Causes of insomnia

The American Psychiatric Association's *Diagnostic and statistical manual of mental disorders* (DSM-III-R, APA 1987) describes insomnias as 'disorders of initiating and maintaining sleep' with nine subcategories.'

1. psychophysiological;

2. psychiatric;

3. drug-induced;

4. associated with sleep induced respiratory impairment such as sleep apnoea;

5. myoclonus and restless legs;

6. medical, toxic, and environmental;

7. childhood onset;

8. unexplained sleep disorders;

9. subjective insomnia not substantiated by observation.

In the author's experience these mainly fall into three categories.

1. medical (including 3, 5, and 6);

2. psychiatric (including 2);

3. psychological (including 1 and 9).

The DSM-III R subcategory no.7 is really a life pattern of poor sleep and does not merit hypnotic drug use as such patients do not really need as much sleep as the average person even if they regret this.

Subcategories 4 and 5 include a ragbag of rare conditions, such as people who wake up every time there is a change in sleep rhythm, e.g. from REM sleep. Sleep apnoea is very rare.

Classification of sleep disorders is important as the patient may just ask for a hypnotic without recognizing that his insomnia may be due to a disease such as depression that can be properly treated by other means. Careless use of a hypnotic in these circumstances can be the beginning of a lifetime use of the drug.

Incidentally, in the writer's practice 20 per cent of a random sample of patients, attending for a consultation not for sleep disturbance and questioned about their sleep, considered themselves poor sleepers although none of these had asked for hypnotics. It seems that the value given to sleep is more important than the actual insomnia and explains the DSM-III R subcategory 9.

It is now well accepted that the approach to sleep disturbance must be based on the cause and, if this is basically a problem of life-style or social situation, then the problem must be addressed rather than simply resorting to drugs. General practice is increasingly moving towards a multidisciplinary primary care team approach, and it is vital that this should be strengthened rather than weakened as a result of new contractual changes. A general practitioner is powerless to deal with social problems that may be fundamental to his patient's insomnia and give rise to a request for tranquillizers or hypnotics. It is far more cost-efficient to look at the source of a problem early on rather than to wait until drug dependence has been established with all the associated misery to patient and family, and subsequent expensive management schemes involving psychologists and long periods of group psychotherapy in one of the many drug withdrawal groups mushrooming all over the country.

Effect of age on sleep needs

It is a well known fact that sleeping tablets are used much more by the elderly, who may overvalue sleep as a means to reduce loneliness and boredom. It is important that patients understand that sleep needs lessen as one gets older (Fig.13.3). Change in the patient's pattern with a daytime nap may be commonplace although the total sleep in 24 is similar to that during adult working life. One of the main reasons why patients end up on long-term hypnotic prescriptions is simply because their expectations for sleep are unrealistic. A few minutes' explanation at the beginning can save the general practitioner endless prescriptions later on—prescriptions that may in the end be used only to prevent the problems of withdrawal rather than promote good sleep (as described in a later section of the methodology for drug withdrawal).

How long does it take to become dependent on hypnotics?

As shown in the graphs for long-term use (Fig.13.2) those who discontinued the drug usually did so within 2 to 4 weeks of the initial prescription. It is now

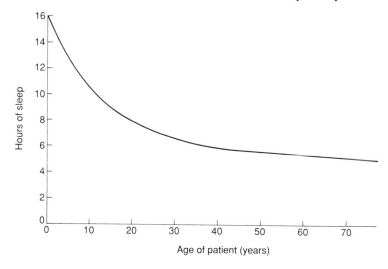

Fig. 13.3. Sleep requirements lessen with age.

recognized that dependence can develop quite early. Oswald (1965) had shown that the EEG (electroencephalogram) changes associated with hypnotic drug usage took about 5 weeks to return to normal after nitrazepam was given at a therapeutic dosage for only 14 days. The advice now commonly given is that hypnotics such as the benzodiazepines should not be given for more than 4 months if dependence is to be avoided (Owen and Tyrer 1983) but most doctors would find it quite difficult to withdraw the drug after even only a month of use.

Should hypnotics be long- or short-acting?

From the dependence point of view there may be little in it, as, whether short- or long-acting, the drug is first taken for its therapeutic aspects and subsequently may be taken to prevent withdrawal symptoms. Short-acting drugs such as clobazam and the slightly longer-acting temazepam can produce a withdrawal effect while in use as the blood levels rapidly fall due to a short half-life (Fig. 13.4; see also Breimer 1978).

Short half-life hypnotics leave the patient fresh on awakening. This accounts for the popularity of temazepam as a hypnotic, but a short half-life can also lead to a shortened sleep, the desire to take another tablet, or to take an increased dose the next night. Most general practitioners will have patients who have escalated their temazepam hypnotic from 10 to 20 mg or to even higher doses. As Breimer also points out, nitrazepam with a very long half-life would continue to produce drowsiness the next day (of course, it does in some people) if it were not for adaptation and tolerance with the likely development of pharmacological dependence.

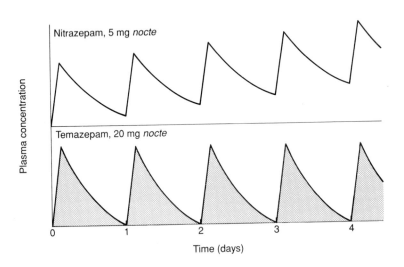

Fig. 13.4. Plasma levels of nitrazepam and temazepam after nightly dosing.

Personality as a factor—can you detect the dependence-prone type?

Certainly in the study carried out by the author in 1971 it was not possible to identify any susceptible personality except for the manipulative hysterical type who is well known to general practitioners for frequent demands for many things and with a low tolerance for any misadventure. However, if we look further towards the field of personal disturbance, as described by Foulds and Hope (1968), there is some evidence that persons scoring highly on the personal disturbance scale were somewhat more disposed to long-term drug usage, and the scale might well be used as a discriminator. For details of this short test, which is not primarily a test of personality, the reader is referred to Foulds (1965).

What alternatives to drugs do we have?

Hollister (1972) quotes Mies van der Rohe's dictum about architecture 'less is more' and applies it to the drug scene in medical practice. I find myself very much in sympathy with this attitude, and drug management of sleep problems should be looked at more as a fine-tuning operation than as a new way of life. If this is to be done, the fundamental problems causing sleep disturbance will have to be dealt with by the right people. This means that doctors must have an easily available team of social workers, counsellors, health visitors, and psychologists. The doctors themselves must look carefully for organic causes of insomnia that are subject to management by eradicating the cause. Of course, there are numerous homely remedies for sleep disturbance ranging from a comfortable bed to a chocolate drink at bedtime. Giblin and Clift (1983) advised the following.

1. Relaxation techniques, possibly using a tape.

2. Information to give a more accurate idea of sleep requirements and sleep-preventing behaviour. Cognitive restructuring should include the concepts that sleep is a natural phenomenon that can be blocked by pain, worry, etc.; that a bad night's sleep is usually followed by a better one; and that it does not help to overvalue sleep. Wakeful periods should be used up with pleasant thoughts about family, hobbies, etc. (Saying one's prayers can also help.)

3. Stimulus control, which means avoiding: television in the bedroom; exciting films before bedtime; or having snacks and cups of tea. Reading is usually not a good idea once one has settled for the night.

All these ideas are equally valuable to the patient endeavouring to withdraw from hypnotics.

Alcohol

It is well known that alcohol can alleviate the withdrawal symptoms from benzodiazepines and cross-tolerance is well established. Indeed, benzodiazepines are used to deal with the withdrawal symptoms in alcoholics. Patients need to be warned of the danger of increasing alcohol intake after the cessation of benzodiazepines.

Prevention rather than treatment

If drug dependence is to be prevented then selective use of the hypnotics in those less vulnerable (e.g. as assessed by the personal disturbance scale) is one approach. It is, however, more important to manage the causes of the insomnia correctly and, as these causes divide into organic, psychiatric, and situational anxiety components, the treatment must be similarly divided. Suffice it to say that most general practitioners are well capable of recognizing an organic cause for insomnia such as dyspnoea. It may take longer to recognize psychiatric illness but treatment of depression in general practice rather than in hospital has become the norm since the advent of effective antidepressant drugs. The general practitioner is at the most disadvantage when coping with situational problems such as marital difficulties, debt, and housing difficulties. Drugs are not the answer here and the use of a social worker to help patients to 'beat the system' and a psychologist to teach them how to react in the adverse circumstances are both important adjuncts to the primary care team. Unfortunately, although the development of primary care teams in general practice has been a most useful, even if patchy, advance it is, in the NHS, increasingly difficult to maintain in the present financial climate. It is the writer's firm opinion that much work needs to be done to establish the value of such team work and, not least, its value in the prevention of iatrogenic drug dependence. In the writer's practice a small survey some years ago showed the value of social worker contact in a small group of patients with situational anxiety problems. Among the group who had social worker contact, benzodiazepines were virtually unused (Table 13.5). It should be emphasized that this was not a controlled trial but it does illustrate the parsimonious use of benzodiazepine drugs including hypnotics that was possible in a practice that made use of the help of a social worker for situational problems such as the following : financial; problems at work; physical or mental handicap; unmarried mother status; social inadequacy; elderly loneliness; alcoholism; organic illness; personality disorder; family relationship problems; marital problems; bereavement.

Problems of relative dosage

It is only in recent years that the relative strength of different benzodiazepine drugs has been established. Drug manufacturers were more likely to stress

Table 13.5. Benzodiazepine usage among patients ($N=25$) making use of the help of social workers

Length of time on drug	No. of females	No. of males
<1 week	5	
1–2 weeks	3	1
2–4 weeks	2	
4–8 weeks	2	
8–16 weeks	1	
Chronic use before and after contact with social worker	15	1
Drug stopped after contact with social worker	2	
No benzodiazepine used at the time	31	12

whether a drug was short-or long-acting or that it was a better anxiolytic, and the simple matter of relative strength was overlooked. This is an important omission as it seems unlikely that a general practitioner would have replaced diazepam 2 mg with lorazepam, 1 mg if he had understood that he was thereby multiplying the benzodiazepine strength by a factor of 5. It is surprising that the *British national formulary*, *vade mecum* of prescribers, did not address this matter. Heather Ashton (1989) has helped general practitioners by giving a useful table of relative doses (Table 13.6).

Recent changes in prescribing practice

It is some years now since the UK government issued a restrictive 'black' list of drugs that could no longer be prescribed under the NHS. The effect of this on

Table 13.6. Relative strengths of benzodiazepines (Ashton 1989)

Benzodiazepine	Relative strength (mg)
Alprazolam	1
Chlordiazepoxide	25
Diazepam	10
Lorazepam	1
Nitrazepam	10
Oxazepam	20
Temazepam	20
Triazolam	0.5

hypnotic prescribing was minimal but it did serve to emphasize that the health authorities were prepared to exercise their right to control prescribing costs, and many of the drugs discontinued were those of unproven value. The start of the PACT scheme whereby general practitioners now receive a complete breakdown of their prescribing costs compared to those of their colleagues along with an analysis as to category gives doctors the chance to note if they are markedly different from their colleagues and may also be an instrument for change in prescribing habits. Lastly, the introduction by some practices of practice formularies means that, in the preparation of such formularies, a drug will need to be justified to one's partners and this also gives an opportunity for the revision of prescribing practice.

Computers are now commonplace in general practice and it is very easy to compile a repeat prescription package. It is incumbent on doctors to incorporate checks to make sure that patients do not slide into drug dependence unbeknown to the doctor. The most important check is simply not to allow repeat prescriptions for hypnotics without a clear understanding of the following.

1. After a few weeks the patient is almost certainly dependent on the drug with ensuing requests for repeat prescriptions.

2. The patient must have a consultation at least every 3 months with a view to negotiating drug withdrawal, or at least establishing need.

The patient who wants to withdraw from hypnotics

The doctor needs to be convinced that it is advantageous to come off the drug before he can convince the patient. It has been shown (Giblin and Clift 1983) that cessation of hypnotics causes no deterioration in sleep latency and, more importantly the patient wakes more refreshed. In general, patients who have undergone a withdrawal programme are delighted. In the study quoted there were no significant changes in feelings of anxiety or depression following drug reduction and the fact that sleep satisfaction continued to be good supports the suggestion that hypnotics in long-term use lose their efficacy (Kales *et al*. 1975). In almost every patient who attempted withdrawal in the author's practice the results were longstanding.

General practitioners would do well to have a personalized stock of advice leaflets on sleep problems and, possibly, relaxation tapes on loan. Contact with a psychologist in the practice is a great advantage, but so also is easy access to someone providing practical help or a shoulder 'to lean on'. Social workers, health visitors, and counsellors are all invaluable additions to the team.

Some patients will prefer to join self-help groups and, indeed, with the new contracts in general practice in the UK such groups could be eligible for health authority funding.

Summary

Dependence on hypnotic drugs can be prevented:

1. by careful selection of patients;

   (a) by avoiding the drug in some personalities;
   (b) by using ancillary help, e.g. social workers to manage situational problems rather than look for a drug solution.

2. by restriction of treatment to no more than 2 weeks.

Dependence can occur with all benzodiazepines but withdrawal effects tend to be more severe with the short-acting ones.

Patients who are drug-dependent can be helped to withdraw within the context of general practitioners consultations. Some guidelines are given.

Patients who withdraw from hypnotics often feel their subsequent sleep is more refreshing.

It is likely that chronic users of hypnotics are obtaining little sleep-producing effect from them.

References

APA (American Psychiatric Association) (1987). *Diagnostic and statistical manual of mental disorders* (3rd edn, revised). American Psychiatric Press, Washington, DC.

Ashton, H. (1989). Helping patients to come off benzodiazepines. *Pulse Magazine*, 22 July 1989, p.50.

Breimer, D.D. (1978). Clinical pharmacokinetic and biopharmaceutical aspects of hypnotic drug therapy. In *Sleep research* (ed. R.G. Priest, A. Pletscher, and J. Ward), Ch.6, p.71. MTP Press, Lancaster, UK.

Clift, A.D. (1972). Factors leading to dependence on hypnotic drugs. *British Medical Journal*, **719**, 614–17.

Clift, A.D. (ed.) (1975). *Sleep disturbance and hypnotic drug dependence*. Excerpta Medica, Amsterdam.

Clift, A.D. (1982). Sleep disturbance in general practice. Paper read to the British Association for the Advancement of Science, Liverpool, 1982.

Clift, A. *et al.* (source of Table 13.1)

Davis, D.R. and Horne, J.a. (1975). Human sleep and individual differences. In *Sleep disturbance and hypnotic drug dependence* (ed. A.D. Clift), p.63. Excerpta Medica, Amsterdam.

Foulds (1965). *Personality and personal illness*. Tavistock, London.

Foulds, G.A. and Hope, K. (1968). *Manual of the Symptom-Sign Inventory*. University of London Press.

Giblin, M.J. and Clift, A.D. (1983). Sleep without drugs. *Journal of the Royal College of General Practitioners*, **33**, 628–33.

Hollister, L.E. (1972). The prudent use of antianxiety drugs. *Rational Drug Therapy*, **6** (3), 5.

Hollister, L.E., Motzenbecker, F.P., and Degan, R.O. (1961). Withdrawal reactions from chlordiazepoxide ('Librium'). *Psychopharmacologia*, **2**, 63–8.

Johnson, J. and Clift, A. (1968). Dependence on hypnotic drugs in general practice. *British Medical Journal*, **4**, 613.

Kales, A., Kales, J.D., Bixler, E.O., and Scharf, M.B. (1975). Effectiveness of hypnotic drugs in prolonged use. *Clinical Pharmacology and Therapeutics*, **18** (30), 356–63.

Marks, J. (1978). *The benzodiazepines: use, overuse, misuse, abuse.* MTP Press, Lancaster, UK.

Merec (1991). Zopiclone, a cyclopyrrolone hypnotic agent. *Merec Bulletin*, Vol. 2 No. 4 April 1991, pp.13–14.

MIMS (Monthly Index Medical Specialties) (1990). Section 3A, Hypnotics, Nov. 1990.

Oswald, I. and Priest, R.G. (1965). Five weeks to escape the sleeping pill habit. *British Medical Journal*, **2**, 1093.

Owen, R. and Tyrer, P. (1983). Benzodiazepine dependence: a review of the evidence. *Drugs*, **25**. 385–98.

Seevers, (1968). Psychopharmacological elements of drug dependence. *Journal of the American Medical Association*, **206**(6), 1263.

Tyrer, P., Owen, R., and Dawling, S. (1983). Gradual withdrawal of diazepam after long term therapy. *Lancet*, **i**, 1402–6.

WHO (World Health Organization Expert Committee on Drug Dependence) (1969). 16th report (WHO Technical Report Series, No.407). World Health Organization, Geneva.

Wilcox, W.H. (1927). The clinical and pathological effects of hypnotic drugs of the barbituric acid and sulphonal groups. *Proceedings of the Royal Society of Medicine, London*, **20** (11), 1479.

Wulff, M.H. (1955). Use and abuse of hypnotics. *Ugeskr. Laeg.*, **117**(50), 1639.

14 Pharmacological differences in the dependence potential of benzodiazepines

Peter Tyrer

Differences between benzodiazepines are relatively small but can be clinically important. Although the differences in dependence potential between the benzodiazepines are sufficiently important to merit a separate chapter in this book, it is important for the reader to realize that the similarities between these drugs are much greater than their differences. Benzodiazepine dependence is a useful common description as the phenomena of cross-tolerance and cross-dependence (i.e. the transfer of tolerance or dependence developed with one drug to another of the same class) are marked with all the benzodiazepines. Although it is frequent to encounter patients in clinical practice who insist that they can only remain free of symptoms if they remain on one named benzodiazepine and cannot therefore change to another, it is likely that a large part of this apparent specificity of action is a psychological one independent of the drug itself. When patients apparently dependent on one benzodiazepine are changed to another at equivalent dosage under double-blind conditions, almost complete cross-dependence is demonstrated (i.e. there is no difference between the withdrawal symptoms of those that change to a new drug and those that stay on the same benzodiazepine; Murphy and Tyrer 1991).

However, these figures apply to patients who have already been taking a single benzodiazepine for many months or years, and it would be wrong to deduce from these data that there are no differences among benzodiazepines in dependence potential, which involves the tendency for patients to desire and persist in taking a drug as well as the nature and extent of withdrawal symptoms on discontinuation.

The uses and classification of the main benzodiazepines are listed in Table 14.1. These demonstrate that benzodiazepines treat a much wider range of conditions than merely anxiety and insomnia (although these account for by far the largest proportion of prescriptions), and the use of these drugs in the treatment of epilepsy and other neurological disorders and in anaesthesia is significant. Clearly, some of the benzodiazepines that are only used on a short-term basis (e.g. midazolam) are much less likely to create dependence than those prescribed in regular dosage by mouth for the treatment of anxiety. Nevertheless, it is worthwhile considering all of them in this review.

Triazolam

Triazolam is the shortest acting of the benzodiazepines used for the treatment of anxiety and insomnia. The elimination half-life of the parent compound is under 3 h and its active metabolites extend this to just over 4 h. This is not an ideal duration of action for a hypnotic but, nonetheless, it has been primarily used for this purpose.

Soon after its introduction to clinical practice there were a series of reports in Holland about its effects, including dependence, where many of the symptoms suggested cognitive and memory impairment (Van der Kroef 1979). Since then, there has been increasing concern about cognitive deficits in the 24 h following the use of triazolam and this is now frequently referred to as the 'triazolam syndrome'. There is now good evidence that triazolam causes significantly more memory impairment than other benzodiazepines (Scharf *et al.* 1988; Greenblatt *et al.* 1989) and, more recently, it has been demonstrated that memory impairment the day after use of triazolam is significantly worse than after either temazepam or placebo (Bixler *et al.* 1991).

Side by side with these reports came other ones suggesting that triazolam was particularly prone to dependence. Animal studies comparing the relative dependences of benzodiazepines and barbiturates have generally shown that triazolam is more likely to induce dependence than other benzodiazepines. In these studies dependence is measured by the animal's wish to receive the drug (i.e. is primarily a measure of the euphoriant effect). Triazolam was more euphoriant than all other benzodiazepines with an effect not far removed from the euphoriant effect of cocaine (Griffiths *et al.* 1985).

Similar studies in man, primarily concentrating on withdrawal symptoms after stopping triazolam, suggested that, after a single dose of triazolam, there was rebound anxiety the next day compared with the response to placebo, and this also indicated dependence (Morgan and Oswald 1982).

The consensus of these findings is that triazolam is not only an extremely potent benzodiazepine that binds readily to benzodiazepine receptors but that it is also more euphoriant and therefore prone to abuse and more likely to lead to severe withdrawal symptoms. These withdrawal symptoms not only include increased anxiety and perceptual disturbance but, more commonly than other benzodiazepines, include confusion, delusions and delirium, and memory impairment. These are all symptoms that are found in benzodiazepine withdrawal (Owen and Tyrer 1983), but are more pronounced with triazolam than with other benzodiazepines. For example, in the latest paper by Bixler *et al.* (1991), after a single dose of 0.5 mg of triazolam the night before one subject could not recall any details of a bus trip that she had made with companions and another tried to leave a grocery store without paying for her purchases. These were not isolated incidents recorded in a few individuals after many years of total drug exposure; they represented findings in a planned research study including 18 subjects with

Table 14.1. Pharmacokinetic data and uses of the most widely used benzodiazepines listed in order of potency

Drug	Active metabolites	Normal daily dosage (mg)	Time to peak plasma levels (h)	Elimination half-life (h)	Main clinical use
Triazolam		0.125–5	1.7	3	Insomnia
Lormetazepam		0.5–1.5	3	10	Insomnia
Alprazolam		0.75–1.5	1	12	Panic
Lorazepam		1–5	2.3	14	Anxiety
Clonazepam		1.5–10	2.3	24	Epilepsy
Diazepam		4–30	1	16	Anxiety, epilepsy, muscle spasm
	Desmethyldiazepam			80	
Nitrazepam		5–15	1.5	30	Insomnia
Clobazam		10–30	1.5	24	Epilepsy*
	N–Desmethylclobazam		40	70	
Midazolam		10–30	0.67	2.4	Premedication anaesthesia†
Temazepam		10–30	0.75	9	Insomnia
Chlordiazepoxide		10–30	1.5	10	Anxiety
	N–Desmethylchlordiazepoxide		10	50	
	N–Desmethyldiazepam		45	80	
Oxazepam		30–90	2	8	Anxiety

* Cannot be prescribed on NHS prescription except for epilepsy.   † Given intravenously.

insomnia who could easily have received triazolam in the normal course of events.

These adverse effects have prompted Oswald (1989) to recommend the withdrawal of triazolam from clinical use. However, although the evidence appears overwhelming, there is some concern that some of these marked symptoms may be related to the fact that triazolam is marketed at a somewhat higher dosage than other benzodiazepines and that this might explain some of the results. Many of the problems of triazolam have been reported with a nighttime dose of 0.5 mg when it is common for 0.125 or 0.25 mg to be used in the treatment of insomnia. If this is true then, if triazolam were marketed in lower dosage regularly, none of these problems would have been found to a greater extent than with other benzodiazepines. However, counteracting this is evidence that, in the lower dosages of 0.125 and 0.25 mg, triazolam is not an effective hypnotic compared with other benzodiazepines (Seidel *et al.* 1986).

It is thus hard to avoid the conclusion that triazolam is a benzodiazepine that should be given rarely, if at all, and, as there is no good evidence that it is superior to other benzodiazepines in any important respect, its continued use in clinical practice should be in doubt.

Lormetazepam, loprazolam, and flunitrazepam

Although only one of these three drugs, lormetazepam, is listed in Table 14.1, they can all be considered together as they have very similar pharmacokinetic properties and are of almost equivalent potency. They are also all used for the treatment of insomnia.

Largely because of the work of Kales and his colleagues (1978) an established system for evaluating the dependence potential of different hypnotic drugs has been developed. A technique commonly used by his group is illustrated in Fig. 14.1. Insomniac subjects are tested in a sleep laboratory before, during, and after withdrawal from an hypnotic drug. Measurements commonly include the electroencephalogram (EEG), which, when measured continuously, allows the total sleep time to be measured; often the electromyogram (EMG) and electro-oculogram (EOG) are measured also. Subjective ratings of the quality of sleep and sleepiness in the morning are also measured. This methodology allows both tolerance and withdrawal symptoms to be measured. Withdrawal symptoms are commonly described as 'rebound insomnia' (Kales *et al.* 1978) but there is qualitatively no difference between this and insomnia experienced as part of a full withdrawal syndrome. A drug that typically causes dependence demonstrates tolerance on repeated usage so that a regular fixed dose is less effective later in the study, followed by a characteristic 'sine-wave' decrease in sleep time which reaches a peak within a few days of withdrawal and then quickly returns to baseline levels (Fig. 14.1).

Lormetazepam (Kales *et al.* 1983*a*) and flunitrazepam (Bixler *et al.* 1977) both led to tolerance and withdrawal symptoms in the form of rebound insomnia 3 days after the drug was withdrawn. Further evidence that this is undoubtedly a drugs-related phenomenon comes from the finding that higher doses of lormetazepam create greater rebound insomnia than do lower doses (Kales *et al.* 1983*a*).

Another index of dependence potential is the relative frequency of abuse. In some countries with comprehensive surveillance of drug prescriptions it is possible to examine the ratio of prescription forgeries and total legal prescriptions. This ratio has been examined in Sweden and the data suggest that flunitrazepam has considerable abuse potential as its forgery/prescription ratio is rising faster than that of other benzodiazepines (Bergman and Lee 1989; Fig. 14.2).

Alprazolam

Alprazolam, like triazolam, is a triazolobenzodiazepine. There have been some suggestions that this chemical nucleus is related to antidepressant as well as to anti-anxiety effects and therefore, that the drug should not be considered to be 'just another benzodiazepine'. Although it is not available on NHS prescription in the UK, it has headed the prescriptions of benzodiazepines (and other psychotropic drugs as well) in the USA for several years. This is because it is primarily marketed for the treatment of panic disorder, an anxious condition that many research workers and psychopharmacologists insist is fundamentally different from other forms of anxiety. Although alprazolam is effective in anxiety, clinical trials have conspicuously failed to compare its efficacy with other benzodiazepines given at equivalent dosage. The dosage issue is an important one, because the recommended

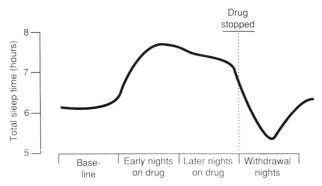

Fig. 14.1. Typical study design for investigation of tolerance and rebound insomnia with a hypnotic drug. The example shows the pattern that is common with short-acting potent benzodiazepines in insomniac patients. After baseline insomnia is demonstrated there is a rapid increase in sleep time after taking the hyptonic, but tolerance begins to develop after a few nights and, immediately after withdrawal, there is rebound (or in this case 'overshoot') insomnia followed by resolution to baseline status.

mean antipanic dose of alprazolam is said to be 6 mg per day, a dosage achieved after gradually increasing the dosage over 3 weeks (Sheehan and Raj 1990). This dose is equivalent to 60 mg of diazepam daily and therefore represents a much higher dosage than that normally recommended.

Patients who take higher doses of benzodiazepines are more prone to dependence so it is not surprising that alprazolam has frequently been implicated in withdrawal reactions. Most studies examining the incidence of withdrawal reactions after stopping alprazolam have shown that approximately one-third of patients have withdrawal symptoms (Pecknold and Swinson 1986; Pecknold *et al.* 1988) even when the drug is withdrawn slowly after relatively short periods of treatment. In personal studies we have found that a similar proportion of patients had withdrawal symptoms with other benzodiazepines apart from alprazolam but most of these had been taking the drug for several years before withdrawal was attempted (Tyrer *et al.* 1981, 1983; Murphy and Tyrer 1991).

In one of the few studies in which alprazolam has been compared with other benzodiazepines during withdrawal Rickels *et al.* (1986) found that alprazolam, together with another potent benzodiazepine, lorazepam, was associated with an earlier more severe withdrawal reaction than were the long-acting benzodiazepines, diazepam and chlorazepate (Fig. 14.3).

Panic attacks

There have also been a number of studies demonstrating other withdrawal phenomena with alprazolam, including withdrawal seizures and amnesic

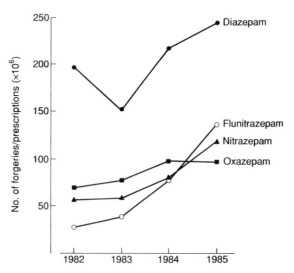

Fig. 14.2. Benzodiazepine prescription forgeries uncovered in Sweden. Reproduced with permission from Bergman and Lee(1989).

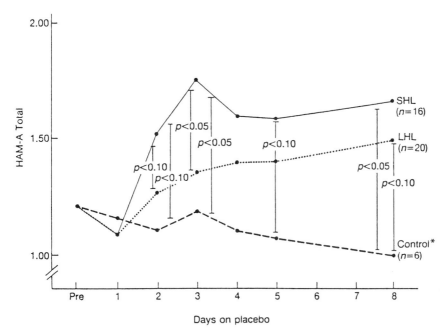

Fig. 14.3. Comparison of withdrawal reponses (HAM-A total scores) between long half-life (LHL) and short half-life (SHL) benzodiazepines and medication controls (*p*-values based on Newman-Keuls statistics; analysis of covariance). Reproduced with permission from Rickels *et al.* (1986).

episodes similar to those already described with triazolam.

It is a matter of some concern that alprazolam continues to be used in such high dosage and for such long periods. It is now regarded as reasonable to prescribe alprazolam and other benzodiazepines long term. In the words of one of the foremost authorities in the USA 'the reality is that most patients with panic disorder have a chronic, relapsing illness that requires chronic medication over many years' (Sheehan and Raj 1990, p. 189). If this type of treatment approach becomes the norm it is hard to avoid the conclusion that the USA is likely to experience much greater problems with benzodiazepine dependence than will other countries where alprazolam is rarely, if ever, used.

Lorazepam

Lorazepam has attracted more attention in the UK with regard to the phenomenon of dependence than any other benzodiazepine, although it is of some interest that in other countries it causes much less concern. Lorazepam is a potent benzodiazepine with no active metabolites that was introduced as a powerful new benzodiazepine with an edge in efficacy over other compounds.

It became popular, possibly because of the 'alprazolam effect' just described. Lorazepam was marketed in doses of between 2 and 10 mg daily and it is only recently that these dosages have been revised downwards. A dose of 10 mg daily lorazepam is equivalent to approximately 100 mg of diazepam (British Medical Association, and Royal Pharmaceutical Society of Great Britain 1991, p. 123) so it is hardly surprising that at first it was viewed as a more powerful drug.

This may explain to some extent why lorazepam appears to be associated with more complaints about dependence in the UK than are other benzodiazepines. It is unlikely to be in a different league in dependence potential from other benzodiazepines but its aggressive marketing in the UK may well have led to its greater use in more anxious patients, those who did not appear to respond to other compounds (probably in lower dosage).

Nevertheless, there is still abundant evidence that lorazepam is more likely to induce dependence and create greater problems of withdrawal than many other benzodiazepines. Subjective effects of lorazepam in acute dosage make it, together with diazepam, more prone to abuse (Griffiths *et al.* 1984), and self-administration experiments in monkeys also show some evidence that lorazepam leads to greater self-administration than many other benzodiazepines (mainly those of long half-life) (Yanagita 1981).

Lorazepam has also been reported to induce amnesia when given by mouth in acute dosage and in this respect it differs from all other benzodiazepines apart from triazolam (McKay and Dundee 1980). Acute dosage studies have also demonstrated that lorazepam impairs complex psychomotor functioning such as that needed in car driving significantly more than other benzodiazepines (Hindmarch and Gudgeon 1980). Since (also in acute dosage) lorazepam appears to create more of the side-effects known to be associated with subsequent dependence (and may even demonstrate symptoms of withdrawal as described previously with triazolam), one might expect to find greater problems following withdrawal after regular prescription. In planning our first study in 1976 we chose lorazepam and diazepam to evaluate the withdrawal problems with benzodiazepines and their possible alleviation by the beta-blocking drug, propranolol. At that time there was little concern about the prescription of benzodiazepines and, of 86 patients identified as being on long-term benzodiazepines unnecessarily, only 40 agreed to take part in the study—32 on diazepam and 8 on lorazepam. Although there was no difference in the severity of withdrawal effects between the two drugs, only one of the eight patients on lorazepam was able to withdraw successfully and one of the other patients had an epileptic seizure during withdrawal (Tyrer *et al.* 1981). However, it is fair to mention that the patients taking lorazepam were taking a mean dose of about 4 mg, compared with 10 mg with diazepam so one might have expected more problems with lorazepam because of its much greater potency.

In more recent work we compared withdrawal symptoms after patients
with putative benzodiazepine dependence (i.e. they had taken their benzodiazepines for more than 6 months and had tried to reduce them but developed
apparent withdrawal symptoms) were randomly assigned to one of three
benzodiazepines—lorazepam, bromazepam, and diazepam in equivalent dosages. After 4 weeks they were withdrawn from their new benzodiazepine over
an 8-week period and their withdrawal symptoms were recorded using the
Benzodiazepine Withdrawal Symptom Questionnaire (BWSQ) (Tyrer et al.
1990). Although overall there were no differences in the incidence and severity
of withdrawal symptoms among the three benzodiazepines, it is of interest that
more patients on lorazepam were unable to complete withdrawal successfully
(10 of 23) compared with those on the other two benzodiazepines (13 of 45).
Of those that completed treatment, patients on lorazepam had somewhat
lower scores on the BWSQ than did patients on bromazepam and diazepam
and, on two of the 20 items on the questionnaire, this achieved significance
(Murphy and Tyrer 1991).

The implication of these findings is that lorazepam is more difficult to
withdraw from than both bromazepam, which has an identical half-life
but is less potent, and diazepam, but lorazepam does not seem to do
this through creating greater withdrawal symptoms. The difference seems
to be that patients on lorazepam are less able to tolerate withdrawal
symptoms with this drug than with other benzodiazepines and the reason why
this should be so is not entirely explained by its potency and elimination
half-life.

Clonazepam

Clonazepam is only used for the treatment of epilepsy. However, all
other benzodiazepines have some anticonvulsant activity and the choice of
clonazepam to treat epilepsy is somewhat arbitrary. There have been very
few problems with clonazepam in clinical practice with regard to dependence
potential. Animal studies involving self-administration of benzodiazepines
generally show clonazepam to be similar to most benzodiazepines in its ability
to maintain the response of self-administration but significantly less so than
lorazepam, alprazolam, midazolam, and triazolam (Griffiths and Ator 1980;
Woods et al. 1987).

Clonazepam accounts for less than 1 per cent of all benzodiazepine
prescriptions but, nonetheless, it is interesting that it has attracted virtually
no attention as a drug of dependence. One possible reason for this is that
it is prescribed for a physical disorder, and most of the patients taking it
do not have significant pathological anxiety or personality characteristics that
are often associated with anxiety, particularly dependent personalities (Tyrer
and Tyrer 1988). It has been argued that personality status is one of the most
important factors determining dependence on benzodiazepines (Tyrer 1989;

Murphy and Tyrer 1991). The low incidence of problems with clonazepam is in keeping with this hypothesis.

Diazepam and chlordiazepoxide

Although diazepam is a short-acting benzodiazepine when given in acute dosage, it is metabolized to desmethyldiazepam (nordiazepam) which has a long half-life of about 80 h (Table 14.1). After regular treatment for more than a week the plasma levels of desmethyldiazepam exceeds that of the parent compound and probably plays the major part in the drug's action.

However, the abuse potential of diazepam is much more related to the parent drug. Diazepam is one of the most lipophilic of benzodiazepines and rapidly enters the brain after being absorbed into the body. One consequence of this is that, when diazepam is given in relatively high dosage, the user can develop a euphoriant 'buzz', which is perceived as pleasant and reinforcing. This explains why diazepam is a relatively popular drug amongst drug abusers where it is taken in dosages approximately 10 times greater than those normally used in clinical practice (which in one recent study of abusers was a mean daily dose of 210 mg; Seivewright *et al.* 1991).

Human studies assessing the reinforcing effect of diazepam have found that it is only when the drug is taken in relatively large dosage that the drug is preferred to placebo (Griffiths *et al.* 1980). In lower doses diazepam does not have this effect (Johanson and Uhlenhuth 1980). However, this issue, which is discussed at much greater length in Chapter 9, this volume, is quite separate from that of low-dose dependence with benzodiazepines. Again, diazepam is often regarded as the bench-mark by which other benzodiazepines should be compared in this respect as, over the years of benzodiazepine prescription, diazepam has exceeded prescriptions of other benzodiazepines for most of the years since 1963. Most of the evidence suggests that diazepam has no special advantages over other benzodiazepines with regard to propensity for withdrawal symptoms. In spite of this, during withdrawal from benzodiazepines, diazepam is often recommended as a substitute benzodiazepine for other ones of greater dependence potential (e.g. Tyrer *et al.* 1981; British Medical Association and Royal Pharmaceutical Society of Great Britain 1991, p. 123).

The major advantages of diazepam for withdrawal purposes are the long half-life of desmethyldiazepam and the many different dosage strengths of the drug. Because diazepam is marketed in 10-, 5-, and 2-mg tablets, each of which can be divided into two without difficulty, it is possible to get reducing programmes allowing daily reductions of half a milligram without much difficulty. Few other benzodiazepines possess this flexibility. However, when the dosage strengths of other benzodiazepines are specially modified to allow reduction in similar stages (a service which is available in many pharmacies irrespective of marketed dosage), no particular benefits of diazepam emerge (Murphy and Tyrer 1991).

Chlordiazepoxide, the original benzodiazepine, can also be considered in the same context as diazepam. Chlordiazepoxide is metabolized to desmethylchlordiazepoxide and desmethyldiazepam, both of which have long elimination half-lives (Table 14.1), so the drug behaves very much like diazepam in long-term dosage. It does not have the same rapid absorption and so is less prone to abuse and for many years has been preferred to other benzodiazepines for detoxification in alcohol withdrawal. This is a reasonable choice, although chlordiazepoxide has somewhat less anticonvulsant activity than diazepam and, if epileptic seizures are expected, than diazepam may be the drug of choice.

Nitrazepam

For many years nitrazepam was the only benzodiazepine marketed as a hypnotic and consequently enjoyed great popularity, not least because of its safety and evidence of prolonged efficacy (Oswald et al. 1982). Nitrazepam also has a place in the treatment of epilepsy, particularly infantile spasms and myoclonic epilepsy. It is most frequently used in paediatric practice.

Nitrazepam was almost the first benzodiazepine to come under serious suspicion of inducing dependence in a paper by Clift (1972) that suggested that amylobarbitone and nitrazepam were similar in creating dependence in general practice. Subsequent experimental studies confirmed that withdrawal problems were found with nitrazepam (Adam et al. 1976). Nitrazepam, for reasons that again relate primarily to marketing policy, has never been available on prescription in the USA and has therefore figured much less often than other hypnotic benzodiazepines in comparisons of withdrawal effects. However, when compared with 14 other hypnotic drugs, nitrazepam, despite its relatively long half-life, is similar to flunitrazepam and lormetazepam in severity of rebound insomnia (Kales et al. 1983a). Nevertheless, midazolam and triazolam produced greater rebound effects and there is reason to believe that the same may be true of the newer non-benzodiazepine hypnotic, zopiclone, which also binds to benzodiazepine receptors (Goa and Heel 1986).

In personal work with my colleague, Dr Siobhan Murphy, we found some interesting differences between withdrawal symptoms in patients who had been on nitrazepam before changing to one of three anxiolytic benzodiazepines, lorazepam, bromazepam, and diazepam, and were then subsequently withdrawn from these after 4 week's treatment (Murphy and Tyrer 1991). All patients in the study had been dependent on other benzodiazepines before being entered into the study, and those who had been dependent on nitrazepam subsequently had greater withdrawal symptoms but were more likely to complete full withdrawal than those taking other benzodiazepines (Murphy 1991). This result is difficult to interpret. It may indicate that patients taking hypnotic benzodiazepines are more persistent in withdrawal practice than those taking anxiolytic equivalents, but it may also be an attribute related to dependence on nitrazepam specifically.

Clobazam

Clobazam is only used in the UK on prescription for the treatment of epilepsy, but in other counties it is used more commonly for the treatment of anxiety. As with the other benzodiazepine marketed primarily for its anticonvulsant activity, clonazepam, there has been little concern about dependence with clobazam. There are some hints that it may be less likely to lead to withdrawal symptoms upon cessation of treatment (Ponciano *et al.* 1981) but more data are necessary before any definite conclusions can be drawn.

Midazolam

Midazolam is a short-acting, water-soluble benzodiazepine that is used for pre-medication and induction of anaesthesia. It is even more lipophilic than diazepam and this explains why it acts almost instantaneously after intravenous dosage. However, in oral doses its half-life is similar to that of triazolam (Table 14.1), and the drug is used as a hypnotic in some countries.

Comparison of midazolam with other benzodiazepines suggests that, in terms of dependence potential, it is almost identical to triazolam. In an initial study in which insomniac patients were treated with midazolam, between 10 and 30 mg at night for 7 days, and then withdrawn from medication suddenly, there was rapid development of tolerance and marked rebound insomnia after withdrawal (Kales *et al.* 1983*b*). There were also reports of amnesia on some days following administration of midazolam, a feature that is common to triazolam. Withdrawal symptoms were much more severe in patients on the higher dose of 30 mg.

In view of these findings it appears to be a mistake to use midazolam as a hypnotic. Its use as an anaesthetic agent is, however, perfectly appropriate and not associated with any dependence potential. The main reason for concern is that intravenous midazolam could be attractive to drug abusers and thus good security is necessary for its supplies.

Temazepam

Temazepam is now the most frequently prescribed benzodiazepine in the UK (Brandon 1990). This reflects its efficacy as a hypnotic, the advantages of its relatively short elimination half-life in reducing hangover effects, and effective marketing policy.

In sleep laboratory studies temazepam has been shown to cause rebound insomnia after discontinuation but this is less severe than that which occurs after stopping other benzodiazepines marketed as hypnotics, including flunitrazepam, lormetazepam, nitrazepam, and triazolam (Mitler *et al.* 1979; Kales *et al.* 1983*a*). This is of some theoretical as well as practical interest, as one might expect that temazepam, with a short elimination half-life, would be prone to more severe withdrawal effects.

These findings suggest that temazepam is nearer to being an ideal hypnotic than any other benzodiazepine, but this conclusion needs to be tempered with a major word of caution. Temazepam is becoming the most popular benzodiazepine for illicit use and, in one recent survey, patients abused temazepam more than all other benzodiazepines added together (Seivewright *et al.* 1991). This is partly explained by temazepam being marketed in liquid form with a gelatine capsule so that the drug can easily be removed for intravenous injection. The manufacturers have attempted to overcome this by making the drug in gel form (Gelthix) but addicts have found that heating up the capsules restores the drug to liquid form. Although temazepam is available in tablet form the absorption of the drug differs from that of the capsule and it is not possible to extrapolate from one to the other.

Oxazepam

Oxazepam was among the first benzodiazepines to be used in clinical practice and yet, despite its long exposure, has been associated with few reports of dependence potential. It shows little evidence of abuse despite being used as the main agent for detoxification in alcohol dependence in several countries (Bliding 1978). Although there have been reports of withdrawal syndromes after stopping the drug in doses within the therapeutic range (Hanna 1972; Pecknold *et al.* 1982; Wilbur and Kulik 1983), these syndromes have not been as severe as those associated with other benzodiazepines.

In the study by Pecknold *et al.* (1982) withdrawal symptoms upon stopping oxazepam after 3 week's treatment were compared with those upon stopping halazepam, a drug that is metabolized to desmethyldiazepam. Despite the fact that oxazepam has a short half-life and therefore might have been expected in comparison with halazepam to have earlier and more serious withdrawal symptoms, it not only showed no difference in the incidence and severity of withdrawal symptoms but at all times had somewhat fewer withdrawal symptoms than halazepam.

Is there a unifying theme to the dependence potential of different benzodiazepines?

There is one characteristic that is more predictive of the dependence potential of different benzodiazepines than any other—potency. This is best indicated by the affinity with which a drug binds with benzodiazepine receptors. Comparison between relative affinities (Fig. 14.4) parallels potency (Table 14.1)

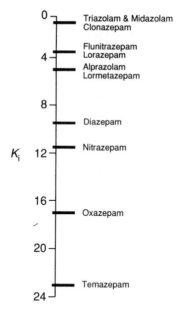

Fig. 14.4. Comparison of binding affinities (K_i) of benzodiazepines. After Arendt *et al.* (1987).

although there are minor variations. Potency now appears to be more important than the pharmacokinetics of elimination half-lives, particularly as it is common for patients on benzodiazepines to withdraw from their drugs slowly and thereby reduce the impact of differences in half-life. Why potency is important in creating dependence is far from clear but it is likely to involve subtle changes at the level of the benzodiazepine receptor. Nutt and his colleagues have suggested that there is a 'receptor shift' from agonist to antagonist activity after prolonged treatment with benzodiazepines, so that there is subsequently reduced sensitivity to conventional agonist benzodiazepines and increased sensitivity to antagonists and inverse agonists (Little *et al.* 1987; Nutt 1990). Although this remains speculative it is a heuristically useful hypothesis that fits many of the known facts and would repay further enquiry.

Acknowledgement

I thank Dr Siobhan Murphy for her collaboration in much of the work described in this chapter.

References

Adam, K., Adamson, L., Brezinova, V., and Hunter, W.M. (1976). Nitrazepam: lastingly effective but trouble on withdrawal. *British Medical Journal*, **1**, 1558–60.

Arendt, R.M., Greenblatt, D.J., Liebisch, D.C., Luu, M.D., and Paul, S.M. (1987). Determinants of benzodiazepine brain uptake; lipophilicity verses binding affinity. *Psychopharmacology*, **93**, 72–6.

Bergman, V. and Lee, D. (1989). Current approaches to measurement of drug use and abuse in Sweden. In *Testing for abuse liability of drugs in humans*, National Institute of Drug Abuse Research Monograph Series, no. 92 (ed. M.W.Fischman and N.K. Mello), pp.267–86. Press Office of the National Institute on Drug Abuse, Rockville, Maryland.

Bixler, E.O., Kales, A., Soldatos, C.R., and Kales, J.D. (1977). Flunitrazepam, an investigational hypnotic drug: sleep laboratory evaluations. *Journal of Clinical Pharmacology*, **17**, 569–78.

Bixler, E.O., Kales, A., Manfredi, R.L., Vgontzas, A.N., Tyson, K.L., and Kales, J.D. (1991). Next-day memory impairment with triazolam use. *Lancet*, **337**, 827–31.

Bliding, A. (1978). The abuse potential of benzodiazepines with special reference to oxazepam. In Pharmacodynamic, pharmacokinetic and clinical aspects on oxazepam and related benzodiazepines (ed. R. Chinnery and A. Sundwall). *Acta Psychiatrica Scandinavica*, **274**, 111–16.

Brandon, S. (1990). Clinical use of benzodiazepines in anxiety and panic disorders. In *Benzodiazepines: current concepts. Biological, clinical and social perspectives* (ed. I. Hindmarch, G. Beaumont, S. Brandon, and B.E. Leonard), pp.111–39. John Wiley, Chichester.

British Medical Association and Royal Pharmaceutical Society of Great Britain (1991). *British National Formulary* Number 21. Pharmaceutical Press, London.

Clift, A.D. (1972). Factors leading to dependence on hypnotic drugs. *British Medical Journal*, **3**, 614–17.

Goa, K.L. and Heel, R.C. (1986). Zopiclone: a review of its pharmacodynamic and pharmacokinetic properties and therapeutic efficacy as a hypnotic. *Drugs*, **32**, 48–65.

Greenblatt, D.J., Harmatz, J.S., Engelhardt, N., and Schader, R.I. (1989). Pharmacokinetic determinants of dynamic differences among three benzodiazepine hypnotics: flurazepam, temazepam, and triazolam. *Archives of General Psychiatry*, **46**, 326–32.

Griffiths, R.R. and Ator, N.A. (1980). Benzodiazepine self-administration in animals and humans: a comprehensive literature review. *National Institute of Drug Abuse Research Monographs Series*, No. 33, 22–36.

Griffiths, R.R., Bigelow, G.E., Liebson, I., and Kaliszak, J.E. (1980). Drug preference in humans: double-blind choice comparison of pentobarbital, diazepam, and placebo. *Journal of Pharmacology and Experimental Therapeutics*, **215**, 649–61.

Griffiths, R.R., Lamb, R.J., Ator, N.A., Roache, J.D., and Brady, J.V. (1985). Relative abuse liability of triazolam: experimental assessment in animals and humans. *Neuroscience and Biobehavioral Reviews*, **9**, 133–51.

Hanna, S.M. (1972). A case of oxazepam (Serenid-D) dependence, *British Journal of Psychiatry*, **120**, 443–5.

Hindmarch, I. and Gudgeon, A.C. (1980). The effects of clobazam and lorazepam on aspects of psychomotor performance and car handling ability. *British Journal of Clinical Pharmacology*, **10**, 145–50.

Johanson, C.E. and Uhlenhuth, E.H. (1980). Drug preference and mood in humans. *Psychopharmacology*, **71**, 269–73.

Kales, A., Scharf, M.B., and Kales, J.D. (1978). Rebound insomnia: a new clinical syndrome. *Science*, **201**, 1039–41.

Kales, J., Bixler, E.O., Soldatos, C.R., Mitsky, D.J., and Kales, A. (1982). Lormetazepam: dose–response studies of efficacy, side-effects, and rebound insomnia. *Journal of Clinical Pharmacology*, **22**, 520–3.

Kales, A., Soldatos, C.R., Bixler, E.O., and Kales, J.D. (1983*a*). Early morning insomnia with rapidly eliminated benzodiazepines. *Science*, **220**, 95–7.

Kales, A., Soldatos, C.R., Bixler, E.O., Goff, P.J., and Vela-Bueno, A. (1983*b*). Midazolam: dose-response studies of effectiveness and rebound insomnia. *Pharmacology*, **26**, 138–49.

Little, H.J., Nutt, D.J., and Taylor, S.C. (1987). Bi-directional effects of chronic treatment with agonists and inverse agonists at the the benzodiazepine receptor complex. *Brain Research Reviews*, **19**, 371.

McKay, A.C. and Dundee, J.W. (1980). The effect of oral benzodiazepines on memory. *British Journal of Alathesia*, **52**, 1247–57.

Mitler, M.M., Carskadon, M.A., Phillips, R.L., Sterling, W.R., *et al.* (1979). Hypnotic efficacy of temazepam; a long-term sleep laboratory evaluation. *British Journal of Clinical Pharmacology*, **8**, 63S–68S.

Morgan, K. and Oswald, I. (1982). Anxiety caused by a short-life hypnotic. *British Medical Journal*, **284**, 942.

Murphy, S.M. (1991). Factors affecting dependence on benzodiazepines. MD Thesis, University of Nottingham.

Murphy, S.M. and Tyrer, P. (1991). A double-blind comparison of the effects of gradual withdrawal of lorazepam, diazepam and bromazepam in benzodiazepine dependence. *British Journal of Psychiatry*, **158**, 511–16.

Nutt, D.J. (1990). Benzodiazepine dependence: new insights from basic research. In *Benzodiazepines: current concepts—biological, clinical and social perspectives* (ed. I. Hindmarch, G. Beaumont, S. Brandon, and B.E. Leonard), pp.19–41. John Wiley, Chichester.

Oswald, I. (1989). Triazolam syndrome 10 years on. *Lancet*, **ii**, 451–2.

Oswald, I., French, C., Adam, K., and Gilliham, J. (1982). Benzodiazepine hypnotics remain effective for 24 weeks. *British Medical Journal*, **284**, 860–3.

Owen, R. and Tyrer, P. (1983). Benzodiazepine dependence: a review of the evidence. *Drugs*, **25**, 385–98.

Pecknold, J.C. and Swinson, R.P. (1986). Taper withdrawal studies with alprazolam in patients with panic disorder and agoraphobia. *Psychopharmacology Bulletin*, **22**, 173–6.

Pecknold, J.C., McClure, D.J., Fleuri, D., and Chang, H. (1982). Benzodiazepine withdrawal effects. *Progress in Neuro-psychopharmacology and Biological Psychiatry*, **6**, 517–22.

Pecknold, J.C., Swinson, R.P., Kuch, K., and Lewis, C.P. (1988). Agoraphobia in panic disorder and agoraphobia: results from a multi center trial. III. Discontinuation effects. *Archives of General Psychiatry*, **45**, 429–36.

Ponciano, E., Relvas, J., Mendes, F., Lameiras, A., *et al.* (1981). Clinical effects and sedative activity of bromazepam and clobazam in the treatment of anxious patients. In *International Congress and Symposium Series*, no. 43, pp.125–32. Royal Society of Medicine Services, London.

Rickels, K., Case, W.G., Schweizer, E.E., Swenson, C., and Fridman, R.B. (1986). Low-dose dependence in chronic benzodiazepine users: a preliminary report on 119 patients. *Psychopharmacology Bulletin*, **22**, 415–17.

Scharf, M.B., Fletcher, K., and Graham, J.P. (1988). Comparative amnesic effects of benzodiazepine hypnotic agents. *Journal of Clinical Psychiatry*, **49**, 134–7.

Seidel, W.F., Cohen, S.A., Bliwise, N.G. *et al.* (1986). Dose-related effects of triazolam and flurazepam on a circadian rhythm insomnia. *Clinical Pharmacology and Therapeutics*, **40**, 314–20.

Seivewright, N., Donmall, M., and Daley, C. (1991). Benzodiazepines in the illicit drug scene—the UK picture and some treatment dilemmas. Paper presented at 2nd International Conference on the reduction of drug related harm, Barcelona.

Sheehan, D.V. and Raj, A. (1990). Benzodiazepine treatment of panic disorder. In *Handbook of anxiety*, Vol. 4 (ed. R Noyes, Jr, M, Roth, and G.D. Burrows), pp.169–206. Elsevier, Amsterdam.

Tyrer, P. (1989). Risks of dependence on benzodiazepine drugs: the importance of patient selection. *British Medical Journal*, **298**, 102–4.

Tyrer, P., Rutherford, D., and Huggett, T. (1981). Benzodiazepine withdrawal symptoms and propranolol. *Lancet*, **i**, 520–2.

Tyrer, P., Owen, R., and Dawling, S. (1983). Gradual withdrawal of diazepam after long-term therapy. *Lancet*, **i**, 1402–6.

Tyrer, P., Murphy, S., and Riley, P. (1990). The Benzodiazepine Withdrawal Symptom Questionnaire. *Journal of Affective Disorders*, **19**, 53–61.

Tyrer, S. and Tyrer, P. (1988). Personnalité et anxiété. *Actualités Médicales Internationales—Psychiatrie*, **79**, (suppl.), 40–2.

Van der Kroef, C. (1979). Reactions to triazolam. *Lancet*, **ii**, 526.

Wilbur, R. and Kulik, A.V. (1983). Abstinence syndrome from therapeutic doses of oxazepam. *Canadian Journal of Psychiatry*, **28**, 298–300.

Woods, J.H., Katz, J.L., and Winger, G. (1987). Abuse liability of benzodiazepines. *Pharmacological Review*, **39**, 251–419.

Yanagita, T. (1981). Dependence producing effects of anxiolytics: psychotropic agents. In *Handbook of experimental psychology*, Vol. 55, part 2. (ed. F. Hoffmeister), pp.395–406. Springer-Verlag, New York.

15 Benzodiazepine use and dependency in the elderly: striking a balance

Raymond J. Ancill and William W. Carlyle

When benzodiazepines were first introduced in the 1960s, they were seen as a modern psychotropic breakthrough because they were clearly both effective anxiolytics and eminently safer than the barbituates that they replaced. This optimism has since been replaced by a growing skepticism and fears regarding side-effects, dependence, and abuse. As a result the prescribing practices have levelled off since the early 1980s and are showing signs of further decline. An attitude held by many physicians that complicates the use of benzodiazepines is that 'a little anxiety is OK'. Many anxious patients may in fact be denied appropriate anxiolytic therapy as a result of these puritanical attitudes (Higgitt 1988).

Epidemiology

Despite these evolving philosophies, benzodiazepine use continues in the elderly population at the same rate as before. In some centres, benzodiazepine use in geriatric patients has not followed the multinational trend towards moderation (Sullivan *et al.* 1988). Indeed, the most likely long-term benzodiazepine user is now the elderly female.

Epidemiological data suggest that up to 20 per cent of elderly people, especially women, experience significant anxiety (Salzman 1990) and as many as 33 per cent of long-term benzodiazepine users are elderly (Mellinger *et al.* 1984). Pure functional anxiety disorders are rare in the elderly and anxiety in any form (primary or secondary) is difficult to differentiate from other psychiatric illnesses, such as depression, or from physical disability and cognitive dysfunction (Salzman 1990). Anxiety often coexists with or is the result of some other underlying disorder (Miller and Whitcup 1986). Anxiety in the elderly is made up of both psychic and somatic components. In geriatric patients the psychic component is often less well expressed while disturbances of behaviour are seen as the primary presenting complaint. This agitation must be differentiated from other disease processes that present with similar behavioural dysfunction. Clinically, it is often extremely difficult to determine whether agitation is the result of underlying illnesses such as hypoglycaemia, hyperthyroidism, delirium, myocardial or cerebral ischaemia, or drug toxicity/withdrawal states. One must diligently search for underlying organic causes of anxiety because, even when present, their associated anxiety component will respond to benzodiazepines. If treatment and investigation is stopped once anxiety control is achieved, the underlying cause will never be adequately acknowledged and treated. Because of their lack of specificity, benzodiazepines are less useful as therapeutic probes as compared to anti-depressants in the treatment of complicated geriatric mood disorders. It is simply not enough to say that a person has an anxiety disorder because they respond to a benzodiazepine. Thus appropriately thorough medical and psychiatric history and examination are required before or during initial benzodiazepine use in order to rule out any underlying organic aetiology for the anxiety state.

Pre-treatment considerations

Despite all their purported risks and deleterious effects, benzodiazepines remain extremely efficacious when appropriately prescribed for the proper indications in the elderly. However, choosing the wrong benzodiazepine, using improper dosage regimes, or using benzodiazepines with less than clear indi-cations will inevitably lead to iatrogenic deterioration. Prescribing in geriatric psychiatry is probably among the least forgiving tasks in medicine because of the tenuous homeostasis of the geriatric patient. Therefore, understanding the implications of benzodiazepine use in this vulnerable population is necessary if we are to avoid these pitfalls and to optimize successful outcome.

Much of the literature on benzodiazepines focuses on their use and effects in the younger adult population. When elderly patients do form the study population, they are usually the 'young old' and the medically healthy, rarely corresponding to the multiply impaired 'geriatric' patient who is 80 years old or more. While little controlled data is available on the impact of benzodiazepines on dementia and other serious chronic medical disor-ders, the clinician is frequently faced with these very patients—multiply ill, multiply treated, anxious, and agitated. In an attempt to minimize ignorance, clinicians must base their treatment decisions on what is known. Once the decision to utilize a benzodiazepine has been made, several factors must be considered before drug choice and implementation. These 'geriatric factors' include pharmacokinetic and pharmacodynamic alterations, the interactions of concomitant illnesses and medications, and altered drug compliance.

Of all the pharmacokinetic changes associated with ageing, the least consistent are those associated with absorption. Declining splanchnic blood flow is essentially offset by diminished gastric motility. Decreased protein binding and greater blood–brain barrier permeability result in higher peak blood flow and probably higher brain benzodiazepine levels. While these factors are important in initial benzodiazepine dosing, significant clinical problems often arise out of long-term treatment. Drug accumulation is the result of declining lean body mass, proportional increases in adipose tissue, and prolonged metabolism and excretion. Routine liver function tests do change little with age but these do not reflect hepatic drug metabolism. The hepatic microsomal system in the geriatric patient is less inducible and the oxidative processes are less efficient. hence long half-life benzodiazepines, such as chlordiazepoxide, diazepam, nitrazepam, and flurazepam, and their active byproducts are metabolized more slowly. However, these changes are less responsible for the declining metabolism when compared to the reduction of hepatic blood flow. This can decline 40–50 per cent by old age and thus even the 'safer' benzodiazepines, such as temazepam, oxazepam, and lorazepam, will probably have a prolonged half-life despite their absence of active metabolites (Omslander 1981; Greenblatt *et al.* 1982). Similarly, renal clearance declines 35–50 per cent in most elderly patients, despite the maintenance of normal values for routine renal function tests. The excretion of active metabolites may be prolonged and add to the risk of drug accumulation.

There were early reports that the incidence of anxiety disorders declined as people aged (Guterman and Eisdorfer 1989). These were based on the monoamine hypothesis of anxiety, whereby potentially anxiogenic neuro-transmitters, such as serotonin and noradrenaline, were seen to decline with age. benzodiazepines, however, exert their effect at the $GABA_A$ receptors and these have also been reported to be reduced in number and sensitivity with advancing age (Steinberg 1990; Warneke 1991). However, this would not explain the increased sensitivity that the elderly show to the sedative and anxiolytic effects of benzodiazepines. It may be that benzodiazepine-induced GABA binding is less affected by ageing than the declines in the noradrenaline and serotonin systems. This would result in a relative increase in the sensitivity to neuronal inhibition with age, and be reflected clinically by increased sedation and other central nervous system toxicities (Nolan and O'Malley 1989; Salzman 1990). While the exact alterations in neuronal sensitivity are unclear, it is clear that changes in the pharmacokinetics do not explain all of the increased sensitivity seen with benzodiazepine use in the elderly. The pharmacodynamic factors await further clarification.

Applying the above principles to benzodiazepine treatment in the elderly will only minimize some of the attendant risks. The patients cannot be seen in isolation from their coexisting medical pathologies as these will have further impact on benzodiazepine efficacy and toxicity. Eighty per cent of those 65 or older will have one or more chronic illnesses (Kusserow 1989). These must be reviewed prior to benzodiazepine use. Chronic illnesses such as cardiovascular, metabolic, hepatic and renal pathologies will not only increase the risk of toxicity, but also may be the underlying cause for the presenting anxiety itself. Chronic obstructive lung disease, for example, has been shown to be associated with anxiety and depression (Karajgi *et al.* 1990). Fluctuating levels of anxiety and panic disorder occur more often in chronic obstructive lung disease patients than in controls. This may be secondary to changes in PCO_2 receptor sensitivity at a central level (Jenike 1989, p. 262). Alternatively, benzodiazepine treatment may worsen underlying physical illness as was reported by Sullivan (1989) in regard to respiratory drive suppression.

Similarly, insomnia, a frequent complaint in geriatric medicine, may be due to benign age-related changes or to more serious events such as congestive heart failure (paroxysmal nocturnal dyspnoea), infection, pain syndromes, or delirium. It is well known that the elderly often have a decline in nocturnal sleep with decreases in stages 3, 4, and REM activity. However, total sleep time over a 24-h period is relatively unchanged compared to that of young adults. Thus, prescribing benzodiazepines for benign sleep disturbances is rarely indicated unless there is evidence of a recent change and impairment in psychosocial functioning. Furthermore, insomnia may be the only presenting symptom of an underlying cardiorespiratory disorder. The onus is on the physician to undertake a thorough history and examination to differentiate primary versus secondary and cause versus effect.

Multiple illness commonly means multiple medications. In 1986, 613 million prescriptions were written in the USA for elderly for elderly patients, converting into 15.5 prescriptions per person for that year (Steinberg 1990). While this number may be disturbing to some health care critics, there is no proper number of medications that a person should be on; one may be too many for some and 10 too few for others. The important aspect is that they must be indicated and regularly reviewed. When prescribing benzodiazepines, all pre-existing medications, prescribed and over the counter, must be known and potential drug interactions predicted whenever possible. The most common type of interaction seen that involves benzodiazepines is additive central nervous system depression which occurs when benzodiazepines are combined with other centrally depressant drugs. Alcohol and other sedative/hypnotic agents, and antidepressants may cause varying degrees of sedation. Benzodiazepine levels and thus effects are increased by concomitant use of cimetidine and estrogen preparations secondary to impaired metabolism. Benzodiazepines are also known to increase the levels of dilantin and digoxin (Bernstein 1988, pp. 348–9).

Treatment compliance is a central aspect of management in all areas of medicine. Non-compliance may play more of a role in geriatric medicine because of the complexity and multiplicity of drug regimes, an aversion to 'pills' resulting from a lack of lifetime exposure to and familiarity with modern medical practices, and varying degrees of cognitive and memory dysfunction. While taking more than prescribed can obviously lead to toxicity, taking less may, for a time, be protective if the particular treatment is not actually required or required but at a lower dose. However, on admission to a care facility or hospital the elderly patient receives all medications at the prescribed dose and frequency. Oversedation and central nervous system toxicity can easily occur and may partly be reflected in the high incidence of delirium seen in hospitalized patients (Francis *et al.* 1990). Therefore, admission is an ideal time to review all prescribed medications and to consolidate treatment.

In summary, physiological alterations, concomitant illness and medications, and individual patient variables such as compliance are significant factors to be aware of when prescribing to the elderly patient. Clinical foresight must be exercised before prescribing benzodiazepines in order to choose the most appropriate agent and thus minimize potential side-effects and toxicity. None of the aforementioned situations or states warrant the 'no benzodiazepine rule' and should merely be acknowledged and made a part of any treatment decision.

Benzodiazepine use in dementia and agitation

As is customary sound medical practice, medications should only be used when there is a targeted illness or disorder warranting treatment. Unfortunately, benzodiazepines are thought to be used indiscriminately by some as behavioural or symptom suppressants (Beardsley *et al.* 1989). Indeed, many elderly patients, especially those in chronic care facilities, have been shown to receive benzodiazepines for poorly defined (if at all) target symptoms. However, what is often not appreciated by critics of medication is the complexity of geriatric disorders and the polymorphic presentation of geriatric illnesses. Cognitive decline, medical illness, and autonomic dysfunction all have an impact on the phenotypic expression of anxiety states. As a result, the usually classic symptom complex of anxiety is frequently absent, being replaced by non-specific agitation, restlessness, and insomnia. The physician must have a high index of suspicion not to overlook anxiety disorders in the demented patient. A comprehensive personal, past, and family psychiatric history are certainly helpful in this regard, as is any past history of benzodiazepine, alcohol, or other substance use. There are situations, however, where even the most careful assessments fail to reveal a cause for the anxiety or agitation. In these instances it is not improper to initiate a trial of benzodiazepines if one is careful to identify and follow the target behaviour(s). This is often the case in dementia, where agitation is felt to reflect the underlying global cognitive impairment. While much has been written about the risks and benefits of benzodiazepine use for dysfunctional behaviour associated with dementia, it is still not a well researched area. Dementia is associated with a number of neurotransmitter changes, many of which are exaggerations of the alterations seen with normal ageing. Altered neurochemistry, neuronal loss, and increased blood–brain barrier permeability result in increased sensitivity to all psychotropics including benzodiazepines; however, in many instances benzodiazepines may still be the safest and most efficacious treatment available. Interestingly, benzodiazepines are often overlooked in the management of agitation in dementia, with antipsychotics being preferred

(Salzman 1987; Ancill and Holliday 1988). On reviewing the studies to date, there is little support for this preference; benzodiazepines have been found to exert a similar efficacy to that of neuroleptics. When one considers the extrapyramidal side-effects, tardive dyskinesia, and atropinic side-effects of antipsychotics, the traditional neuroleptic preference is even less supported. While benzodiazepines are not without a side-effect profile, they are generally safer than neuroleptics when used judiciously and they do not have the inherent long-term risks associated with neuroleptics. Furthermore, in the absence of psychosis, neuroleptics are often chosen to sedate or tranquillize the agitated patient, something that high-potency agents do very poorly. Despite this, haloperidol is one of the most frequently prescribed medications in long-term care facilities (Buck 1988). The reasons for this choice are lacking and appear to be based more on folklore than medical fact. Benzodiazepines are tranquillizing, have anxiolytic efficacy, and, even in the elderly, continue to have a high margin of safety.

So what is wrong with benzodiazepines?

Issues of dependency, abuse, and withdrawal

There has been a growing concern in the adult literature that benzodiazepines may evoke physiological tolerance and psychic dependence leading to medication abuse. There is, however, no consistent clinical evidence to support an association of diminished anxiolytic efficacy with long-term use (Warneke 1991). Tolerance may develop to the hypnotic effects within a number of weeks, especially if rapidly eliminated drugs are used (Teboul and Chouinard 1991). Because of the organicity of geriatric anxiety, patients are more likely to receive these medications on a chronic basis. There is no evidence to suggest that long-term users have a greater likelihood of developing dependence than short-term users (Garvey and Tollefson 1986). Physiological tolerance does occur but, despite their widespread use, very little clinical abuse is seen (Warneke 1991). In a comparison of other substances of abuse in adults, Dupont's (1988) 12-month survey showed that 73.5 per cent use alcohol, 36.6 per cent smoke, 15.3 per cent use marijuana, 6.3 per cent cocaine, 4.0 per cent stimulants, 1.4 per cent hallucinogens, but only 3.5 per cent use benzodiazepines or other tranquillizers. While there is some data on substance misuse in the elderly (Schweizer *et al.* 1989), there is little evidence of dose escalation with long-term use. Tolerance to the anti-anxiety effects of benzodiazepines is not clinically seen (Owen and Tyrer 1983; Schopf 1983), and they are rarely used to achieve disinhibition or a 'high' (Warneke 1991). When benzodiazepines are abused, it is usually in association with other drugs, in a vain attempt to self-medicate other functional disorders such as depression, or to prevent withdrawal during abstinence from the primarily abused agent (Warneke 1991). Given the paucity of other treatment options, the chronic nature of geriatric anxiety, and the availability of more dangerous substances (alcohol), there is little to support the 'no benzodiazepine' premise when faced with a chronically agitated or anxious patient. Physicians' fears of causing dependency are simply not warranted. One must be wary, however, when prescribing benzodiazepines to patients with a history of alcohol or other substance abuse (Warneke 1991). Even here, treatment should not be categorically denied and each case should be assessed on its individual merit and risks.

Despite the prevalence of benzodiazepine use in the elderly, withdrawal syndromes have not been well studied. Physiological tolerance is the cause of withdrawal syndromes and, because of pharmacokinetic and pharmaco-dynamic changes in the elderly, they may present somewhat atypically. A frequent problem in assessing withdrawal is its coexistence with rebound symptoms and/or the recurrence of pre-treatment anxiety. The severity of the latter two syndromes vary with the dose of benzodiazepine used, the duration of treatment, its half-life, and, inversely, with the rate of discontinuation. These symptoms do not represent dependence. Rebound symptoms occur gradually upon discontinuation while withdrawal often evokes new symptoms—dysphoria, depersonalization, nausea, tremor, headache, and perceptual distortions—and usually occurs in the ensuing days to weeks (Teboul and Chouinard 1991). While there are reports of more severe withdrawal symptoms in the elderly, recent evidence refutes this (Schweizer *et al.* 1989). Withdrawal, rebound, and recurrence can all be minimized by conservative dosage tapering of 25 per cent of the pre-termination dose per week (Ancill *et al.*, in press). Benzodiazepine accumulation and prolonged half-life may be of some benefit during the tapering process by prolonging drug removal. This can also, however, delay the onset of discontinuation-related symptoms and can make it less obvious to the clinician that there are withdrawal events.

The chronic anxiety states seen among the elderly should result in the clinician anticipating long-term use but not absolutely expecting it. With this often comes an increased risk of withdrawal. Thus, it may be advantageous to discuss with the patient the risks of entering into long-term benzodiazepine use and arrive at a mutual understanding of the target symptoms of treatment and the perceived goal. The need for benzodiazepines should be regularly reviewed and cautious dosage reductions undertaken once target symptoms are controlled. In many physicians the fears of patient dependence often overshadow the consequences of not treating. This attitude leaves the patient to their own devices to control their distressing symptoms by any means available to them (Warneke 1991). The consequences of self-treatment and mental suffering are less visible to the clinician and may inadvertently reinforce the 'benefit' of not treating. So, while there may be some evidence associating chronic benzodiazepine use with physical dependence and tolerance, the issues of psychological dependence remain obscure. One must weight the small risk of dependence against the implications of withholding treatment. Rifkin (1990) summarized the dilemma well by stating that 'while benzodiazepine abuse does occur and abrupt withdrawal of therapeutic doses can cause withdrawal symptoms, even seizures, to conclude from these two facts that therapeutic use leads to abuse is false logic and bad clinical judgement.'

Benzodiazepine side-effects in the elderly

All medications used in psychiatry have side-effects, and nowhere is this more true than for the geriatric patient. Because of their physiological changes, medical infirmity, and multiple medications they not only experience more frequent side-effects than younger benzodiazepine users, but also some unique and potentially lethal complications as well. What is a mild and tolerable side-effect in the young can be extremely serious for the elderly (Steinberg 1990). Benzodiazepines are known to be central nervous system depressants and this may well be the result of altered benzodiazepine receptor sensitivity compounded by drug accumulation (Salzman 1990). The cerebral side-effects of oversedation, incoordination, ataxia, and slurred speech are well recognized, but effects on psychomotor speed and cognitive functioning are less well appreciated. A 'pseudodementia' has been attributed to benzodiazepines, resulting from oversedation and memory impairment; this was reversible on discontinuation of the associated drug (Ancill *et al.* 1987). Reports of impaired short- and long-term memory have been described (Jenike 1989, p. 260), and there is a suggestion that benzodiazepines interfere with memory consolidation. High-potency, short-acting agents (e.g. triazolam, lorazepam) appear to be more likely to affect memory processes. Alternatively, some investigators have found that cognitive performance and recall are enhanced with benzodiazepine control of anxiety (Jenike 1989, p. 261). Memory dysfunction appears to be dose-related (Jenike 1989, p. 261) and, at moderate doses in the absence of oversedation, is not a significant problem. In contrast, long-acting benzodiazepines, while able to cause cognitive impairment, tend to do so insidiously and are less likely to be identified. Long-term treatment and accumulation of these agents can mimic dementia. Only removal of the agent can differentiate a pseudodementia from the true state (Salzman 1990). The risk of cognitive and psychomotor impairment from benzodiazepines must be weighed against the cognitive side-effects of other medications used in this age group. Agitation in dementia is often treated with neuroleptics and their anticholinergic effects are well known to impair cognition. When the additional neuroleptic risks of extrapyramidal side-effects, neuroleptic malignant syndrome, irreversible tardive dyskinesia, and postural hypotension are taken into account, the benefit of neuroleptics over benzodiazepines is less than clear. Trials of benzodiazepines in agitation associated with dementia reveal similar efficacy to that of neuroleptics—both are successful in less than 50 per cent of cases (Salzman 1987).

Another common concern for physicians treating agitated demented patients is the risk of further disinhibition and aggravation of their aggressive behaviour. While the incidence of this is increased when the patient has cognitive impairment or head injury, the risk is still less than 1 per cent (Jenike 1989, p. 261). A conservative estimate that puts the risk of tardive dyskinesia from neuroleptics at 15 to 20 per cent seems to be somehow more acceptable. The indifferent attitude towards tardive dyskinesia on the part of physicians may be the result of the delayed onset of this condition and the perception that 'the patient will be somebody else's problem by then'.

Patients receiving benzodiazepines have frequently been reported to experience more falls and hip fractures than patients not receiving psychotropics (Ray *et al*. 1987). Ray *et al*. (1989) further state that there is a difference in relative risk between fractures secondary to falls in those using long —as opposed to short half-life benzodiazepines, (1.7 versus 1.1 per cent, respectively). However, Jacobs and Das (1990) emphasized that, while 211 000 hip fractures occur in the USA each year, less than 6 per cent of these occur in patients taking long-acting benzodiazepines and 20.6 per cent occur in patients receiving other psychotropic medications. So, while it makes pharmacological and clinical sense that long half-life benzodiazepine users may be more at risk for falls and fractures owing to oversedation and accumulation, this risk cannot be viewed in isolation from the risk associated with other psychotropic drugs. Not prescribing benzodiazepines for fear of causing falls is simply not justified as the alternative is one of equal or greater risk. Each individual situation must be assessed, focusing on the risk factors for falls; gait, walking aids, degree of mental/cognitive impairment, postural hypotension, and environment to name just a few.

Benzodiazepine choice

It has taken much discussion to reach the point of actual benzodiazepine choice. Before discussing the merits and risks of individual agents some general comments are needed. First, following the identification of the target symptoms, a decision is needed regarding the likely duration of treatment to be required. Many elderly have chronic anxiety and may require long-term treatment. Others continue to receive chronic treatment, despite having only temporary or short-term benzodiazepine need. Second, in geriatric treatment, it is easier to determine those benzodiazepines to be avoided than those to be used. There are no data suggesting that benzodiazepines have any differences in therapeutic efficacy but they do differ in their relative propensity towards anxiolysis and sedation. As such, some agents are marketed primarily as hypnotics; however, these too have anxiolytic activity. Third, initial geriatric dosages for benzodiazepines should be roughly one-third of those used for younger patients. The clinician should titrate the dose more slowly, allowing for the longer half-lives and time to reach steady state. Yet, contrary to many opinions, there are no definitive data on a unique geriatric dose. The limits should be defined by monitoring the response of target symptoms as viewed against any emergent side-effects. The final dose achieved in the geriatric patient may not be any different to that used in younger patients. What should be different is the rate of the titration phase. In addition, owing to the longer half-lives, it may be possible to give even the short-acting agents twice or thrice daily instead of following the more common three or four time daily schedules. Overall, the principle of 'start low, go slow, and review often' is a fundamental one.

While serum half-lives reflect the time needed to eliminate one-half of a given dose from the body, they do not necessarily equal the half-lives of the benzodiazepines within the central nervous system. They offer only a rough guide and are of some use where full diurnal effect is not required. In insomnia the half-life of the drug chosen should reflect the sleep disturbance. Initial insomnia may be best treated with triazolam, while middle and terminal sleep disturbances are better treated with mid-duration agents such as temazepam. The latter has a longer half-life than triazolam and aids in sleep maintenance while minimizing the risk of rebound insomnia, possible amnesic effects, and daytime sedation. Flurazepam, marketed as an hypnotic, has a half-life of up to at least 100 in the elderly (Bernstein 1988, p. 59) and is more likely to accumulate than temazepam owing to its hepatic oxidation. Temazepam has no active intermediates and is inactivated directly by hepatic conjugation.

In terms of daytime anxiety lorazepam is often chosen because of its multiroute preparations, absence of active metabolites, and relatively short half-life. However, there are reports emerging (Salzman 1990; Ancill *et al.* 1987, 1991) that lorazepam is associated with more central nervous system toxicity, ataxia, and memory impairment, which may reflect its high lipophilicity and preferential accumulation in the brain.

Alprazolam may be a useful alternative to neuroleptics in the management of the behavioural disturbances, agitation, and pacing that are seen with dementia (Salzman 1987; Ancill 1990). Alprazolam is a potent anxiolytic that is oxidized by the liver and that has a short half-life. It is not prone to accumulation and does not appear to cause the degree of central nervous system toxicity that has been associated with lorazepam (Ancill *et al.* 1991). However, alprazolam's short half-life and the need for multiple daily dosing has led some, with good success, to use clonazepam for behavioural disorders associated with cerebral vascularities and Alzheimer's disease (Jones and Chouinard 1985).

Alternatives to benzodiazepines

The growing interest in geriatric anxiety disorders and the dissatisfaction, deserved or not, with benzodiazepines has led to the development of some novel agents and new indications for others.

One new compound, the azapirone buspirone, is a non-benzodiazepine anti-anxiety agent. It has partial serotonin agonist properties affecting the 5-HT_{1A} receptor with no effect on the 5-HT_2 receptor sites. In the general population, it has been shown to be as efficacious as diazepam in controlling generalized anxiety (Rickels *et al.* 1982) but not useful in panic disorder, obsessive–compulsive disorder, or insomnia (Jenike 1989, p. 264). No dosage adjustment is required for the elderly patient and it may take more than a week to have its full effect (Steinberg 1990). It has no cross-tolerance with benzodiazepines so care must be exercised when switching from a benzodiazepine to buspirone in order to avoid precipitating rebound or withdrawal reactions. While no double-blind, controlled trials have been conducted in this population, buspirone may prove useful in the geriatric patient because of the absence of sedation, tolerance, discoordination, and minimal interaction with other concomitantly prescribed medications (Steinberg 1990; Salzman 1990). Buspirone may be of benefit in diminishing the mild-to-moderate degrees of agitation associated with dementia, without the toxicities of neuroleptics and benzodiazepines. While the authors of this chapter have had some open-trial success with buspirone in these clinical situations, it appears that it works either very well or not at all. The pharmacological mechanisms for this are not well understood and further direct comparisons are needed with both benzodiazepines and neuroleptics.

Antihistamines such as diphenhydramine and hydroxyzine have non-specific sedative properties and are of some use in the short-term management of insomnia. But, because of rapid physiological tolerance to their hypnotic properties and their risk of precipitating anticholinergic delirium, they offer little long-term benefit (Salzman 1990). They may be of some additional use in the treatment of anxiety associated with severe chronic obstructive lung disease, although buspirone would appear to be a better choice where respiratory function is compromised. Benzodiazepines carry significant risks for these patients owing to their ability to suppress respiratory drive and further escalate anxiety symptoms.

Somatic symptoms of anxiety, such as tachycardia, palpitations, tachypnoea, tremulousness, and diaphoresis, are mediated by the sympathetic nervous system. Some researchers believe that anxiety states result from the patient's sensitivity and interpretation of these symptoms (Omslander 1981). It is suggested that beta-blockers may alleviate this type of anxiety in the elderly when the somatic symptoms are prominent (Salzman 1988). Their use in the elderly is somewhat limited by the prevalence of physical contraindications such as chronic obstructive lung disease, asthma, congestive heart failure, bradycardia, and the significant risks in the elderly of heart block and postural hypotension. Low doses of propranolol, 5 to 10 mg once to four times daily, may be effective for geriatric anxiety states, but more experience is needed to better establish the dosage range (Salzman 1990).

Lastly, anxiety is a frequent concomitant symptom of endogenous geriatric depression. If depression is the primary diagnosis, then the anxiety will probably respond in parallel to direct treatment of the depression (Jenike 1989, p. 266). Caution must be exercised when assessing insomnia in the elderly. Overlooking a depressive illness and treating the anxiety or insomnia as the primary problem will result in a perpetuation of the depressive illness and increase the risks inherent in an untreated mood disorder.

Conclusion

Despite our limited understanding of benzodiazepine physiology in the geriatric patient, these agents continue to prove themselves as safe and effective in the treatment of anxiety and related disorders. As a group benzodiazepines do carry significant risks but these must be weighed against both the consequences of not treating and the risks associated with alternative agents, which may carry significant risks themselves. Controlled trials are needed not only to assess the differences between benzodiazepines, but also to address the dependence and abuse fears so prevalent in the media and in the medical community itself. Fear of dependency should not result in therapeutic nihilism. There is a place for the proper use of benzodiazepines in the elderly. Indeed, striking this balance is perhaps what geriatric psychiatry is all about. The best clinical decisions must balance the patient and his history against the medications and their risk/benefit ratio. This is no small task when prescribing benzodiazepines to the elderly and requires patience, knowledge, and a consistent, flexible, and vigilant approach.

References

Ancill, R.J. (1990). Benefits and risks of benzodiazepines in the geriatric patient: striking the balance. *Psychiatry*, **4**,(1), 3–5.

Ancill, R.J. and Holliday, S.G. (1988). The assessment and management of dysfunctional behavior in the cognitively impaired elderly. *Psychiatry*, April, 20–4.

Ancill, R.J., Embury, G.D., MacEwan, G.W., and Kennedy, J.S. (1987). Lorazepam in the elderly—a retrospective study of the side effects in 20 patients. *Journal of Psychopharmacology*, **2**, 126–7.

Ancill, R.J., Carlyle, W.W., Liang, R.A., and Holliday, S.G. (1991). Agitation in the demented elderly: a role for benzodiazepines? *International Clinical Psychopharmacology*, **6**, 141–6.

Beardsley, R.S., Larson, D.B., Burns, B.J., Thompson, J.W., and Kamerow, D.B. (1989). Prescribing of psychotropics in elderly nursing home patients. *Journal of the American Geriatric Society*, **37**(4), 327–30.

Bernstein, J.G. (1988). *Handbook of drug therapy in psychiatry* (2nd edn). PSG Publishing Co, Littleton.

Buck, J.A. (1988). Psychotropic drug practice in nursing homes. *Journal of the American Geriatric Society*, **36**(5), 409–18.

Dupont, R.L. (1988). Abuse of benzodiazepines: the problems and the solutions. A report of a committee of the Institute for Behavior and Health, Inc. *American Journal of Drug and Alcohol Abuse*, **14** (suppl.), 1–69.

Francis, J., Martin, D., and Kapoor, W.N. (1990). A prospective study of delirium in hospitalized elderly. *Journal of the American Medical Association*, **263**(8), 1097–101.

Garvey, M. and Tollefson, G. (1986). Prevalence of misuse of prescribed benzodiazepines in patients with primary anxiety disorder or major depression. *American Journal of Psychiatry*, **143**(12), 1601–3.

Greenblatt, D.J., Sellers, E.M., and Shader, R.I. (1982). Drug disposition in old age. *New England Journal of Medicine*, **306** (18), 1081–8.

Guterman, A. and Eisdorfer, C. (1989). Other psychiatric conditions of the elderly. In *Comprehensive textbook of psychiatry*, Vol. 2 (5th edn) (ed. H.I. Kaplan and B.J. Sadock), pp.2031–2. Williams and Wilkins, Baltimore.

Higgitt, A. (1988). Indications for benzodiazepine prescriptions in the elderly. *International Journal of Geriatric Psychiatry*, **3**, 239–43.

Jacobs, J. and Das, A. (1990). Benzodiazepines and hip fracture. *Journal of the American Medical Association*, **263**,(24), 3260–1.

Jenike, M.A. (1989). Anxiety disorders of old age. In *Geriatric psychiatry and psychopharmacology*, pp.248–71. YearBook Medical Publishers, Chicago.

Jones, B. and Chouinard, G. (1985). Clonazepam in the treatment of recurrent symptoms of depression and anxiety in a patient with systemic lupus erythematosus. *American Journal of Psychiatry*, **142** (3) 354–5.

Karajgi, B., Rifkin, A., Doddi, S., and Ravindra, K. (1990). The prevalence of anxiety disorders in patients with chronic obstructive pulmonary disease. *American Journal of Psychiatry*, **147** (2), 200–1.

Kusserow, R.P. (1989). *Medicare drug utilization review*. Department of Health and Human Services, January.

Mellinger, G.D., Balter, M.B., and Uhlenhuth, E.H. (1984). Prevalence and correlates of the long-term regular use of anxiolytics. *Journal of the American Medical Association*, **251**, 375–9.

Miller, G.D., Whitcup, S. (1986). Inappropriate prescribing of benzodiazepines in depressed elderly patients. *Journal of Clinical Psychopharmacology*, **6**, 384–5.

Nolan, L. and O'Malley, K. (1989). Adverse drug reactions in the elderly. *British Journal of Hospital Medicine*, **41**, 447–57.

Omslander, J.G. (1981). Drug therapy in the elderly. *Annals of Internal Medicine*, **94**, 711–22.

Owen, R.T. and Tyrer, P. (1983). Benzodiazepine dependence: a review of the evidence. *Drugs*, **25**, 385–98.

Ray, W.A., Griffin, M.R., Schaffner, W., Baugh, D.K., and Melton, L.J. (1987). Psychotropic drug use and the risk of hip fracture. *New England Journal of Medicine*, **316**, 363–9.

Ray, W.A., Griffin, M.R., and Downey, W. (1989). Benzodiazepines of long and short elimination half-life and the risk of hip fracture. *Journal of the American Medical Association*, **262** (23), 3303–7.

Rickels, K., Weisman, K., Norstad, N., Singer, M., Stoltz, D., Brown, A., and Danton, J. (1982). Buspirone and diazepam in anxiety: a controlled study. *Journal of Clinical Psychiatry*, **43** (12), 81–6.

Rifkin, A. (1990). Benzodiazepines for anxiety disorders. Are the concerns justified? *Postgraduate Medicine*, **87** (1), 209–19.

Salzman, C. (1987). Treatment of the elderly agitated patient. *Journal of Clinical Psychiatry*, **48** (Suppl.5), 19–22.

Salzman, C. (1988). Treatment of agitation, anxiety and depression in dementia. *Psychopharmacology Bulletin*, **24**, 39–42.

Salzman, C. (1990). Anxiety in the elderly. *Journal of Clinical Psychiatry*, **51** (Suppl. 10) 18–21.

Schopf, J. (1983). Withdrawal phenomenon after long term administration of benzo-diazepines: a review of recent investigations. *Pharmacopsychiatrica*, **16**, 1–8.

Schweizer, E., Case, W.G., and Rickels, K. (1989). Benzodiazepine dependence and withdrawal in elderly patients. *American Journal of Psychiatry*, **146** (4), 529–31.

Steinberg, J.R. (1990). Prescription drug impairment in the elderly. *Drug Therapy Supplement*, August, 83–100.

Sullivan, R.J. (1989). Respiratory depression requiring ventilatory support following 0.5 mg triazolam. *Journal of the American Geriatric Society*, **37** (5), 450–2.

Sullivan, C.F., Copeland, J.R.M., Dewey, M.E., Davidson, I.A., McWilliam, C., Saunders, P., *et al.* (1988). Benzodiazepine usage amongst the elderly: findings in the Liverpool Survey. *International Journal of Geriatric Psychiatry*, **3**, 289–92.

Teboul, E. and Chouinard, G. (1991). A guide to benzodiazepine selection. Part III: Clinical aspects. *Canadian Journal of Psychiatry*, **36** (3), 62–73.

Warneke, L.B. (1991). Benzodiazepines: abuse and new use. *Canadian Journal of Psychiatry*, **36** (3), 194–205.

16 Benzodiazepines in general practice

Richard J. Simpson

The current view of benzodiazepines from a general practice perspective is a bleak one. After two decades, the 1960s and 1970s, during which this class of compound appeared to be safe and efficacious, practitioners have seen their use restricted in the 1980s. There is now the prospect of litigation by hundreds of users who believe they are dependent or have been damaged.

The slowness with which the profession has responded to the growing volume of careful research into dependency is a sorry reflection of our collective failure to conduct adequate self-audit where it matters, i.e. in primary care. The benzodiazepines are just one more group in the list of compounds following a similar path. The amphetamines were finally restricted in 1968, 29 years after the first publication warning of their dangers, and the barbiturates in the early 1970s, a similar length of time after warnings about their dangers.

The first warnings of the problems to come date from the early 1960s, only a few years after the introduction of the first benzodiazepine. Unnecessary use of hypnotics and inappropriate prescribing for the treatment of depression were demonstrated in the 1970s. However, the extent and nature of the dependency problem were not identified until late in that decade. Wells (1973), reporting on the elimination of barbiturate prescribing from his practice, substituted nitrazepam. The excess of unnecessary hypnotic takers, even at that time, was indicated by his achievement of a reduction of 41 per cent in the overall prescribing of hypnotics. Similarly, Clift (1972) reduced the long-term taking of hypnotics from 32 to 8 per cent, again mainly by the reduction of barbiturates.

Wilks (1975, 1980) published analyses of his practice's psychotropic pre-scribing in 1971–72 and again in 1975. He was advocating in his 1971–72 survey that there should be a reduction in both the variety of psychotropics and, particularly, in the use of barbiturates and minor tranquillizers. Consequent reduction (see Table 16.1) concurred almost exactly with the author's own unpublished analyses, carried out on his own practice by the Pharmacy Department of Heriot Watt University for the years 1972 and 1977. These figures supported the need for a more rational view of prescribing, both in reducing benzodiazepines prescribed as hypnotics and as anxiolytics, and for an increased use of antidepressants.

In examining problems with benzodiazepines, we then need to ask the following questions.

Table 16.1 Changes in prescribing levels of hypnotics and tranquillizers*

Study	Year	N	Prescriptions for							
			Hypnotics/ barbiturates		Non-barbiturates		Tranquillizers		Antidepressants	
			No. (10³)	%	No. (10³)	%	No. (10³)	%	No. (10³)	%
England & Wales†	1970	908	276	30.4	152	16.7	366	40.3	114	12.6
England†	1975	750	148	19.7	214	28.5	214	28.5	174	23.2
Wilks‡	1971	438	65	14.8	21	4.8	174	39.7	178	40.6
Wilks‡	1976	345	10	2.9	15	4.3	98	28.4	222	64.3
Simpson§	1972	497	50	10.1	50	10.1	203	40.9	194	39.0
Simpson§	1977	446	15	3.4	35	7.9	100	22.4	296	66.4

* Modified from Wilks (1980).   † Source: national Prescription Authority (1970, 1975)   ‡ Source: Wilks (1975, 1980).
§ Unpublished data from the author's own practice.

- Why did it take so long to recognize the dependency problem?

- How did the drug come to be used inappropriately in so many cases?

- Do we now understand the full extent and the nature of its chronic use?

- Could this happen again with a further class of compounds, or indeed be happening at this very time?

Wright (1991) states 'Much of our knowledge of the action and relative value of psychotropic drugs is derived from hospital based trials. It is therefore important to investigate the reason for the initial prescription and use of psychotropic drugs, the effectiveness of these drugs, and the impact of such factors as the patient's personality and the therapeutic setting in which medicaments are prescribed.'

In the same editorial Wright reminds us that the overwhelming majority of psychiatric illness and psychological problems are seen and managed by general practitioners alone.

There are many problems facing general practitioners in managing mental ill health. These include the relative paucity of postgraduate training in psychiatry; it is still possible to be 'fully' vocationally trained in general practice without ever doing any formal postgraduate training in psychiatry. Furthermore, despite the curriculum advocated by the Joint Committee of the Royal Colleges of Psychiatry and General Practice in 1978, much of the training that is available is lacking in relevance to primary care.

Even if general practitioners had the personal skills and training, we would still lack the time to undertake most therapies other than pharmaceutical ones. Furthermore, it must be recognized that, even where a clear psychiatric diagnosis exists, the possibilities for referral to such resources as community psychiatric nurses, community nurse therapists, and clinical psychologists are severely limited. These problems of resources are compounded by the fact that the general practitioner is faced with an enormous range of human distress from the clearly identifiable diagnosis that fits either the International Classification of Diseases (ICD-9) or the *Diagnostic and statistical manual of mental disorders* (DSM-III R; APA 1987) to the much more common distress symptoms, associated either with the patient's current situation or with anxiety generated through the threat of physical disease. The ICD and DSM-III R are inadequate for describing the daily problems seen in primary care. Problem tallies analysed from data presenting to a practice of 30 000 in Southampton and the authors own practice of 5 500 in Bridge of Allan (see Table 16.2) show something of this reality.

In meeting the challenge of the benzodiazepines, simple replacement of these drugs by others, as the barbiturates were replaced by the benzodiazepines, will not be enough. Understanding the problems faced by those of us in primary care may help to prevent a repetition of past problems.

In offering a view of the use and overuse of this class of compounds in UK

Table 16.2. Problem tallies in general practice*

	Prevalence (no./1000)
Anxiety	74
Social problems	30
Drinking problems†	26
Acute depression	26
Bereavement	25
Sleep problems	21
Marital problems	20
Over-anxious problems	15
Neurosis	15
Behavioural problems	12
Enuresis	11
Unhappiness	10
Social dependency	10
Domestic problem	9
Psychosexual problems	8
Marital breakdown/divorce	7
Speech problems	6
Housing problems	5
Psychosis	4
Relationship problems	4
Miscellaneous	78
	——
	338

Total prevalence of all problems 416 per 1000

* Source: Simpson (1989).
† This was the Scottish Centre rate—the Southampton rate was less than 10.

general practice, the timing is important since the prescribing habits of general practitioners in the 1990s are undoubtedly changing. The high point of UK use was reached around 1980 and has been dropping ever since. In the 1990s use will be further curtailed under the varied influences of new instructions on the appropriate use of benzodiazepines from the Committee on the Safety of Medicines (1988), the statement on appropriate use from the Royal College of Psychiatrists (1988), and, not least, from anticipated law suits being brought by long-term users against pharmaceutical companies and general practitioners.

It is possible, but not probable, that new long-term benzodiazepine users will not be added to the present cohort in this decade. However, as will be seen from the general practitioner and community research reviewed, this cohort is predominantly elderly and major misuse should decline naturally with their eventual demise.

Patient characteristics

It is important to recognize that, of the many hundreds of research studies
on benzodiazepine use and abuse published, the overwhelming majority
have drawn on unrandomized and often self-selected populations. Thus, in
describing withdrawal, both in terms of those features that may well be new
symptoms characteristic of dependency and those that are more typical of
rebound or re-emergence of pre-treatment states, the average age of those
studied was between 30 and 50 years. This falls well short of the mean age
of users in the community. Age is not the only factor where specialist studies
fail to reflect accurately the realities of general practice in the UK or the
community at large.

Table 16.3 is a summary of the findings in four UK general practices (six
published papers): Salinsky and Dore (1987); Rodrigo *et al.* (1988) and King
et al. (1990); Catalan *et al.* (1988), Simpson *et al.* (1990*a*) and Forth Valley
GP Research Group (1990). Also summarized for comparison is Mellinger *et
al.*'s (1984) American report of the 1979 National Survey on psychotherapeutic
drug use.

Age of users

These studies confirm that users in general practice are typically older and
start benzodiazepine use at a later age than is generally portrayed. This
is not surprising if one refers back to Skegg *et al.*'s (1977) analysis of
psychotropic prescribing. They reported on an Oxfordshire practice where
33 per cent of women aged 45–59 received a psychotropic drug in 1 year
and, more relevant to this chapter, the long-term use was reflected in 12.9
per cent of the women receiving more than five repeat prescriptions. Williams
(1982), looking prospectively at the prescribing of six general practitioners,
described an age of more than 45 years as one of the variables associated
with longer-term use. These four studies do not readily lend themselves to
a meta-analysis. Nevertheless, the figures of current age all confirm a group
predominantly in their sixties. Previously published age-related rates from our
own work (see Table 16.4) show the substantial usage in ageing groups.

It is therefore not accidental that this view from general practice should
come after the chapter examining effects in the elderly. It is the risk/benefit
analysis for that elderly group, and each individual therein, that must be
undertaken before general practitioners can go beyond assisting those who,
following discussion, volunteer to be withdrawn from drugs.

Usage patterns

The number of specialist papers reporting on dependence and withdrawal over
the past 10 years attest to the growing concern of psychiatrists about long-term
users. There can be no doubt about the existence of a dependency in some
patients but, before embarking on a withdrawal programme in the elderly

Table 16.3. General practice and community studies of long-term benzodiazepine, hypnotic, or anxiolytic users

Sample (no. patients)		Length of prescription		Original reason		Female patients (%)	Age now		Factors	Patient views	
Psychotropic drugs	Total	Years	%	Reason	%		Years	%	Factors	View	%
Study 1 (UK: Salinsky and Dore 1987)*											
96	6000	>5	72	Anxiety	66	81	>45	82	Chronic physical illness	Helpful	79
		>10	44	Crisis†	60		>55	60	Loss of father (>18 patients)	Intend to stop	41
Study 2 (UK: Rodrigo et al. 1988; King et al. 1990)‡											
84	4000	5 (average)		Insomnia	61	76	>40	8		Had tried to stop in previous year	66
				Anxiety	15			41			
Study 3 (UK: Catalan et al. 1988)§											
318	8442	3–5	21			74	>50	71	Psychiatric diagnosis (30 of 70)	Help with sleep	80
		6–10	40				>65	33		Calming effect	56
										Had tried to stop in previous years	58
										Wanted to stop	50
Study 4 (UK: Forth Valley GP Research Group 1990; Simpson et al. 1990a)¶											
445	17000	>6	50			77	>49	18	Physical ill health (cardiovascular)	'Vital or very important or help to cope'	81
		8 (average)					64 average; (SD, 14 years)			Not concerned about medicine	41
Study 5 (USA: Mellinger et al. 1984)*											
3161‡‡						61	'Older'		Somatic ill health (cardiovascular) Emotional distress		

* Anxiolytics only; 45% had stopped at follow-up.   † This included 19% bereavement.
‡ 80% of prescriptions started by general practitioner.   § Psychotropic drugs >1 year. There was a control sample of 70. 56% were on anxiolytics.
¶ The average age of starting benzodiazepines was 47 years.   ** A community study of psychotropics.   ‡‡ 11% of the general population.

Table 16.4. Age-band prevalence rates of long-term benzodiazepine users

| Age (years) | Age distribution | | | | Rate of benzodiazepine users (per 1000) |
| | Practice population | | Benzodiazepine users | | |
	No.	%	No.	%	
20–9	2605	22	3	(<1)	1
30–9	2237	19	22	(5)	10
40–9	2033	17	53	(12)	26
50–9	1795	15	67	(15)	37
60–9	1646	14	133	(30)	81
70–9	948	8	115	(26)	121
80–9	392	3	49	(11)	125
90+	102	<1	3	(<1)	29
Totals	11758		455		

* Source: Simpson *et al.* (1990*b*).

similar to that undertaken with barbiturates in the late 1960s and early 1970s, general practitioners need a clearer definition of this patient population.

The 1979 National Survey reported by Mellinger in 1984 was undertaken by the National Institute for Mental Health as part of a broader programme looking at psychotropic drugs in the population at large. 3161 people aged 18–79 were interviewed personally. The study showed that 11 per cent had used anxiolytics in the previous 12 months. (This was thought to be an under reporting by about 2 per cent, the correction being assessed by previous validity studies.) Of this 11–13 per cent, 84 per cent used benzodiazepines. Detailed analysis of this group, however, indicated the following:

- 80 per cent had used these drugs for less than 4 months;

- 67 per cent for less than 4 weeks;

- 62 per cent for less than 2 weeks.

Moreover, the common pattern was occasional use, never more than a day or two at a time, though this pattern did not clarify how frequently this intermittent use occurred. Of all the anxiolytic users, 15 per cent i.e. 1.7 per cent of the total population sample, were long-term regular users (more than 12 months). This is less than the 2.6 per cent reported by the author in his late 1980s study (Simpson *et al.* 1990).

Physical morbidity in users

Mellinger *et al.* (1984) compared long-term users to short-term users (less than 12 months) and non-users. He found clear differences with respect to age (long-term users being older) and sex (there were more females). The measurement of 'emotional' problems used PSYDIS a 17-item check-list derived from the Hopkins Symptom Check-list, scoring for mood depression, mood anxiety, anergia, and impaired cognitive functioning. Both long- and short-term users had more and higher scores than non-users for anxiety and depression with long-users more likely to score high on both. However, the factor that distinguished these three groups most sharply was neither age nor sex nor emotional distress, but somatic health. Furthermore, somatic health differences remained strong even after controlling for age. Two other American studies, one a major community survey by Uhlenhuth *et al.* (1978) and the other a review of physicians' prescribing patterns (Balter and Levine 1973), commented on the interaction of emotional distress preceded or aggravated by a primary diagnosis of physical disorder. In Cooperstock and Leonard's (1979) biased sample in Canada, 53 per cent indicated somatic problems and coping with them as the initial reason for prescriptions.

On this side of the Atlantic this evidence of associated somatic ill health was supported by Williams in his review in 1978, which correlates evidence of substantial physical morbidity and psychotropic drug prescription. Williams himself commented that many of the community and general practitioners studies on which he drew had flaws.

Salinsky and Dore's (1987) open study of 6000 patients in a London practice noted high levels of physical morbidity. Catalan *et al.* (1988) in reviewing an Oxfordshire practice of 8442 patients where prescribing reflected the national pattern for all classes of compound, described the use of hospital services comparing 70 index patients (long-term users) with matched controls. He found that, although there were no differences in the preceding 12 months with respect to admissions or surgery, there was a significant excess for users of general hospital out-patient appointments. Hospital attendance differences could not be accounted for by any excess use of emergency treatment facilities since this sample did not show raised levels of road traffic accidents or accidents at home or at work in the index group. Rodrigo *et al.* (1988) in a similar approach reported that 33 per cent of men and 30 per cent of women in the long-term user group consulted a hospital physician or surgeon in the year prior to the study, a higher rate than predicted for this population.

The Forth Valley GP Research Group (Simpson 1990*a*) examined three practices in the Central Region of Scotland. Four hundred and forty-five patients out of a total practice population of 17 000 were identified as long-term users. A random subsample of 205 was matched for age and sex to controls who were not currently prescribed benzodiazepines. Both groups' records were examined for somatic illness over the previous 25 years and allocated by one experienced general practitioner (who was blind to user or non-user status) to either a major or minor episode (excluding trivial illness). The allocation was based on the need for in-patient treatment, referral, investigation, long-term non-psychotropic medication, and/or permanent disability. The consistency of allocation was checked independently by another researcher. Finally, all lists were rechecked against original records to ensure against omissions. Table 16.5 shows the differences that were significant.

The benzodiazepine group had experienced significantly more episodes of major (p <0.001) and minor (p <0.01) somatic illness than controls. When all major and minor episodes were combined, 32 per cent of the benzodiazepine group had seven or more episodes compared to 16 per cent of non-users.

The prevalence of cardiovascular problems shown in Table 16.5 is supported by Rodrigo *et al.*'s (1988) uncontrolled study showing non-psychotropic drugs as being used by 63 per cent of men and 30 per cent of women, with one in five using more than three medications, most commonly for cardiovascular problems. Williams's (1978) review showed that the psychotropic drug most likely to be prescribed was a minor tranquillizer, and that cardiovascular disease was the category of illness most likely to be associated with psychotropic use.

Psychiatric morbidity in users

All the evidence, from both specialist and general practitioner papers, point to the fact that around half of all the long-term user group do not appear to be suffering from a diagnosable psychiatric disorder. The remainder either have a disorder for which benzodiazepines are not the treatment of choice, such as depression, or are suffering from anxiety or panic disorder, which is inadequately controlled by the benzodiazepines.

The underdiagnosis of depression in general practice is well recognized. The

Table 16.5. Physical morbidity among long-term users of benzodiazepines and age-and sex-matched controls in general practice*

		Users (n=205)	Controls (n=205)	Significance p
Cardiovascular	(Major)	145	68	<0.001
Gastrointestinal	(Major)	88	46	<0.005
	(Minor)	102	50	<0.001
Genitourinary	(Major)	70	41	<0.01
	(Minor)	104	70	<0.05
Respiratory	(Major)	30	8	<0.01
Central nervous	(Major)	16	5	<0.05
Ear, nose and throat	(Minor)	61	38	<0.05

* Source: Simpson *et al.* (1990*a*).

inappropriate treatment of individual depressive symptoms such as insomnia, irritability, and psychic or somatic anxiety with benzodiazepines is a major cause for concern.

An example illustrating many of the worst-features of this mis-prescribing is in depression following childbirth. Cooperstock and Leonard (1979) in Canada and others such as Sclare (private communication) in Glasgow reported that the first year after childbirth was a time at which benzodiazepines were more frequently prescribed. Bryce Pitt (1968, 1975) showed substantial underdiagnosis of depression throughout the first year after childbirth. His criteria of depression were strict, and a slightly looser definition would substantially raise his figures of 10 per cent at 14 days and 3 per cent at the end of the first year.

The author has seen two cases remanded following infanticide and a number of other cases of child assault where misprescribing of benzodiazepines to depressed mothers was implicated as a factor in reducing self-control without alleviation of the depression.

The re-emergence of generalized anxiety disorder (GAD) or panic disorder also occurs. While antidepressant treatment may be useful for the undiag-nosed depression, this class of drug is not yet widely accepted as first-line therapy for GAD or panic disorder in general practice. Of greater proven value is cognitive–behavioural therapy (CBT). Power *et al.*'s (1990) report of 101 DSM-III GAD patients who were not currently on benzodiazepines, in a five-way study of placebo, diazepam, and CBT alone and in combination (i.e. group 4 = placebo + CBT; group 5 = diazepam + CBT) showed definite superior benefits for CBT at the end of a 6-week treatment period. Moreover, the benefits were sustained for the CBT alone and CBT + diazepam groups at 6-month follow-up. Power *et al.*'s study also confirmed the findings of many other studies that a 3-week taper-off after 6 weeks of diazepam therapy of normal therapeutic dosage showed no withdrawal effects.

Patient attitudes

The interaction of the views of the general practitioner as the main prescriber and those of the patient needs elucidation. The current public attitude of patients towards general practitioners' use of benzodiazepines is perhaps best shown by the illustration taken from Hilary Prentice's (1991) Release publication (Fig. 16.1).

Evidence from Cartwright's (1967; Cartwright and Anderson 1981) reviews of general practice in 1964 and 1977 showed that patients were more likely in the 1970s than in 1964 to perceive their doctor as being, 'too inclined to resort to a prescription'. By 1977 those holding this view of their doctor outnumbered those who perceived him as being reluctant to resort to the prescribing pad. Two other UK reports worth mentioning here are one by Marks (1983) reporting a doubling of the proportion of psychotropic prescriptions that were long-term repeats from 30 per cent in 1967 to 60 per cent in 1977: also Drury's (1982) observations showed that there was a marked rise in the number of repeats being issued unseen, i.e. without face-to-face consultation. Mellinger *et al.*'s (1984) USA study is somewhat at odds with this finding, showing that the gap between visits in the USA was only 4–6 months on average. Much of the evidence points towards a growth in prescribing that is repeated and poorly supervised, at least in the UK.

The pressures of pending litigation have produced a major change in approach to benzodiazepine prescribing. Most general practitioners will by now have offered their long-term users the opportunity of stopping. Many will also have recorded interviews where any continued use followed specific advice to stop. In doing so, albeit for defensive reasons, doctors are supporting the desire of a sizeable proportion of their patients to stop. Salinsky and Dore

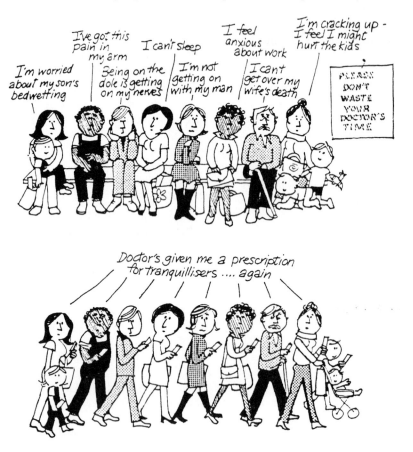

Fig. 16.1. An appropriate illustration reproduced with permission from Prentice (1991).

(1987) showed that 41 per cent had the intention to stop with 66 per cent of his sample having attempted to stop in the previous year. King *et al.* (1990) and Rodrigo *et al.* (1988) found that 50 per cent of their samples wanted to stop and 58 per cent had tried to stop in the previous year. The Forth Valley GP Research Group (1990) found that 41 per cent were very willing or fairly willing to stop. However, this last sample was probably biased towards those willing to stop in its method of selection and, despite this bias, 77 per cent did express concern that their medication might indeed be stopped.

Withdrawal

General practitioners will also have abandoned much of the routine unseen prescribing of benzodiazepines in favour of face-to-face consultations however brief. There is good evidence from Jones's (1990) study that even elderly patients will respond to direct offers of support. In his study 43 per cent decreased their medication and 41 per cent were able to stop with a variety of measures of support offered.

However, care is essential in managing patient's reduction or stopping of medicine. A case quoted in the *British Journal of Psychiatry* (1984) illustrates the dangers of sudden cessation.

A 54 year old woman who had taken diazepam for many years stopped taking the drug and became depressed and anxious. In the supermarket she stole some ice cream cones and 'immediately felt better', she went on to steal some butter. On this and other occasions the exitement of stealing gave dramatic relief of her withdrawal symptoms. She made no attempt to conceal her thefts, however, waiting outside the stores till apprehended.

In contrast, even the most difficult patients can sometimes benefit enormously from withdrawal. The author in a recent placebo-controlled trial had one such case.

A 44-year-old man who had been on lorazepam for 12 years had been markedly agoraphobic even on treatment. As the taper-off regime progressed he withdrew to bed and finally refused to emerge from beneath the bed covers even for food. He was admitted to hospital, completed his withdrawal with some difficulty, and recovered. He enthusiastically talks about the 'new colour' in his life contrasting this with his previous grey existence.

This case, while more extreme than most, was a theme in a significant group of those withdrawing in this unpublished study.

Prescribing of benzodiazepines

General practitioners must resist the temptation to alleviate temporary distress by using benzodiazepines. Situations such as bereavement or loss are unpleasant but natural; they require time and empathic support, not drugs.

One further method of prescribing may become more widespread with patients being encouraged to use a benzodiazepine only at times of stress or anxiety. This linkage of stress to the ingestion of a 'relieving pill' does not seem appropriate. Indeed, it involves avoiding more appropriate antistress measures and, in its very linkage, creates a basis for psychological dependency. The development of health promotion stress-management clinics may be useful in breaking this chain. Where prescribing is to continue a new openness is desirable and again this meets the wishes of patients. Levy and Clayton (1986) reviewed the attitude of patients towards doctors' prescribing habits and found that what patients wanted from their doctor was verbal and written information about the nature and cause of their illness and its natural history and prognosis, as well as about the alternative therapies available. This information should be in addition to an explanation of the nature of the drug being prescribed and the expected benefits and limitations of drug therapy. It is perhaps time then that we moved to a more sophisticated approach with our patients, in discussing a reasoned risk/benefit analysis.

Perhaps the growing involvement of nurses, also now being advocated, will allow us to develop these alternative non-pharmaceutical strategies and allow us to bury the image in Fig. 16.1. However, I suspect that compassion, poor training, insufficient time, lack of alternative resources, and the skill of the pharmaceutical industry will continue to seduce us into reaching for the prescribing pads.

Acknowledgement

My thanks go to Mrs Vivien Swanson, research administrator of the Forth Valley GP Research Group and Christine Simpson, for checking this manuscript.

References

APA (American Psychiatric Association) (1987). *Diagnostic and statistical manual of mental disorders* (3rd edn, revised). American Psychiatric Press, Washington, DC.

Balter, M. B. and Levine, J. (1973). Character and extent of psychotherapeutic drug usage in the USA. In *Proceedings of Vth World Congress of Psychiatry*. Excerpta Medica, Amsterdam. 1973.

British Journal of Psychiatry (1984). A case report. *British Journal of Psychiatry*, **145**, 552–4.

Cartwright. A. (1967). *Patients and their doctors—a study of general practice*. Routledge and Keegan Paul, London.

Cartwright, A. and Anderson, R. (1981). *General practice revisited*. Tavistock Press, London.

Catalan, J., Gath, D. H., Bond, A., Edmonds, G., Martin, P., and Ennis, J. (1988). General practice patients on long term psychotropic drugs. *British Journal of Psychiatry*, **152**, 399–405.

Clift, A. D. (1972). Factors leading to dependence on hypnotic drugs. *British Medical Journal*, **3**, 614–17.

Committee on the Safety of Medicines (1988). Benzodiazepines: dependence and withdrawal symptoms. *Current Problems*, no. 21.

Cooperstock, R. and Leonard, H. L. (1979). Some social meanings of tranquilliser use. *Sociology of Health and Illness*, **1**, 331–7.

Drury, V. W. M. (1982). Repeat prescribing: a review. *Journal of the Royal College of General Practice*, **32**, 42–5.

Forth Valley GP Research Group (1990). The concerns of patients. Psychological ill-health and attitudes to benzodiazepine use and withdrawal among long-term benzodiazepine users. *Scottish Medicine*, **10** (3), 15–17.

Jones, D. (1990). Weaning elderly patients off psychotropic drugs in general practice. *Health Trends*, **1**(22), 164–6.

King, M. J., Gabe, J., Williams, P., and Rodrigo, E. K. (1990). Long-term use of benzodiazepines: the views of patients. *Journal of the Royal College of General Practitioners*, **40**, 194–6.

Levy, B. and Clayton, S. (1986). Drug prescribing and patients' views. *Journal of the Royal College of General Practitioners*, **36**, 169–70.

Marks, J. (1983). Benzodiazepines—for good or evil. *Neuropsychobiology*, **10**, 115–7.

Mellinger, G. D., Balter, M. B., and Uhlenhuth, E. H. (1984). Prevalence and correlates of the long-term regular use of anxiolytics. *Journal of the American Medical Association*, **251**, 375–9.

Pitt, B. (1968), Depression following childbirth. *British Journal of Psychiatry*, **114**, 1325.

Pitt, B. (1975). Depression following childbirth. *British Journal of Psychiatry*, Special Issue No. 9, p.40.

Power, K. G., Simpson, R. J., Swanson, V., Wallace, L., Feistner, A., and Sharp, D. (1990). A controlled comparison of cognitive behaviour therapy, diazepam, and placebo, alone and in combination, for the treatment of generalised anxiety disorder. *Journal of Anxiety Disorders, USA*, **4**, 267–92.

Prentice, H. (1991). *Trouble with tranquillisers*. (revised version). Release Publications Ltd, London.

Rodrigo, E. K., King, M. B., and Williams, P. (1988). The health of long-term benzodiazepine users. *British Medical Journal*, **296**, 603–6.

Royal College of General Practioners (1978). *Some aims for training for general practice*. Occasional Paper 6.

Royal College of Psychiatrists (1988). Benzodiazepines and dependence. 'A College Statement'. *Bulletin of the Royal College of Psychiatrists*, **12**, 107–8.

Salinsky, J. V. and Dore, C. J. (1987). Characteristics of long-term benzodiazepine users in general practice. *Journal of the Royal College of General Practitioners*, **37**, 202–4.

Simpson, R.J. (1984). Psychological illness in general practice. In *General practice medicine* (ed. J H Barber), p.289. Churchill Livingstone, Edinburgh.

Simpson, R. J., Power, K. G., Wallace, L. A., Butcher, M. H., and Simpson, E. C. (1990*a*). Controlled comparison of the characteristics of long-term benzodiazepine users in general practice. *Journal of the Royal College of General Practitioners*, **40**, 22–6.

Simpson, R.J., Power, K.G., and Swanson, V. (1990*b*). Age-hand prevalence rates of long-term benzodiazepine users. *Journal of the Royal College of General Practitioners*, **40**, 168–9.

Skegg, D. C. G., Doll, R., and Perry, J. (1977). Uses of medicines in general practice. *British Medical Journal*, **1**, 1561–3.

Uhlenhuth, E. H., Balter, M. B., and Lipman, R. B. (1978). Minor tranquillisers: clinical correlates in an urban population. *Archives of General Psychiatry*, **35**, 650–5.

Wells, F. O. (1973). Prescribing barbiturates drug substitutes in general practice. *Journal of the Royal College of General Practitioners*, **23**, 164–7.

Williams, P. (1978). Physical ill-health and psychotropic drug prescription—a review. *Psychological Medicine*, **8**, 683–93.

Williams, P., Murray, J., Clare, A. (1982). A longitudinal study of psychotropic drug prescription. *Psychological medicine*, **12**, 201–6.

Wilks, J. M. (1975). A year's survey of the use of psychotropic drugs in general practice. *Journal of the Royal College of General Practioners*, **25**, 731–44.

Wilks, J. M. (1980). Psychotropic drug prescribing: a self-audit. *Journal of the Royal College of General Practioners*, **30**, 390–5.

Wright, A. (1991). Editorial: General practitioners and psychiatry an opportunity for research. *Journal of the Royal College of General Practitioners*, **41**, 223–4.

17 Pharmacological alternatives to benzodiazepine therapy of anxiety disorders

Edward Schweizer and Karl Rickels

Anxiety may manifest as a transient situational response to stress, a secondary reaction to a medical condition, or as a primary anxiety disorder. If one restricts oneself to the latter, lifetime prevalence estimates in the USA for aggregate anxiety disorders have been reported to be as high as 14 per cent (Robins and Regier 1990). Primary anxiety disorders such as generalized anxiety disorder (GAD), panic disorder, and social phobia are frequently chronic conditions that may benefit from long-term treatment. The prevalence and frequent chronicity of anxiety disorders, and the physical dependence liability of benzodiazepines, together provide a strong impetus for establishing the safety and efficacy of alternative pharmacological and psychological treatments for anxiety. This chapter will give a brief summary of the pharmacological alternatives to the benzodiazepines for the treatment of anxiety disorders. Before turning to the newer, non-benzodiazepine anxiolytics, we would like to briefly review the instances in which drugs other than benzodiazepines are indicated for the treatment of anxiety disorders.

The choice of non-benzodiazepine alternative therapy based on diagnosis

Two important considerations guide the choice of drug used to treat anxiety: (1) the specific anxiety diagnosis; and (2) the presence or absence of a co-morbid diagnosis. Insufficient attention to identifying the type of anxiety disorder with which we are confronted may lead to inappropriate choice of a benzodiazepine and, therefore, may result in inadequate or partial treatment response. A review of the literature on 'detection' rates for various anxiety disorders, whether among psychiatrists or non-psychiatrists, is beyond the scope of this chapter, but is generally agreed to be only fair-to-poor. A patient presenting with psychological and physical symptoms of anxiety may have any of several different diagnoses for which benzodiazepines have not been established as efficacious.

Obsessive–compulsive disorder, (OCD) whose lifetime prevalence in the USA is estimated at over 2 per cent (Robins and Regier 1990), frequently presents with anxiety symptoms. Benzodiazepines may have a marginal role as adjunctive therapy in OCD. A growing number of controlled studies (Fontaine and Chouinard 1985; 1988; Goodman *et al.* 1989; Trimble 1990; Clomipramine Collaborative Study Group 1991) suggest that serotonin re-uptake-inhibiting antidepressants such as clomipramine, fluoxetine, and fluvoxamine are especially efficacious. There are no published controlled studies demonstrating efficacy for benzodiazepines in *simple phobia*, which appears to be more responsive to behavioural therapy. *Social phobia*, with a lifetime prevalence of approximately 2 per cent (Robins and Regier 1990), has been called the 'most neglected' anxiety disorder. Preliminary evidence suggests a role for benzodiazepines such as clonazepam (Davidson *et al.* 1991), but there is more evidence of efficacy from the monoamine oxidase (MAO) inhibitor class of antidepressants—both phenelzine and the newer MAO_A antidepressant moclobemide (Liebowitz *et al.* 1988). There is a large literature on non-benzodiazepine alternatives for the treatment of *panic disorder*, most notably the tricyclic antidepressants such as imipramine and the MAO inhibitor antidepressants such as phenelzine. (Sheehan *et al.* 1980; Zitrin *et al.* 1983) *Posttraumatic stress disorder* (PTSD), which has been increasingly recognized as a frequent sequel of traumatic events such as rape and non-sexual assault, is characterized by sleep depressive and dissociative symptoms in addition to prominent symptoms of anxiety and panic. Pilot studies suggest that PTSD may partially respond to benzodiazepines (Davidson *et al.* 1991), but equally convincing (or rather, equally unconvincing) evidence has been reported for response to various tricyclic (Davidson *et al.* 1990) and MAO inhibitor (Hogben and Cornfield 1981; Davidson *et al.* 1987; Shestatsky *et al.* 1988) antidepressants.

As can be seen, the presence of anxiety symptomatology may be a necessary, but is certainly not a sufficient condition to warrant prescription of a benzodiazepine. For OCD, simple phobia, social phobia, and PTSD alternative pharmacological treatments are frequently the treatments of choice. Neglecting to carefully establish a specific anxiety diagnosis will in many instances lead to an inappropriate prescription of a benzodiazepine.

It is only drug therapy for GAD that, until recently, has been almost the exclusive province of the benzodiazepines. But here again, attention to the presence of a co-morbid diagnosis provides a clinical indication that may favour the use of an alternative agent over that of a benzodiazepine.

The choice of non-benzodiazepine alternative therapy based on co-morbidity

Anxiety disorders have a high co-morbidity, especially with affective illness, alcoholism, and Axis II personality disorders. This co-morbidity consists both of the *current* co-occurrence of an anxiety or non-anxiety disorder (cross-sectional co-morbidity), and the development of a second non-anxiety disorder at some point during the course of the anxiety illness (longitudinal co-morbidity). Longitudinal co-morbidity for GAD, panic disorder, OCD, and social phobia are all estimated to be substantial (Barlow *et al.* 1986; Master *et al.* 1990; Robins and Regier 1990), perhaps 50 per cent or higher. For this reason, any benzodiazepine therapy that extends beyond acute treatment requires periodic re-evaluation as to diagnosis. Cross-sectional co-morbidity also occurs in a substantial subgroup of patients suffering from anxiety disorders. As has been noted often, persons seeking treatment generally are found to have more co-morbid diagnoses than patients with an illness who are untreated in the community. The Epidemiological Catchment Area (ECA) community survey (Robins and Regier 1990) found that 21 per cent of all anxiety disorder diagnoses were currently complicated by an affective illness. Eighty per cent of the persons diagnosed with an anxiety disorder in this large (18 000+) sample were receiving no treatment, suggesting that this might be a low estimate for cross-sectional co-morbidity compared to that observed for patients in treatment. If one examines only GAD, perhaps one-third of GAD patients suffer from a concurrent depression and perhaps an equal proportion suffer from a concurrent 'other' anxiety disorder, e.g. panic or social phobia. In either instance an antidepressant might be considered as an alternative to the benzodiazepines.

GAD is also commonly diagnosed in patients suffering from Axis II personality disorders—not only the 'anxious' cluster, but also antisocial personality and borderline personality disorder (Tyrer *et al.* 1983; Weiss *et al.* 1983; Koenigsberg *et al.* 1985). Finally, the ECA survey found that 17 per cent of all anxiety disorder diagnoses were complicated by alcohol dependence or abuse. This appears to be higher for panic disorder and social phobia and lower for GAD (Hirschfield *et al.* 1990; Meyer *et al.* 1990). Benzodiazepines may be relatively contraindicated in anxious patients with co-morbid alcoholism—due to the likelihood of increased euphoric effects (Ciraulo *et al.* 1989)—or personality disorders—due to a possible increase in dependence and withdrawal liability (Rickels *et al.* 1988b).

As can be seen, co-morbidity in patients with anxiety disorders may discourage use of a benzodiazepine or may encourage use of an alternative agent that is likely to be more effective. Much more controlled research needs to be conducted on the treatment of these mixed anxiety states. Current pharmacological treatment studies tend to either exclude patients with co-morbidity, or to include them without carefully defining the co-morbid illness. For now we must rely on clinical experience, but this experience, coupled with reasonable (though unconfirmable) inferences from existing treatment studies of individual 'pure' anxiety disorders, suggests that MAO inhibitor, tricyclic, and serotonin-selective antidepressants have a prominent role in the treatment of anxiety, and offer a safe and efficacious alternative to the benzodiazepines.

Pharmacological alternatives to the benzodiazepines for the treatment of 'pure' generalized anxiety

Even after the diagnostic winnowing suggested above, the clinician will be left with a group of generalized anxiety patients with no significant panic, phobic, or obsessive–compulsive symptoms. This group of patients can be well-managed on benzodiazepines, but what are the treatment alternatives, and how do they compare in safety and efficacy to the benzodiazepines? The non-benzodiazepine 'anxiolytics' can be divided, for the sake of discussion, into four general categories of drugs: (1) drugs of historical interest (e.g. alcohol, opiates, barbiturates, neuroleptics) whose availability generally preceded that of the benzodiazepines; (2) drugs active at serotonin receptors (e.g. the azapirones, but also 5-HT_2 and 5-HT_3 compounds); (3) drugs active at the benzodiazepine receptor (e.g. partial agonists, etc.); and (4) miscellaneous other drugs.

Drugs of historical interest

Prior to the introduction of benzodiazepines, barbiturates were the most widely prescribed anxiolytics. Interestingly, barbiturates also appear to work as anxiolytics through a modulation of GABAergic transmission (Haefely and Polc 1986). But, unlike benzodiazepines, which have been hypothesized to work primarily by increasing the probability of chloride channel opening (Chan and Farb 1985), barbiturates act through a separate allosteric site to increase channel opening *time*. The problems with barbiturate anxiolytics have been well-reviewed in the past and include greater cognitive and psychomotor toxicity per unit 'dose' of anxiolytics, a narrower therapeutic window, greater overdose lethality, and greater dependence and withdrawal liability.

In the centuries prior to the introduction of the barbiturates, alcohol was the mainstay of anxiolytics. It also, and not surprisingly, has modulatory effects on GABAergic transmission, along with a well-documented host of other problems, not the least of which are its high abuse potential and extensive organ toxicity. The opiates also appear to have an anxiety-reducing effect, possibly in part mediated through their inhibitory modulation of the β-adrenergic system. Throughout the last half of the nineteenth century laudanum, an opiate/alcohol concoction, was one of the most widely taken patent medicines—in many cases, no doubt, for its anxiolytic properties.

In this century a variety of other medications have been used as anxiolytics in the pre-benzodiazepine era, including bromides, antihistamines, and, more readily recently, meprobomate and low-dose neuroleptics.

Drugs active at serotonin receptors

Twenty years ago it was first suggested (Wise *et al.* 1972) that the anxiolytic effect of the benzodiazepines was mediated, at least in part, by a serotonergic mechanism. Since then other studies (Tye *et al.* 1979; Cook and Sepinwall 1980; Thiebot *et al.* 1982) have confirmed a role for the serotonergic system in benzodiazepine anxiolytics. It was only a small step from these studies to an examination of the efficacy of directly acting serotonergic drugs.

The serotonin receptor system, as our knowledge of it has evolved, has come to appear exceedingly complex, with multiple receptor subtypes. The serotonin-selective drugs that have been most extensively studied as anxiolytics consist of: (1) the partial agonists of the 5-HT_{1A} receptor, primarily drugs belonging to the class of azapirones; (2) the 5-HT_3 receptor antagonists; and (3) the 5-HT_2 receptor antagonists. The drugs evaluated in the most depth have been the azapirones, such as buspirone (the only one marketed worldwide), gepirone, ipsapirone, tandospirone, and zalospirone.

We will review in some detail the anxiolytic profile of *buspirone*—both because it is representative of the 5-HT_{1A} class of drugs and because it is the first marketed non-benzodiazepine anxiolytic. It should be noted that there are subtle differences in neurochemical and pharmacodynamic properties among the different azapirones, although the clinical significance of these differences, if any, is unknown. For example, gepirone has fivefold less affinity for 5-HT_{1A} receptors than does buspirone (Blier and DeMontigny 1990). Buspirone appears to have partial agonist effects at the D_2 dopamine receptor, being primarily active at presynaptic sites, while gepirone, ipsapirone, and enciprazine do not appear to have any dopaminergic receptor activity. In acute, relatively high doses, buspirone and gepirone (the latter at a dose of ≥ 20 mg) have been found in human subjects to increase plasma levels of growth hormone and prolactin (Cowen *et al.* 1990). After chronic use of similar high daily dosages of buspirone, plasma levels of growth hormone, prolactin, and cortisol remained unchanged (Cowen *et al.* 1990). Finally, Lesch *et al.* (1989) noticed a dose-related increase in growth hormone and plasma cortisol levels but not prolactin levels with ipsapirone. Whether these differences in receptor and neuroendocrine effects among the azapirones may translate into different clinical activity is too early to say. This is not surprising, since clinical research on this class of compounds is still in the early phases of attempting to broadly establish clinical efficacy.

The evidence for buspirone's clinical efficacy in the acute treatment of generalized anxiety disorder (GAD; DSM-III -R) rests on a series of studies dating from 1979, when Goldberg and Finnerty (1979) published the first controlled comparison of buspirone versus diazepam versus placebo in a pilot study of 54 anxious out-patients. Since that time, at least a dozen double-blind controlled studies have been published comparing the efficacy of buspirone in daily dosages of 15–25 mg, in studies usually lasting 4–6 weeks, with diazepam (Feighner *et al.* 1982; Rickels *et al.* 1982; Wheatley 1982; Olajide and Lader, 1987; Pecknold *et al.* 1989), clorazepate (Cohn *et al.* 1986a; Rickels *et al.* 1988a), lorazepam (Cohn and Wilcox 1986), alprazolam (Cohn and Wilcox 1986), clobazam (Bohm *et al.* 1990), and oxazepam (Strand *et al.* 1990). Unfortunately, many of the studies were not placebo-controlled.

As has been often noted, the onset of action of buspirone tends to be slower than that of the benzodiazepines, with many patients taking 1–3 weeks to respond (Rickels *et al.* 1988*a*). It is interesting to note that the somatic, and not psychic, symptoms of anxiety account primarily for the perceived slow onset of clinical improvement. Quite conceivably, buspirone's lack of sedating properties may contribute to the drug's slower and more gradual onset of anxiolytic action, since the somatic aspects of anxiety, particularly insomnia, improve during buspirone treatment only after the patient's psychic anxiety has decreased. Because of this, buspirone does not appear to be the drug of first choice to treat 'transient anxiety' or to be used on an 'as needed' basis. In such cases the benzodiazepines are preferable; on the other hand buspirone may well be preferred in the long-term therapy of chronic GAD patients because of its lack of physical dependence (Rickels *et al.* 1988*a*).

The side-effect profile of buspirone compares favourably to that of the benzodiazepines. It includes dizziness, headache, and nausea as the most common complaints in patients treated with buspirone, while drowsiness and fatigue are the most common complaints in patients treated with benzodiazepines. It should be noted that all adverse effects noted for buspirone occurred at a frequency of less than 10 per cent. Severe side-effects are rare in buspirone treatment, and the therapeutic index of the drug is fairly high. There have been no reported fatalities in overdoses involving buspirone. Yet hypertensive crises have been reported where buspirone was administered together with MAO inhibitor antidepressants (Gelenberg 1990).

Since buspirone does not interact with the benzodiazepine–GABA receptor complex, it differs from the benzodiazepine anxiolytics in several clinically important ways. First, buspirone does not generally cause drowsiness (Newton *et al.* 1986). Second, it does not impair psychomotor function and does not impair driving skills (Mattila *et al.* 1982; Moskowitz and Smiley 1982). Buspirone also causes no impairment in vigilance or attention, nor does it appear to have any adverse effects on memory or cognition, as is observed with the benzodiazepines (Lister 1985; Lucki *et al.* 1987). Buspirone does not have any anti-epileptic activity but, then again, abrupt discontinuation after long-term use does not appear to pose a risk of seizures. It does not have any demonstrable abuse potential (Cole *et al.* 1982), and co-administration with alcohol or other sedatives has no additive effect on psychomotor impairment (Griffith *et al.* 1986; Mattila *et al.* 1982). Finally, unlike the occasional patient on benzodiazepines (Rosenbaum *et al.* 1984), buspirone has not been shown to cause aggressive behaviour (Rickels *et al.* 1982); in fact, it may reduce aggression.

A clinician might favour use of buspirone over a benzodiazepine in the following cases: (1) if the patient is in some occupation in which impairment of psychomotor function or attention would be especially detrimental; (2) in a patient suffering from chronic anxiety; (3) in patients who need their daily alcoholic beverage, as no negative buspirone/alcohol interactions exist; or (4) in someone who appears to need maintenance of long-term anxiolytic therapy, because (as discussed below) buspirone appears to have no dependence or withdrawal liability.

Buspirone might also offer an advantage in patients suffering from mixed anxiety and depression. Mixed anxiety–depressive states are frequently observed in non-psychiatric medical practices, but have been the subject of much less research than GAD. Unlike most benzodiazepines, buspirone has been shown to have antidepressant properties (Robinson *et al*. 1990). Preliminary reports suggest similar antidepressant efficacy for gepirone (Jenkins *et al*. 1990; Rausch *et al*. 1990) and ipsapirone (Heller *et al*. 1990).

The 5-HT_2 and 5-HT_3 receptor ligands have been much less well studied clinically compared to the 5-HT_{1A} compounds. Nonetheless there is a growing body of preclinical research (Fozard 1984; Fake *et al*. 1987; Tyers *et al*. 1987; Butler *et al*. 1988; Jones *et al*. 1988; Gleeson *et al*. 1989; for a review see Costall *et al*. 1990), some of it contradictory (e.g. File and Johnston 1989), that suggests that these agents might have anxiolytic effects. This preclinical research also suggests that anxiolysis might be achieved by these compounds without either cognitive or psychomotor impairment, and without significant dependence and withdrawal liability. Most preclinical work has been done with the 5-HT_3 antagonists such as ondansetron, zacopride, ICS 205–930, and MDL 72222. Ondansetron is already marketed for the control of chemotherapy-related nausea, but it is also being studied, along with the other 5-HT_3 antagonists, in current phase II and phase III clinical trials for anxiety relief.

Drugs active at the benzodiazepine receptor

The risks associated with classical benzodiazepines—sedation, psychomotor impairment, cognitive impairment, dependence, and withdrawal liability—are often felt to be counterbalanced by their unusual efficacy as anxiolytics, an efficacy not nearly matched, some might argue, by the serotonergic anxiolytics, especially in speed of onset of clinical effect. Because of this, much research in the past decade has been devoted to finding agents that are active at the benzodiazepine–GABA receptor system, but that have a reduced adverse effect profile. Several promising drugs that appear to fit this bill are currently in development. They are loosely grouped together as 'partial agonists' due to their lower intrinsic activity at the benzodiazepine receptor (Haefely *et al*. 1990). Intrinsic activity refers to the capacity of a compound to activate the benzodiazepine receptor, which in turn modulates GABA-mediated chloride ion flux. Full agonists such as diazepam achieve a maximal pharmacological effect before all the receptors are occupied (Miller *et al*. 1987). Another promising avenue of anxiolytic drug development, but one that is not as far advanced, is the use of mixed benzodiazepine agonist–antagonist drugs. Clinical use of such drugs would be analogous to the use of mixed agonist–antagonist opiates.

At this point it is unclear if the (apparently) more favourable clinical profiles of the current partial agonists are due to their lower intrinsic activity at the benzodiazepine receptor, or to a hypothesized (Sanger *et al.* 1991) selectivity for the 'omega subtype' of the benzodiazepine receptor. Far too little is currently known about the regional distribution of benzodiazepine–GABA$_A$ receptors, or what their native composition or conformational states are, to make any confident statements that explain clinical effect. Studies do clearly suggest, however, that treatment with partial agonists does *not* result in GABA$_A$ receptor tolerance or down-regulation as is observed with full agonists such as diazepam or alprazolam (Feely *et al.* 1989; Miller *et al.* 1990; Miller and Heller 1991). This makes it likely that the dependence and withdrawal liability of these partial benzodiazepine agonists will be much lower than those of currently available agents. Some of these newer drugs have fairly high potency, for example, bretazenil which has a 10-fold higher affinity for the benzodiazepine receptor than diazepam (Haefely *et al.* 1990). Other partial agonist or drugs acting on the benzodiazepine receptor that are being studied clinically are alpidem (Casacchia *et al.* 1989; Diamond *et al.* 1991; Morselli 1990), F68205 (Tricklebank *et al.* 1990), suriclone, and the beta-carboline abecarnil (Ballenger *et al.* 1991). However, much more research is needed to establish both the efficacy and the safety of these agents.

Miscellaneous drugs

The antidepressants, as mentioned earlier in this chapter, have an important role to play in the treatment of several of the anxiety diagnoses, for example, panic disorder and social phobia. But is there any evidence that they might serve as alternatives to the benzodiazepines for the treatment of *generalized* anxiety? The answer may be a qualified 'yes'. Kahn *et al* (1986) have reported that tricyclic antidepressants were as efficacious as benzodiazepines in a diagnostically heterogeneous population of anxious patients. Our group has reported a preliminary analysis of a carefully diagnosed group of GAD patients, in which care was taken to exclude concomitant depression and panic disorder, that found that imipramine was comparable in efficacy, though slower in onset of action, to diazepam (Rickels *et al.*, in preparation). If subsequent studies corroborate this finding, we may have to (again) rethink our current dogma that states that tricyclic antidepressants treat panic disorder but not GAD.

A variety of other drugs that are not active at either benzodiazepine–GABAergic or serotonergic sites may have potential as anxiolytics. These include drugs that are active at central and peripheral systems also implicated as potential substrates of anxiety, for example, the central and peripheral β-adrenergic system, the purinergic adenosine receptor system, and the brain CCK-B (cholecystokinin B) receptor system.

Theophylline compounds such as caffeine and aminophylline have well-documented anxiogenic effects, apparently mediated by their antagonism of the inhibitory adenosinergic system. Adenosine agonist drugs have been suggested as potential anxiolytics (Williams 1983), though no clinical trials in humans have been published.

Brain CCK-B receptors are part of another recently characterized and widely distributed anxiogenic/arousal system. Several potent CCK-B antagonists (e.g. PD 134308 and PD 135158 of Parke-Davis and L-365, 260 of Rhone-Poulenc) have shown significant anxiolytic activity in animal models (Costall *et al.* 1991; Hughes *et al.* 1991 Rataud *et al.* 1991; Singh *et al.* 1991). There is no evidence of anxiolytic effect from compounds active at the CCK-A receptor. Preliminary results suggest that these CCK-B antagonist compounds have much less prominent sedative effects, less psychomotor impairment, and less dependence and withdrawal liability than the benzodiazepines. Their efficacy and safety will, however, need to be tested extensively in phase II and phase III clinical trials before a judgement can be made about their anxiolytic merits compared to those of currently marketed benzodiazepines.

The β-adrenoceptor antagonists are another example of a class of drugs, not directly active at the benzodiazepine receptor, that have shown some benefit as anxiolytics. Though they have been available for a long time and though they have enjoyed wide clinical use, especially among non-psychiatric physicians, there is little in the way of controlled studies to suggest that 'beta-blockers' are as potent anxiolytics for either generalized or panic anxiety as are the benzodiazepines (Turner 1991). They appear to be most beneficial in treating the autonomic and somatic symptoms commonly observed in anxiety. Their clinical role should probably be limited to adjunctive use, or as second-line drugs in such disorders as social phobia or panic disorder (Liebowitz *et al.* 1988).

The lesson from such drugs as the β-adrenoceptor and CCK-B antagonists is that both preclinical and clinical researchers must be alert to the anxiolytic potential of compounds originally studied for other indications. Another recent example of this is the metabolites of the steroid hormone progesterone, which have been shown in pilot studies to have possible sedative/anxiolytic potential (Crawley *et al.* 1986; Majewska *et al.* 1986; Peters *et al.* 1988; Powell and Barrett 1991). This is not surprising since there appears to be an allosteric site for steroids that modulates GABAergic transmission.

Conclusion

In conclusion, we are far from an exhaustive understanding of the neural substrates of anxiety. As understanding proceeds, so will the introduction of alternative anxiolytic drugs. Conversely, serendipitous discovery of anxiolytic effects from drugs marketed for other indications may well open wholly unexpected avenues into the brain. From a heuristic standpoint, the unusual efficacy, safety, and clinical dominance over the past 3 decades of the benzodiazepines has been a mixed blessing. On the one hand, this class of drugs has pointed us in directions that have helped illuminate brain mechanisms—making anxiety arguably the best understood of all psychiatric disorders at a molecular level. On the other hand, the very dominance of the benzodiazepines has, perhaps until recently, discouraged a vigorous pursuit of other, possibly equally important, neural substrates that are crucial to both anxiogenesis and anxiolysis.

Acknowledgement

This paper was supported in part by USPHS Research Grant MH08957.

References

Ballenger, J.C., McDonald, S., Noyes, R., Rickels, K., Sussman, N., Woods, S., Patin, J., Singer, J. (1991). The first double-blind, placebo-controlled trial of a partial benzodiazepine agonist abecarnil (ZK 112–119) in generalized anxiety disorder. *Psychopharmacology Bulletin*, **27**(2), 171–9.

Barlow, D.H., DiNardo, P.A., Vermilyea, B.B., Vermilyea, J., and Blanchard, E.B. (1986). Co-morbidity and depression among the anxiety disorders. *Journal of Nervous and Mental Disorders*, **174**, 63–72.

Blier, P. and De Montigny, C. (1990). Differential effect of gepirone on presynaptic and postsynaptic serotonin receptors: single-cell recording studies. *Journal of Clinical Psychopharmacology*, **10**, 13S–20S.

Bohm, C., Placchi, M., Stallone, F., Gammans, R.E., Alms, D.R., Shrotriya, R.C., and Robinson, D.S. (1990). A double-blind comparison of buspirone, clobazam, and placebo in patients with anxiety treated in a general practice setting. *Journal of Clinical Psychopharmacology* **10**, 38S–42S.

Butler, A., Hill, J.M., Ireland, S.J., Jordon, C.C., and Tyers, M.B. (1988), Pharmacological properties of GR 38032F, a novel antagonist at 5-HT$_3$ receptors. *British Journal of Pharmacology*, **94**, 397–412.

Casacchia, M., Farolfi, A., Priore, P., Magni, G., Stratta, P., Cesana, B., and Rossi, A. (1989). A double-blind, placebo-controlled study of alpidem, a novel anxiolytic of imidazopyridine structure, in chronically anxious patients. *Acta Psychiatrica Scandinavica*, **80** (2), 137–41.

Chan, C.Y. and Farb, D.H. (1985). Modulation of neurotransmitter action: control of the γ-aminobutyric acid response through the benzodiazepine receptor. *Journal of Neuroscience*, **5**, 2365–73.

Ciraulo, D.A., Barnhill, J.G., Ciraulo, A.M., Greenblatt, D.J., and Shader, R.I. (1989). Parental alcoholism as a risk factor in benzodiazepine abuse: a pilot study. *American Journal of Psychiatry*, **146**, 1333–5.

The Clomipramine Collaborative Study Group (1991). Clomipramine in the treatment of patients with obsessive–compulsive disorder. *Archives of General Psychiatry*, **48**, 730–8.

Cohn, J.B. and Wilcox, C.S. (1986). Low-sedation potential of buspirone compared with alprazolam and lorazepam in the treatment of anxious patients: a double-blind study. *Journal of Clinical Psychiatry*, **47**, 409–12.

Cohn, J.B., Bowden, C.L., Fisher, J.G., and Rodos, J.J. (1986*a*), Double-blind comparison of buspirone and clorazepate in anxious patients. *American Journal of Medicine*, **80**, 10–16.

Cohn, J.B., Wilcox, C.S., and Meltzer, H.Y. (1986*b*). Neuroendocrine effects of buspirone in patients with generalized anxiety disorder. *American Journal of Medicine*, **80** (3B), 36–40.

Cole, J.O., Orzack, M.H., Beake, B., Bird, M., and Bar-Tal, Y. (1982). Assessment of the abuse liability of buspirone in recreational sedative users. *Journal of Clinical Psychiatry*, **43**, 69–75.

Cook, L. and Sepinwall, J. (1980). Relationship of anticonflict activity of benzo-diazepines to brain receptor binding, serotonin and GABA. *Psychopharmacology Bulletin*, **16**, 30–2.

Costall, B., Naylor, R.J., and Tyers, M.B. (1990). The psychopharmacology of 5-HT$_3$ receptors. *Pharmacological Therapeutics*, **47**, 181–202.

Costall, B., Domeney, A.M., Hughes, J., Kelly, M.E., Naylor, R.J., Wood-ruff, G.N. (1991). Anxiolytic effects of CCK-B antagonists. *Neuropeptides*, **19** (suppl.), 65–73.

Cowen, P.J., Anderson, I.M., and Graham-Smith, D.G. (1990). Neuroendocrine effects of azapirones. *Journal of Clinical Psychopharmacology*, **10**, 21S–25S.

Crawley, J.N., Glowa, J.R., Majewska, M.D., and Paul, S.M. (1986). Anxiolytic activity of an endogenous adrenal steroid. *Brain Research*, **390**, 382–5.

Davidson, J.R.T., Walker, J.I., and Kilts, C.D. (1987). A pilot study of phenelzine in post-traumatic stress disorder. *British Journal of Psychiatry*, **150**, 252–5.

Davidson, J.R.T., Kudler, H., Smith, R., Mahorney, S.L., Lipper, S., Hammett, E., Saunders, W.B., and Cavenar, J.O. (1990). Treatment of posttraumatic stress disorder with amitriptyline and placebo. *Archives of General Psychiatry*, **47**, 259.

Davidson, J.R.T., Ford, S.M., Smith, R.D., and Potts, N.L.S. (1991). Long-term treatment of social phobia with clonazepam. *Journal of Clinical Psychiatry*, **52** (11), 16–20.

Diamond, B.I., Nguyen, H., O'Neal, E., Ochs, R., Kaffeman, M., and Borison, R.L. (1991). A comparative study of alpidem, a nonbenzodiazepine, and lorazepam in patients with nonpsychotic anxiety. *Psychopharmacology Bulletin*, **27** (1). 67–71.

Fake, C.S., King, F.D., and Sanger, G.J. (1987). BRL 43694: a potential novel 5-HT$_3$ antagonist. *British Journal of Pharmacology*, **91**, 335P.

Feely, M., Boyland, P., Picardo, A., Cox, A., and Gent, J.P. (1989). Lack of anticonvulsant tolerance with RU 32698 and RO 17–1812. *European Journal of Pharmacology*, **164**(2), 377–80.

Feighner, J.P., Merideth, C.H., and Henrickson, G.A. (1982). A double-blind comparison of buspirone and diazepam in outpatients with generalized anxiety disorder. *Journal of Clinical Psychiatry*, **43**, 103–7.

File, S.E. and Johnston, A.L. (1989). Lack of effects of 5HT$_3$ receptor antagonists in the social interaction and elevated plus-maze tests of anxiety in the rat. *Psychopharmacology*, **99**(2), 248–51.

Fontaine, R. and Chouinard, G. (1985). Fluoxetine in the treatment of obsessive – compulsive disorder. *Progress in Neuro-psychopharmacology and Biological Psychiatry*, **9**, 605–8.

Fontaine, R. and Chouinard, G. (1988). Fluoxetine in the treatment of obsessive – compulsive disorder. In Proceedings of the 141st annual meeting of the

American Psychiatric Association; May 12, 1988; Montreal, Canada, Symposium paper no. 23.

Fozard, J.R. (1984). MDL 72222, a potent and highly selective antagonist at neuronal 5-hydroxytryptamine receptor. *Naunyn-Schmiedeberg's Archives of Pharmacology*, **326**, 36–44.

Gelenberg, A.J. (1990). Buspirone–MAOI interaction. *Biological Therapies in Psychiatry Newsletter*, **13**, 36.

Gleeson, S., Ahlers, S.T., Mansbach, R.S., Foust, J.M., and Barrett, J.E. (1989). Behavioral studies with anxiolytic drugs. VI. Effects on punished responding of drugs interacting with serotonin receptor subtypes. *Journal of Pharmacology and Experimental Therapeutics*, **250**, 809–17.

Goldberg, H.L. and Finnerty, R.J. (1979). The comparative efficacy of buspirone and diazepam in the treatment of anxiety. *American Journal of Psychiatry*, **136**, 1184–7.

Goodman, W.K., Price, L.H., Rasmussen, S.A., Delgado, P.L., Heninger, G.R., and Charney, D.S. (1989). Efficacy of fluvoxamine in obsessive-compulsive disorder; a double-blind comparison with placebo. *Archives of General Psychiatry*, **46**, 36–44.

Griffith, J.D., Jasinski, D.R., Casten, G.P., and McKinney, G.R. (1986). Investigation of the abuse liability of buspirone in alcohol-dependent patients. *American Journal of Medicine*, **80**, 30–5.

Haefely, W. and Polc, P. (1986). Physiology of GABA enhancement by benzodiazepines and barbiturates. In *Benzodiazepine–GABA receptors and chloride channels: structural and functional properties* (ed. R.W. Olsen and J.C. Venter), pp.97–133. Alan R. Liss, New York.

Haefely, W., Martin, J.R., and Schoch, P. (1990). Novel anxiolytics that act as partial agonists at benzodiazepine receptors. *Trends in Pharmacological Sciences*, **11**(11), 452–6.

Heller, A.H., Beneke, M., Kuemmel, B., Spencer, D., and Kurtz, N.M. (1990). Ipsapirone: evidence for efficacy in depression. *Psychopharmacology Bulletin*, **26**, 219–22.

Hirschfield, R.M.A., Hasin, D., Keller, M.B., Endicott, J., and Wunder, J. (1990). Depression and alcoholism: comorbidity in a longitudinal study. In *Comorbidity of mood and anxiety disorders* (ed. J.D. Maser and C.R. Cloninger), Chapter 18. American Psychiatric Press, Washington, D.C.

Hogben, G.I. and Cornfield, R.B. Washington, D.C. (1981). Treatment of traumatic war neurosis with phenelzine. *Archives of General Psychiatry*, **38**, 440–5.

Hughes, J., Hunter, J.C., and Woodruff, G.N. (1991). Neurochemical actions of CCK underlying the therapeutic potential of CCK-B antagonists. *Neuropeptides*, **19** (suppl.), 85–9.

Jenkins, S.W., Robinson, D.S., Fabre, L.F., Andary, J.J., Messina, M.E., and Reich, L.A. (1990). Gepirone in the treatment of major depression. *Journal of Clinical Psychopharmacology*, **10**(3), 77S–85S.

Jones, B.J., Costall, B., Domeney, A.M., Kelly, M.E., Naylor, R.J., Oakley, N.R., and Tyers, M.B. (1988). The potential anxiolytic activity of GR 38032F, a 5-HT$_3$ receptor antagonist. *British Journal of Pharmacology*, **93**, 985–93.

Kahn, R.J., and McNair, D.M., Lipman, R.S., Covi, L., Rickels, K., Downing, R., Fisher, S., and Frankenthaler, L.M. (1986). Imipramine and chlordiazepoxide in depressive and anxiety disorders. II. Efficacy in anxious outpatients. *Archives of General Psychiatry*, **43** 79–85.

Koenigsberg, H.W.S., Kaplan, R.D., Gilmore, M.M., and Cooper, A.M. (1985). The relationship between syndrome and personality disorder in DSM-III: experience with 2,462 patients. *American Journal of Psychiatry*, **142**, 207–12.

Lesch, K.-P., Rupprecht, R., Poten, B., Muller, U., Sohnle, K., Fritze, J., and Schulte, H.M. (1989) Endocrine responses to 5-hydroxtryptamine-1A receptor activation by ipsapirone in humans. *Biological Psychiatry*, **26**, 203–5.

Liebowitz, M.R., Gorman, J.M., Fyer, A.J., Campeas, R., Levin, A.P., Sandberg, D. *et al.* (1988). Pharmacotherapy of social phobia: an interim report of a placebo-controlled comparison of phenelzine and atenolol. *Journal of Clinical Psychiatry*, **49**, 252–7.

Lister, R.G., (1985). The amnesic action of benzodiazepine in man. *Neuroscience and Biobehavioral Reviews*, **9**, 87–94.

Lucki, I., Rickels, K., Giesecke, M.A., and Geller A. (1987). Differential effects of the anxiolytic drugs, diazepam and buspirone, on memory function. *British Journal of Clinical Pharmacology*, **23**, 207–11.

Majewska, M.D., Harrison, N.L., Schwartz, R.D., Barker, J.L., and Paul, S.M., (1986). Steroid hormone metabolites are barbiturate-like modulators of the GABA receptor. *Science*, **232**, 1004–7.

Maser, J.D., and Cloninger, C.R. (ed.) (1990). *Comorbidity of mood and panic Disorders*. American Psychiatric Press, Washington, DC.

Mattila, M.J., Aranko, K., Seppala, T. (1982). Acute effects of buspirone and alcohol on psychomotor skills. *Journal of Clinical Psychiatry*, **43**, 56–60.

Meyer, R.E., and Kranzler, H.R. (1990). Alcohol abuse/dependence and comorbid anxiety and depression. In *Comorbidity of mood and anxiety disorders* (ed. J.D. Maser and C.R. Cloninger), Chapter 17. American Psychiatric Press, Washington, DC.

Miller, L.G., Greenblatt, D.J., Paul, S.M., and Shader, R.I., (1987). Benzodiazepine receptor occupancy *in vivo*: correlation with brain concentrations and pharmacodynamic actions. *Journal of Pharmacology and Experimental Therapeutics*, **240**, 516–22.

Miller, L.G., Galpern, W.R., Greenblatt, D.J., Lumpkin, M., and Shader, R.I. (1990). Chronic benzodiazepine administration. VI. A partial agonist produces behavioral effects without tolerance or receptor alterations. *Journal of Pharmacology and Experimental Therapentics*, **254**, 33–8.

Miller, L.G., and Heller, J. (1991). Chronic exposure to a benzodiazepine partial agonist does not alter GABAA receptor function in cultured neurons. *European Journal of Pharmacology*, **199**(1), 111–113.

Morselli, P.L. (1990). On the therapeutic action of alpidem in anxiety disorders: an overview of the European data. *Pharmacopsychiatry*, **23**(3), 129–34.

Moskowitz, H. and Smiley, A. (1982). Effects of chronically administered buspirone and diazepam on driving-related skills performance. *Journal of Clinical Psychiatry*, **43**, 45–55.

Newton, R.E., Marunycz, J.D., and Alderdice, M.T. (1986). Review of the side-effect profile of buspirone. *American Journal of Medicine*, **80**, 17–21.

Olajide, D. and Lader, M. (1987). A comparison of buspirone, diazepam, and placebo in patients with chronic anxiety states. *Journal of Clinical Psychopharmacology*, **7**, 148–52.

Pecknold, J.C., Matas, M., Howarth, B.G., Ross, C., Swinson, R., Vezeau, C., and Ungar, W. (1989). Evaluation of buspirone as an antianxiety agent: buspirone and diazepam versus placebo. *Canadian Journal of Psychiatry*, **34**, 766–71.

Peters, J.A., Kirkness, E.F., Callachan, H., Lambert, J.J., and Turner, A.J. (1988). Modulation of the GABAA receptor by depressant barbiturates and pregnane steroids. *British Journal of Pharmacology*, **94**(4), 1257–69.

Powell, K.R. and Barrett, J.E. (1991). Evaluation of the effects of PD 134308 (CI-988), a CCK-B antagonist on the punished responding of squirrel monkeys. *Neuropeptides*, **19** (suppl.), 75–8.

Rataud, J., Darche, F., Piot, O., Stutzmann, J.M., Bohme, G.A., and Blanchard, J.C. (1991). Anxiolytic effect of CCK-antagonists on plus-maze behaviour in mice. *Brain Research*, **548**(1–2), 315–17.

Rausch, J.L., Ruegg, R., and Moeller, F.G. (1990). Gepirone as a 5-HT1A agonist in the treatment of major depression. *Psychopharmacology Bulletin*, **26**, 169–73.

Rickels, K., Weisman, K., Norstad, N., Singer, M., Stoltz, D., Brown, A., and Danton, J. (1982). Buspirone and diazepam in anxiety: a controlled study. *Journal of Clinical Psychiatry*, **43**, 81–6.

Rickels, K., Schweizer, E., Csanalosi, I., Case, W.G., and Chung, H. (1988*a*). Long-term treatment of anxiety and risk of withdrawal: prospective comparison of clorazepate and buspirone. *Archives of General Psychiatry*, **45**, 444–50.

Rickels, K., Schweizer, E., Case, W.G., and Garcia-España, F. (1988*b*). Benzodiazepine dependence, withdrawal severity, and clinical outcome: effects of personality. *Psychopharmacology Bulletin*, **24**(3), 415–20.

Robins, L. and Regier, D.A. (ed.) (1990). *Psychiatric disorders in America.* Free Press, New York.

Robinson, D.S., Rickels, K., Feighner, and J., Fabre, L.F., Gammans, R.E., Shrotriya, R.C., Alms, D.R., Andary, J.J., and Messina, M.E. (1990) Clinical effects of the 5-HT$_{1A}$ partial agonists in depression: a composite analysis of buspirone in the treatment of depression. *Journal of Clinical Psychopharmacology*, **10**(3), 67S–76S.

Rosenbaum, R.F., Woods, S.W., Groues, J.E., and Klerman, G.L. (1984). Emergence of hostility during alprazolam treatment. *American Journal of Psychiatry*, **141**, 792–3.

Sanger, D.J., Perrault, G., Morel, E., Joly, D., and Zivkovic, B. (1991). Animal models of anxiety and the development of novel anxiolytic drugs. *Progress in Neuro-psychopharmacology and Biological Psychiatry*, **15**(2), 205–12.

Sheehan, D.V., Ballenger, J., and Jacobsen, G. (1980). Treatment of endogenous anxiety with phobic, hysterical, and hypochondriacal symptoms. *Archives of General Psychiatry*, **37**, 51–9.

Shestatsky, M., Greenberg, D., and Lerer B. (1988). A controlled trial of phenelzine in post-traumatic stress disorder. *Psychiatry Research*, **24**, 149–55.

Singh, L., Lewis, A.S., Field, M.J., Hughes, J., and Woodruff, G.N. (1991). Evidence for involvement of the brain cholecystokinin B receptor in anxiety. *Proceedings of the National Academy of Sciences, USA*, **88**, (4), 1130–3.

Strand, M., Hetta, J., Rosen, A., Sorenson, S., and Malmstrom, R., Fabian, C., Marits, K., Vetterskog, K., Liljestrand, A-G., and Hegen, C. (1990). A double-blind controlled trial in primary care patients with generalized anxiety: a comparison between buspirone and oxazepam. *Journal of Clinical Psychiatry*, **51**, (suppl. 9), 40–5.

Thiebot, M.H., Hamon, M., and Soubrie, P. (1982). Attenuation of induced-anxiety in rats by chlordiazepoxide: role of raphe dorsalis benzodiazepine binding sites and serotonergic neurones. *Neuroscience*, **7**, 2287–94.

Tricklebank, M.D., Honore, T., Iversen, S.D., Kemp, J.A., Knight, A.R., Marshall, G.R., Rupniak, N.M., Singh, L., Tye, S., and Watjen, F. (1990). The pharmacological properties of the imidazobenzodiazepine, FG 8205, a novel partial agonist at the benzodiazepine receptor. *British Journal of Pharmacology*, **101** (3), 753–61.

Trimble, M.R., (1990). Worldwide use of clomipramine. *Journal of Clinical Psychiatry*, **51** (8), 51–4.

Turner, P. (1991). Clinical psychopharmacology of beta-adrenoceptor antagonism in treatment of anxiety. *Annals of the Academy of Medicine, Singapore*, **20**, (1), 43–5.

Tye, N.C., Everitt, B.J., and Iversen, S.D. (1979). The effects of benzodiazepines and serotonergic manipulations on punished responding. *Neuropharmacology*, **18**, 689–95.

Tyers, M.B., Costall, B., Domeney, A.M., Jones, B.J., Kelly, M.E., Naylor, R.J., and Oakley, N.R. (1987). The anxiolytic activities of 5-HT$_3$ receptor antagonists in laboratory animals. *Neuroscience Letters*, **29** (suppl.), S68.

Tyrer, P., Casey, P., and Gall, J. (1983). Relationship between neurosis and personality disorder. *British Journal of Psychiatry*, **142**, 404–8.

Weiss, J.M.A., Davis, D., Hedlund, J.L., and Cho, D.W. (1983). The dysphoric psychopath: a comparison of 524 cases of antisocial personality disorder with matched controls. *Comprehensive Psychiatry*, **24**, 355–69.

Wheatley, D. (1982). Buspirone: multicenter efficacy study. *Journal of Clinical Psychiatry*, **43**, 92–4.

Williams, M. (1983). Anxioselective anxiolytics. *Journal of Medical Chemistry*, **26**, 620–8.

Wise, C.D., Berger, B.D., and Stein, L. (1972). Benzodiazepines: anxiety-reducing activity by reduction of serotonin turnover in the brain. *Science*, **177**, 180–3.

Zitrin, C.M., Klein, D.F., Woerner, M.G., and Ross, D.C. (1983). Treatment of phobias: I. Comparison of imipramine, hydrochloride and placebo. *Archives of General Psychiatry*, **40**, 125–38.

18 Psychological alternatives to taking benzodiazepines

Ann Hackmann

In considering alternatives to benzodiazepines one needs first to consider the range of problems for which they are prescribed. In addition to their use in the wide range of anxiety disorders, reactive depression, and stress reactions, they may also be prescribed for psychosomatic disorders including hypertension, asthma, gastrointestinal problems, and eczema. They may also be offered to people suffering from sexual problems, sleep disorder, chronic pain, headaches, premenstrual syndrome, and epilepsy (Lader and Davies 1985). Alternative psychological approaches are also available and can be effective in all these conditions (for a summary see Hawton *et al.* 1989). In this chapter an attempt is made to describe some of these alternatives and to evaluate their effectiveness, both intrinsically and relative to benzodiazepines, where this evidence is available.

A general model for understanding how individuals react to what they perceive as difficult situations is sketched out in Fig. 18.1. This illustrates the way in which an individual's reaction to an event, which could be a psychological event or a physical event like the beginnings of a headache or the aura of an epileptic fit, will be determined by their appraisal of the event and of their ability to cope with it. Obviously, these will be very much influenced by previous experiences, and the effect of the individual's perception of his or her previous reactions to these experiences.

In turn, these appraisals will lead to a tendency to react in certain ways. Emotional reactions will be accompanied by changes in physiological arousal and muscle tension. These could include the somatic manifestations of anxiety or the chronic over-arousal that can lead to a variety of psychosomatic complaints. These reactions are then perceived by the individual, who will then include them in appraisals of the self and may take them as worrying evidence that he or she is ill, incompetent, or out of control in some way, which heightens anxiety.

The person's perception of the situation will also give rise to a tendency to react in particular ways. If they see themselves as being in danger, they will wish to avoid the situation or behave within it in ways which they believes will prevent the worst from happening. Unfortunately, to the extent to which a person avoids the situation, they will also miss the opportunity to find

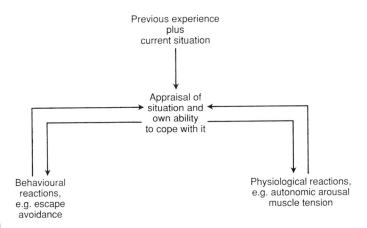

Fig. 18.1

out what really would have happened if they had stayed in the situation or had not employed the strategies they believe prevented 'the worst' from happening (Salkovskis 1991). Finally, if a person's appraisals of the situation and of their ability to cope with it are not accurate, their reaction to it will be inappropriate, and the problem is unlikely to be resolved. Some of the strategies a person mistakenly uses may also make the situation worse. All of these activities and their effects will again feed back into the basic appraisal, and can lead to a decrease in confidence.

These three aspects, i.e. physiological arousal, behavioural reactions, and cognitive appraisals, form the backbone for various psychological treatments that may be given as an alternative to benzodiazepines.

Psychological treatments as alternatives to benzodiazepines

Methods of decreasing physiological arousal

Originally, full-blown progressive muscular relaxation was taught to patients with anxiety problems and psychosomatic disorders (Jacobsen 1938) and used either to bring down the level of background tension, or paired with imagined feared situations in an attempt to de-condition the associated anxiety (Wolpe and Lazarus 1966). Attempts were also made in the laboratory to use tailored biofeedback techniques for psychosomatic problems. Eventually, studies led to the conclusion that much abbreviated relaxation procedures could be as effective as either of the above approaches. For example, a brief relaxation procedure has been found to be useful as part of the treatment of insomnia (Borkovec 1982).

Modern relaxation techniques have become much more like active coping skills, and are taught in such a way that they can actually be used in the actual stressful situation to bring about reductions in physiological arousal and muscle tension.

The most researched application is that of applied relaxation, well described by Ost (1987) and Hawton *et al.* (1989). Several sessions are spent teaching the patient to relax well in a comfortable chair. Then, in subsequent sessions they are taught to relax more and more rapidly in increasingly naturalistic postures. The last phase of treatment involves going into feared situations and applying the relaxation technique unobtrusively and rapidly as soon as the first sign of increased arousal occurs.

The successful application of this technique to a range of problems is discussed in a special edition of the *Scandinavian Journal of Behaviour Therapy* (Ost 1988). It has been shown to be effective (often in controlled trials with follow-up data) in the treatment of dental phobia, claustrophobia, social phobia, agoraphobia, panic disorder, tension headaches, epilepsy, non-ulcer dyspepsia, tinnitus, hypertension, chronic pain, and asthma (Gentry 1984). In the psychosomatic disorders patients were trained to spot the first signs of the problem coming on, and again to apply the relaxation technique rapidly.

Another technique often taught to anxious patients early in treatment in order to give them a strategy to control arousal and hence to perceive themselves as being more in control is that of distraction. Patients are taught to shift their attention away from an internal focus (e.g. awareness that they are starting to blush or shake) to an external focus so that they pay attention to people and things around them. This typically reduces anxiety, at least temporarily, and hence decreases arousal. It is a strategy that has been used as part of anxiety-management training for social phobia and generalized anxiety disorder (Butler *et al.* 1984, 1987).

Patients can also be taught to increase arousal in, for example, the atypical phobia we call blood/injury phobia. Here a brief initial increase in heart rate and blood pressure is followed by a sudden drop, and often by fainting. In this case applied tension, in which the muscles of the arms, legs, and torso are tensed until the blood pressure rises, is effective. As in applied relaxation patients learn to spot the earliest signs of changed physiological reaction in the phobic situation. They then apply tension rather than relaxation to reverse the reaction. Again patients gain an enhanced sense of being in control, and often become less vulnerable to responding in a pathological way in the situation, so that they no longer need to use the special technique (Ost and Sterner 1987).

Methods of changing behavioural reactions to difficult situations in order to alleviate distress

As mentioned above, appraising a situation as difficult, and one's resources to cope with it as inadequate tend to lead to escape or avoidance. A major platform in cognitive behaviour therapy has been to effect exposure so that anxiety will decrease when there are no feared consequences. Exposure has played an important part in the treatment of phobias (Wolpe 1961; Paul 1966), social phobia (Butler *et al.* 1984); (Mattick and Peters 1988), agoraphobia

(Mathews *et al.* 1981), obsessions (Foa and Godstein 1978; Rachman and Hodgson 1980), and generalized anxiety disorder (Butler *et al.* 1991). There is a vast literature on how best to carry out exposure, and the main guidelines have been that practice should be graduated, repeated, and prolonged and that tasks should be clearly specified in advance. Once again, this work is described and summarized by Hawton *et al.* (1989).

Exposure alone has been shown to be a very effective treatment in a number of disorders. For example, it has been shown that specific phobias can be very successfully treated in one long exposure session and remain well at 1-year follow-up (Ost 1989; Ost *et al.* 1991). Mathews *et al.* 1981 have demonstrated that the majority of agoraphobics do well with a home-based exposure programme involving only a few hours of therapist time, and gains are maintained at 2-year follow-up (Munby and Johnston 1980). Exposure treatment has also been shown to be significantly more effective than being on the wait-list for social phobics, and gains are maintained at follow-up (Butler *et al.* 1984; Mattick and Peters 1988; Butler 1989), although these studies indicate that the effects of exposure may be potentiated by adding anxiety-management procedures, which enhance the sense of being in control, or by cognitive procedures (see the next section).

Exposure also forms part of the cognitive behavioural treatment for sexual problems (Masters and Johnson 1970; Hawton 1985). A ban is put on sexual intercourse and a graded series of exercises is introduced with increasing degrees of intimate physical contact.

Recently, the cognitive aspects of phobias have been brought into focus. People are asked to consider exactly what drives their fears and what predictions they are making in specific phobic situations. After exposure these can be re-evaluated. In this way cognitive procedures help the patient to assimilate the new information collected during exposure, and to potentiate the change in thinking that appears to be required for stable long-term change (Goldfried and Robins 1983; Kendall 1984).

For some years there has been an increasing emphasis in exposure treatment on encouraging the patient to really focus on the feared situation and to concentrate on what is actually happening instead of being preoccupied with fears of what might happen and trying to focus away from it. This is in line with the attention that has recently been given to subtle forms of avoidance within the feared situation (Salkovskis 1991). It has been noted that, even when they are in the phobic situations, patients tend to do a number of things that prevent disconfirmation of their belief that something awful will happen. For example, in an agoraphobic with fears of losing control or collapsing, these could include keeping their behaviour under tight control in case they went berserk and ran out of the situation, or stiffening their legs or hanging on to a shopping trolley to prevent themselves from collapsing or falling. In therapy patients are asked to drop these subtle forms of avoidance while carrying out exposure.

This method of combining cognitive procedures with brief exposure should be particularly effective in bringing about belief change without repeated or prolonged exposure being necessary. Thus exposure sessions could be devised in the manner of behavioural experiments, intended as an information-gathering exercise directed towards invalidating threat-related interpretations. The element of response prevention has also been important in the treatment of obsessional neurosis where patients are asked to drop their rituals while exposing themselves to feared situations (Meyer 1966; Rachman and Hodgson 1980).

Another important element of attention to behaviour is in the stimulus control aspect of therapy that forms part of the treatment of eating disorders and sleep problems. In the case of eating disorders the timing and content of meals are planned and eating is made a 'pure' experience, so that the person feels that their eating is back under their control and not cued by irrelevant stimuli such as feeling miserable (Garner and Bemis 1982; Fairburn 1988). Similarly, in the treatment of insomnia, regular times for going to bed and getting up are introduced, no activities other than rest or sleeping are carried out in bed, and the patient gets up for a while if they are not asleep after 20 min (Lacks 1987). The use of relaxation techniques for sleep problems has already been described (Borkovec, 1982) and cognitive procedures (discussed later) can also be used to deal with worry about background problems and about sleep itself (Haynes *et al.* 1981; Kirmil-Gray *et al.* (1985).

Behavioural patterns that arise from negative appraisal of the self may, in certain situations, also play a part in maintaining depression. Depressed patients often fall into a pattern of not bothering to do things because they do not expect either to succeed at them or to enjoy themselves. One of the first aspects to be tackled is to plan activities that will increase both their sense of mastery and the amount of pleasure they experience in order to prevent the initiation of a vicious circle of demoralization (Beck *et al.* 1979). Similarly, anxiety-management treatment for patients with generalized anxiety disorder often includes planning to increase pleasurable and rewarding activities that will help to re-build confidence (Butler *et al.* 1991), and time management skills can be taught to patients with chaotic life-styles to help them get more of a sense of their life being under their own control.

Ways of changing negative appraisals of situations and of one's resources to cope with them

Another way of helping individuals to change their appraisals is, of course, to work on them directly. Cognitive therapy is based on Beck's model of the emotions (Beck 1967, 1976). The central notion in this model is that it is not events *per se* but rather peoples' interpretation of them that is responsible for the production of feelings such as anxiety and/or depression. In depression the important interpretations relate to the element of loss, in anxiety they relate to perceptions of danger, and in pathological anxiety there are overestimates of the danger inherent in any situation. Not only external events may be seen as a source of danger but also internal events, such as the symptoms of anxiety themselves. There is also a reciprocal relationship between external events and these perceptions of danger. For example, once an individual has labelled a situation as dangerous, he or she tends to selectively scan and interpret situations in ways that augment his or her sense of being in danger.

The main focus of cognitive therapy is to help people to identify their negative thoughts and then to challenge and test them out. A wide range of procedures are used to help patients evaluate and modify their negative thoughts. Detailed descriptions of these are given in Beck *et al.* (1979, 1985*a*) and Burns (1980). Two main ways of challenging negative beliefs are through discussion techniques, which may provide new information or a framework for re-evaluating previously held information, and behavioural experiments to test out these beliefs. As mentioned above, the most effective way to conduct exposure therapy may be to view it as a definite series of behavioural experiments in which predictions are made and tested. The use of non-exposure-related behavioural experiments can be illustrated by the case of a woman who experienced frightening panic attacks in which she thought she was seriously ill. Reproduction of all her symptoms by voluntary hyperventilation (Clark *et al.* 1985; Clark 1986) allowed her to see that her symptoms could simply be the result of stress-induced hyperventilation and not be dangerous.

As well as modifying the particular thoughts that occur in anxiety-provoking situations, cognitive therapy also aims to modify dysfunctional assumptions. These are general beliefs that predispose individuals to negative automatic thoughts. A typical set of dysfunctional assumptions might be, 'I am inadequate unless I succeed; all my past successes count for nothing unless I succeed; nobody will love me if I do not succeed.' Therapist and patient work together to produce rational responses to such assumptions as these, and a plan for change.

Cognitive therapy has been shown to be effective in the treatment of depression (e.g. Kovacs *et al.* 1981; Beck 1985*b*, generalized anxiety (Butler *et al.* 1991), panic and agoraphobia (Clark *et al.* 1985; Salkovskis *et al.* 1986; Sokol-Kessler and Beck 1987; Beck 1988; Clark *et al.* 1990), social phobia (Mattick and Peters 1988; Butler *et al.* 1989), hypochondriasis (Salkovskis and Warwick 1986), and stress (Beck 1984). It has also been used as a part of the treatment of other disorders, such as eating disorders (Fairburn 1988) and obsessions (Salkovskis and Warwick 1988). Another strategy for helping patients deal more effectively with stresses is to offer problem-solving treatment (D'Zurilla and Goldfried 1971; Duckworth 1983; Hawton *et al.* 1989; Nezu *et al.* 1989). This involves clearly specifying problems and agreeing on goals and the necessary steps to achieve them, and then tackling these in a step-wise way and evaluating progress as time goes by. Again this approach can be used in conjunction with other cognitive or behavioural techniques.

Summary of the psychological alternatives to benzo-diazepines

An attempt has been made to give a broader view of the psychological alternatives to benzodiazepines in a wide spectrum of disorders ranging from anxiety, stress, and depression through disorders of sleep, eating, and sexuality, and on into psychosomatic problems such as gastrointestinal disorders and hypertension and even on to the alleviation of chronic pain and epilepsy. In some cases the work described is still at an exploratory stage, but in other areas there are well controlled outcome studies with long-term follow-up results that are robust. The studies described here belong in the tradition of cognitive behaviour therapy but it will be apparent that many of the techniques described are also present in the fields of non-directive psychotherapy and counselling. The overall picture presented here may give an opportunity for understanding which techniques may be suited to particular aspects of problems presented.

Comparing the effectiveness of benzodiazepines and psychological alternatives

There have not been a great many studies in which benzodiazepines have been tested against psychological alternatives. In a study by Catalan *et al.* (1984) 91 patients with minor affective disorders, thought suitable for anxiolytic medication by their general practitioners, were allocated either to treatment by the general practitioners with a benzodiazepine of his choice, or by brief counselling, simply involving explanation of the symptoms, explanation of the underlying problems and ways of dealing with them, and the reasons for not prescribing drugs, if appropriate. Improvements were similar and parallel in the two groups on all measures, and the non-drug group did not make increased demands on the doctor's time. Sixty per cent of each group recovered in 4 weeks, and a further 10 per cent within 28 weeks.

In a recent study (Catalan *et al.*, 1991) the 30 per cent of this mixed group of patients who did not show improvement after 4 weeks were looked at in more detail. Half were given four sessions of problem-solving treatment by a psychiatrist, and half received treatment as usual by the general practitioner (which could include psyochotropic medication). The degree of improvement was greater in the problem-solving group at the end of treatment and 16 weeks later, and the problem-solving group patients made fewer visits to the general practitioner and were less likely to request medication, during the follow-up period. They also rated their treatment more highly than the control group did, on various measures. A further study will look at the feasibility of teaching this simple problem-solving treatment to general practitioners.

Until recently, little research has been done on the usefulness of benzo-diazepines in panic and agoraphobia (Marks 1983). Three early studies combined diazepam with exposure-based therapy (Marks *et al.* 1972; Johnston and Gath 1973; Hafner and Marks 1976). In two studies slight temporary gains were observed, but, in the only study to follow up the patients for a month, the gains were lost. Similar results were obtained by Chouinard *et al.* (1982), using alprazolam for generalized anxiety disorder and panic disorder. Diazepam was used in high doses in panic disorder and agoraphobia in a study by Noyes *et al.* (1984) with good effect in the 2-week period studied. However, a cross-over design in which patients switched to propanolol (which was far less effective) precluded any follow-up.

A number of studies have reported a success with high-potency drugs such as clonazepam and alprazolam in uncontrolled trials. One of the few properly controlled trials with follow-up results is the Upjohn cross-national collaborative panic study (Ballenger *et al.* 1988; Pecknold *et al.* 1988). Five hundred patients with panic disorder were given large doses of alprazolam (up to 10 mg a day or placebo). Sixty per cent were panic-free on alprazolam after 8 weeks, compared with 30 per cent of the placebo group. Relief was often obtained after a few days. However, there was a 90 per cent relapse rate, and 30 per cent had more severe 'rebound' panic attacks than they had had before admission to the study. Difficulties in discontinuing benzodiazepines are discussed elsewhere in the literature (e.g Fontaine *et al.* 1984; Sheki and Patterson 1984; Fyer *et al.* 1987) and also in this volume.

In another study of panic disorder Klosko *et al.* (1990) compared high doses of alprazolam with a panic control treatment comprising exposure, interoceptive exposure, relaxation, and cognitive therapy. Results in the panic control treatment group were significantly better than in the placebo or wait list condition, while the alprazolam showed results that did not significantly differ from those of either the panic control treatment or placebo. Posttest measures were in some cases taken when patients were still taking alprazolam, since they were allowed to resume previous dosages if they experienced any difficulty when starting to take medication, which many of them did.

Another recent large study (Marks and Swinson 1990) looked at the effects of combining up to 5 mg of alprazolam or placebo with either relaxation or exposure in the treatment of panic disorder with agoraphobia over 8 weeks. Up to week 8 the effect of alprazolam was moderate and the effect of exposure was strong, although neither had a significant effect on panic. Results did not support giving alprazolam for longer, since there was little improvement between weeks 4 and 8. After taper there was no alprazolam effect and during follow-up (at week 43) alprazolam was worse than placebo. In contrast, exposure without drug yielded marked improvement, which persisted to week 43. It is worth noting that recent trials of cognitive therapy for panic with and without agoraphobia yield an 85–95 per cent success rate in terms of numbers of patients free of panic after treatment, and at 1- to 2-year follow-up (Clark *et al.* 1985, 1990; Salkovskis *et al.* 1986; Sokol-Kessler and Beck 1987; Beck 1988).

In the field of generalized anxiety disorder there are many studies on the effectiveness of benzodiazepines, well summarized by Barlow (1988). He concludes that the effects of benzodiazepines compared with those of placebo appear to be fairly marginal and short-lived. For example, in a study by Shapiro *et al.* (1983) significant drug effects were apparent at 1 week but not thereafter. Early psychological treatment for this disorder also showed fairly weak effects; however, more recent studies (e.g. Barlow *et al.* 1984; Borkovec *et al.* 1987; Butler *et al.* 1991) showed significantly greater effects and continued improvements during the follow-up period.

One of the few studies to directly compare benzodiazepines and cognitive therapy in generalized anxiety disorder was that of Lindsay *et al.* (1987). Lorazepam was compared with two different types of cognitive behaviour therapy over a period of 4 weeks. In the lorazepam group there was a marked initial improvement, which declined as the trial progressed and was minimal at the end. Cognitive behavioural therapy patients continued to improve throughout treatment, and gains persisted at 3-month follow-up despite the fact that the cognitive therapy treatment was perhaps not given in an optimal way, or for an adequate length of time. There do not seem to have been any studies on the effectiveness of benzodiazepines in social phobia.

The effects of benzodiazepines on sleep have been widely researched (see Parkes 1985; Davies 1991) but not compared with the effects of psychological treatments. Benzodiazepines have been shown to be effective in the short term, although their effects begin to decline after about 12 days. There may be some difficulty in titrating the dose in such a way as to avoid morning insomnia and anxiety with short-acting drugs, or sedation and impairment the next day with long-acting drugs. Certain groups of people with health problems should not take them and, on discontinuation, there may be rebound insomnia and withdrawal symptoms. Psychological treatments have none of these disadvantages and may be useful even for chronic hypnotic users, who still have persistent sleep problems (Davies 1991).

There has also been little research on the effectiveness of benzodiazepines in the treatment of simple phobias, possibly because there has been near-unanimity amongst workers on the likely effectiveness of exposure alone. A few studies (e.g. Whitehead *et al.* 1978; Sartory 1983) have examined the potential contribution of benzodiazepines. Occasionally, transient beneficial effects have been noted, but the conclusion is that drugs do not contribute to exposure-based therapy, and may even hinder its effects, possibly because of state-dependent learning (e.g. Sartory 1983). These unpromising results are echoed in animal studies where, typically, higher doses of drugs have been used.

Two main effects have been noted in the animal work. Benzodiazepines tend to block both the partial reinforcement and the partial punishment effects (Gray 1982). If these effects are construed as habituation effects and if exposure therapy is seen as guided habituation to phobic stimuli, then it follows that these anti-anxiety drugs might also be expected to block the effects of behaviour therapy. Taub *et al.* (1977) carried out an experiment with rats to mimic the effects of combining behaviour therapy and drug treatment. Rats learned to avoid shock by jumping on to a ledge. There was then a brief exposure to the grid floor, without shock, and with the ledge retracted. Three days later the rats were retested without shock, to see to what extent their avoidance response had been affected by the exposure session. There was a significant reduction in avoidance in the undrugged rats who had had the exposure session, relative to the control group who had not. This effect was attenuated in the rats given drugs such as chlordiazepoxide.

Conclusion

In the short term, benzodiazepines have a significant effect on a wide range of psychological and somatic symptoms. In this chapter alternative forms of psychological treatments for a range of similar problems have been discussed. The evidence, where it is available, suggests these treatments appear to be as effective, or more effective, than benzodiazepines in the early phases of treatment. As therapy progresses, the effectiveness of the benzodiazepines tends to decline and, at follow-up, gains may be lost, while in the psychological treatment groups gains tend to be maintained or improved upon during follow-up periods of up to 2 years.

In view of the fact that psychological treatments do not have side-effects or withdrawal or rebound effects, and do not affect other aspects of functioning, they should be the first treatment to be given, where it is possible to offer a choice. This would appear to be particularly true if the problem is a chronic one, rather than an acute reaction to temporary stress.

References

Ballenger, J.C., Burrows, G., Du Pont, R., Lesser, I., Noyes, R., Pecknold, J., Riskin, A., and Swinson, R. (1988). Alprazolam in panic disorder and agoraphobia: Results from a multicenter trial: 1. Efficacy in short term treatment. *Archives of General Psychiatry* **45**, 413–22.

Barlow, D.H. (1988). *Anxiety and its disorders.* Guilford Press, New York.

Barlow, D.H., Cohen, A.S., Waddell, M.T., Vermilyea, B.B., Klosko, J.S., Blanchard, E.B., and DiNardo, P.A. (1984). Panic and generalised anxiety disorders: nature and treatment. *Behaviour Therapy*, **15**, 431–49.

Beck, A.T. (1967). *Depression: clinical, experimental and theoretical aspects.* Harper and Row, New York.

Beck, A.T. (1976). *Cognitive therapy and the emotional disorders.* International Universities Press, New York.

Beck, A.T. (1984). Cognitive approaches to stress. In *Principles and practice of stress management* (ed. R. Woolfolk and P. Lehrer), pp.255–305. Guilford Press, New York.

Beck, A.T. (1988). Cognitive approaches to panic disorder: theory and therapy. In

Panic: psychological perspectives (ed. S. Rachman and J.D. Maser), pp.91–110. Lawrence Erlbaum Associates, New Jersey.

Beck, A.T., Rush, A.J., Shaw, B.F., and Emery, G. (1979). *Cognitive therapy of depression*. Guilford Press, New York.

Beck, A.T., Emery, G., and Greenberg, R.L. (1985*a*). *Anxiety disorders and phobias: a cognitive perspective*. Basic Books, New York.

Beck, A.T., Hollon, S.D., Young, J.E., Bedrosian, R.C., and Budenz, D. (1985*b*). Treatment of depression with cognitive therapy and amitryptine. *Archives of General Psychiatry*, **42**, 142–8.

Borkovec, T.D. (1982). Insomnia. *Journal of Consulting and Clinical Psychology*, **50**, 880–95.

Borkovec, T.D., Mathews, A., Chambers, A., Ebrahimi, S., Lytle, R., and Nelson, R. (1987). The effects of relaxation training with cognitive or non-directive therapy and the role of relaxation-induced anxiety in the treatment of generalised anxiety. *Journal of Consulting and Clinical Psychology*, **55**, 883–8.

Burns, D. (1980). *Feeling good*. New American Library, New York.

Butler, G. (1989). Issues in the application of cognitive and behavioural strategies to the treatment of social phobia. *Clinical Psychology Review*, **9**, 91–106.

Butler, G., Cullington, A., Munby, M., Amies, P., and Gelder, M. (1984). Exposure and anxiety management in the treatment of social phobia. *Journal of Consulting and Clinical Psychology*, **52**, 642–50.

Butler, G., Cullington, A., Hibbert, G., Klimes, I., and Gleder, M. (1987). Anxiety management for persistent generalised anxiety. *British Journal of Psychiatry*, **151**, 535–42.

Butler, G., Fennell, M., Robson, P., and Gelder, M. (1991). Comparison of behaviour therapy and cognitive behaviour therapy in the treatment of generalised anxiety disorder. *Journal of Consulting and Clinical Psychology*, **59**(1), 167–75.

Catalan, J., Gath, D., Edmonds, G., and Ennis, J. (1984). The effects of non-prescribing in general practice: I. Controlled evaluation of psychiatric and social outcome. *British Journal of Psychiatry*, **144**, 593–603.

Catalan, J., Gath, D.H., Anastasiades, P., Bond, S.A.K., Day, A., and Hall, L. (1991), Evaluation of a brief psychological treatment for emotional disorders in primary care, *Psychological Medicine*, **21**, 1013–18.

Chouinard, G., Annable, L., Fontaine, R., and Solyom, L. (1982). Alprazolam in the treatment of generalized anxiety and panic disorders: A double-blind placebo controlled study. *Psychopharmacology*, **77**, 229–33.

Clark, D.M. (1986). A cognitive approach to panic. *Behavioural Research and Therapy*, **24**, 461–70.

Clark, D.M. and Beck, A.T. (1988). Cognitive approaches. In *Handbook of anxiety disorders* (ed. C.G. Last and M. Hersen), pp.362–85. Pergamon Press, New York.

Clark, D.M., Salkovskis, P.M., and Chalkley, A.J. (1985). Respiratory control as a treatment for panic attacks. *Journal of Behaviour Therapy and Experimental Psychiatry*, **16**, 23–30.

Clark, D.M., Gelder, M.G., Salkovskis, P.M., Hackmann, A., Middleton, H., and Anastadiades, P. (1990). Cognitive therapy for panic: comparative efficacy. Paper presented at the annual conference of the American Psychiatric Association, May 15th, New York.

Davies, D.R. (1991). A comparison of hypnotic and non-hypnotic users in the group therapy of insomnia. *Behavioural Psychotherapy*, **19** 193–204.

Duckworth, D. (1983). Evaluation of a prgramme for increasing the effectiveness of personal problem-solving. *British Journal of Psychology*, **74**, 119–27.

D'Zurilla, T.J., and Goldfried, M.R. (1971). Problem solving and behavior modification. *Journal of Abnormal Psychology*, **78**, 107–26.

Fairburn, C. (1988). The current status of psychological treatments for bulimia nervosa. *Journal of Psychosomatic Research*, **32**, 635–45.

Foa, E.B. and Goldstein, A. (1978). Continuous exposure and strict response prevention in the treatment of obsessive–compulsive neurosis. *Behavior Therapy*, **9**, 821–9.

Fontaine, R., Chouinard, G., and Annable, L. (1984). Rebound anxiety in anxious patients after abrupt withdrawal of benzodiazepine treatment. *American Journal of Psychology*, **141**, 848–52.

Fyer, A., Liebowitz, M., Gorman, J., Compeas, R., Levin, A., Davies, S., Goetz, D., and Klein, D. (1987). Discontinuation of alprazolam treatment in panic patients. *American Journal of Psychiatry*, **144**, 303–8.

Garner, D.M. and Bemis, K.M. (1982). A cognitive–behavioral approach to anorexia nervosa. *Cognitive Therapy and Research*, **6**, 123–50.

Gentry, W.D. (1984). *Handbook of behavioral medicine*. Plenum Press, New York.

Goldfried, M.R. and Robins, C. (1983). Self-schema, cognitive bias, and the processing of therapeutic experiences. In *Advances in cognitive–behavioral research and therapy*, Vol. 2 (ed. P.C. Kendell), pp.33–80. Academic Press, New York.

Gray, J.A. (1982). *The neuropsychology of anxiety*. Clarendon Press, Oxford.

Hafner, R.J. and Marks, I.M. (1976). Exposure in vivo of agoraphobics: contributions of diazepam, group exposure and anxiety evocation. *Psychological Medicine*, **6**, 71–88.

Hawton, K. (1985). *Sex therapy: a practical guide*. Oxford University Press, Oxford.

Hawton, K., Salkovskis, P.M., Kirk, J., and Clark, D.M. (1989). *Cognitive behaviour therapy for psychiatric problems a practical guide*. Oxford University Press, Oxford.

Haynes, S.N., Adams, A., and Franzen, M. (1981). The effects of pre-sleep stress on sleep-onset insomnia. *Journal of Abnormal Psychology*, **90**, 601–6.

Jacobsen, E. (1938). *Progressive relaxation*. University of Chicago Press, Chicago.

Johnston, D. and Gath, D. (1973). Arousal levels and attribution effects in diazepam assisted flooding. *British Journal of Psychiatry*, **123**, 463–6.

Kendall, P.C. (1984). Cognitive processes and procedures in behavior therapy. In *Annual review of behavior therapy; theory and practice*, Vol. 10. (ed. C.M. Franks, G.T. Wilson, P.C. Kendall, and K.D. Brownell), pp.123–63. Guilford Press, New York.

Kirmil-Gray, K., Eaglestone, J.R., Thorensen, C.E., and Zatcone, V.P. (1985). Brief consultation and stress management. Treatment for drug-dependant insomnia: effects on sleep-quality, self-efficacy and daytime stress. *Journal of Behavioural Medicine*, **8**, 79–99.

Klosko, J.S., Barlow, D.H., Tassinari, R., and Cerny, J.A. (1990). A comparison of alprazolam and behavior therapy in treatment of panic disorder. *Journal of Consulting and Clinical Psychology*, **58** (1), 77–84.

Kovacs, M., Rush, A.J., Beck, A.T., and Hollon, S.D. (1981). Depressed outpatients tested with cognitive therapy or pharmacotherapy: one year follow-up. *Archives of General Psychiatry*, **38**, 33–9.

Lacks, P. (1987). *Behavioural treatment for persistent insomnia*. Pergamon, New York.

Lader, M.H. and Davies, H.C. (1985). *Drug treatment of neurotic disorders: focus on alprazolam*. Churchill Livingstone, New York.

Lindsay, W.R., Gamsu, C.V., McLaughlin, E., Hood, E.M., and Espie, C.A. (1987). A controlled trial of treatments for generalised anxiety. *British Journal of Clinical Psychology*, **26**, 3–15.

Marks, I.M. (1983). Comparative studies on benzodiazepines and psychotherapies. *L'Encéphale*, **9**, 23–30.

Marks, I.M. and Swinson, R.P. (1990). Results of London/Toronto comparative studies: alprazolam and exposure for panic disorder and agoraphobia. *Journal of Psychiatric Research*, **24**, (suppl. 1), 100–1.

Marks, I.M., Viswanthen, R., and Lipsedge, M.S. (1972). Enhanced extinction of fear by flooding during waning diazepam effect. *British Journal of Psychiatry*, **121**, 493–505.

Masters, W.H. and Johnson, V.E. (1970). *Human sexual inadequacy*. Churchill, London.

Mathews, A.M., Gelder, M.G., and Johnston, D.W. (1981). *Agoraphobia: nature and treatment*. Guilford Press, New York.

Mattick, R.P. and Peters, L. (1988). Treatment of severe social phobia: effects of guided exposure with and without cognitive restructuring. *Journal of Consulting and Clinical Psychology*, **56**, 251–60.

Meyer, V. (1966). Modification of expectations in cases with obsessional rituals. *Behavioral Research and Therapy*, **4**, 273–80.

Munby, M. and Johnston, D.W. (1980). Agoraphobia: the long-term follow-up of behavioral treatment. *British Journal of Psychiatry*, **137**, 418–27.

Nezu, A.M., Nezu, C.M., and Perri, M.G. (1989). *Problem-solving therapy for depression*. John Wiley, New York.

Noyes, R., Anderson, D.J., Clancy, M., Crowe, R.R., Slymen, D.J., Ghoneim, M.M., and Hinrichs, J.V. (1984). Diazepam and proponalol in panic disorder and agoraphobia. *Archives of General Psychiatry*, **41**, 287–92.

Ost, L.G. (1987). Applied relaxation: description of a coping techniques and review of controlled studies. *Behavioral Research and Therapy*, **25**, 397–410.

Ost, L.G. (1988). Applied relaxation: description of an effective coping techniques. *Scandinavian Journal of Behaviour Therapy*, **17**, 83–96. [Special issue on applied relaxation.]

Ost, L.G. (1989). One session treatment for specific phobias. *Behavioral Research and Therapy*, **27**, 1–7.

Ost, L.G. and Sterner, U. (1987). Applied tension: a specific behavioural method for treatment of blood phobia. *Behavioral Research and Therapy*, **25**, 25–30.

Ost, L.G., Salkovskis, P.M., and Kellstrom, K. (1991). One-session therapist-directed exposure vs. self-exposure in the treatment of spider phobia. *Behavior Therapy*, **22**, 407–22.

Parkes, J.D. (1985). Drugs and the treatment of insomnia. In *Sleep and its disorders*, pp.437–56. W.B. Saunders Company, Philadelphia.

Paul, G.L. (1966). *Insight vs. desensitisation in psychotherapy*. Stanford University Press, California.

Pecknold, J.C., Swinson, R.P., Kuch, K., and Lewis, C.P. (1988). Alprazolam in panic disorder and agoraphobia: Results from a multicentre trial: 3. Discontinuation effects. *Archives of General Psychiatry*, **45**, 429–36.

Rachman, S.J. and Hodgson, R. (1980). *Obsessions and compulsions*. Prentice Hall, Englewood Cliffs, New Jersey.

Salkovskis, P.M. (1991). The importance of behaviour in the maintenance of anxiety and panic: a cognitive account. *Behavioural Psychotherapy*, **19**, 6–19.

Salkovskis, P.M. and Warwick, H.M.C. (1986). Morbid preoccupations, health anxiety and reassurance: a cognitive behavioural approach to hypochondriasis. *Behavioral Research and Therapy*, **24**, 597–602.

Salkovskis, P.M. and Warwick, H.M.C. (1988). Cognitive therapy of obsessive compulsive disorder. In *The theory and practice of cognitive therapy* (ed. C. Perris, I.M. Blackburn, and H. Perris), pp.376–95. Springer-Verlag, Heidelberg.

Salkovskis, P.M., Jones, D.R.O., and Clark, D.M. (1986). Respiratory control in the treatment of panic attacks: replication and extension with concurrent measurement of behaviour and pCO_2. *British Journal of Psychiatry*, **148**, 526–32.

Sartory, G. (1983). Benzodiazepines and the behavioural treatment of phobic anxiety. *Behavioural Psychotherapy*, **11**, 204–17.

Shapiro, A.K., Streuning, E.L. Shapiro, E., and Milearek, J. (1983). Diazepam: how much better than placebo? *Journal of Psychiatric Research*, **17**, 51–73.

Sheki, M. and Patterson, M. (1984). Treatment of panic attacks with alprazolam and propranolol. *American Journal of Psychiatry*, **141**, 900–1.

Sokol-Kessler, M.S. and Beck, A.T. (1987). Cognitive therapy for panic disorder. Paper presented at the 140th Annual Meeting of the American Psychiatric Association, May 9–14, Chicago, Illinois.

Taub, J., Taylor, P., Smith, M., Kelly, K., Becker, B., and Reid, L. (1977). Methods of deconditioning persisting avoidance: drugs as adjuncts to response prevention. *Physiological Psychology*, **5**, 67–72.

Whitehead, W.E., Robinson, A., Blackwell, B., and Stutz, R. (1978). Flooding treatment of phobias: Does chronic diazepam increase effectiveness? *Journal of Behaviour Therapy and Experimental Psychiatry*, **9**, 219–25.

Wolpe, J. (1961). The systematic desensitisation of neurosis. *Journal of Nervous and Mental Disorders*, **132**, 189–203.

Wolpe, J., and Lazarus, A.A. (1966). *Behavior therapy techniques*. Pergamon, New York.

19 Psychological treatments for benzodiazepine dependence

Susan Golombok and Anna Higgitt

General approaches

Psychological approaches to the treatment of benzodiazepine dependence have focused on tailoring behavioural and cognitive anxiety-management techniques to the needs of long-term benzodiazepine users in combination with a gradual reduction of drug intake. Behavioural techniques are based on models that are derived from learning theory, in which symptoms such as anxiety are considered to be learned, either as a result of classical conditioning, in which an association builds up between a particular stimulus and an anxiety response, or as a result of operant conditioning, in which it becomes rewarding for the patient to avoid situations in which he or she feels anxious. The aim of behaviour therapy is for the patient to 'unlearn' the anxiety response. The most common behavioural techniques used in anxiety are the exposure therapies, in which the patient is exposed to the stimuli that produce anxiety until he or she becomes desensitized to them and the anxiety response no longer occurs. Although the anxiety experienced by patients withdrawing from benzodiazepines is to some extent pharmacologically based, the principles of exposure therapy remain applicable.

Cognitive theorists hold the view that symptoms such as anxiety result from disturbances in thinking, and that people who are anxious misinterpret harmless events as threatening and overestimate danger in any situation. Therapeutic techniques based on this approach are aimed at identifying and modifying the thoughts that appear to cause anxiety in order to help the patient develop a more realistic way of perceiving his or her environment.

It is generally accepted that gradual reduction of benzodiazepine intake is more likely than stopping the drug abruptly to lead to abstinence in the long term. The rationale behind this approach is that withdrawal symptoms will be minimized thus enabling patients to become desensitized to these unpleasant symptoms rather than overwhelmed by them. Gradual withdrawal also gives an opportunity to learn and practise alternative coping strategies for anxiety that can replace drug taking. Although the exact procedures used for gradual reduction of drug intake differ to some extent from study to study, the general approach is described by Higgitt *et al.* (1985, 1987). During a baseline period, patients are requested to keep to their existing dose and to divide their daily intake into three or four equal portions to be taken at fixed times of the day. This is to break the habit of pill-taking in response to specific cues. The patients are also asked to monitor their subjective need for benzodiazepines at the times of pill-taking to help in the planning of their withdrawal programme. Higgitt *et al.* (1985) argue that reduction of medication should not follow a rigid programme. Instead, the rate of reduction of drug intake should be titrated against the patient's withdrawal symptoms. Dose reduction begins by asking patients to omit the daily dose that they feel they could most easily do without. As treatment progresses, further doses are reduced beginning with the one that is least difficult to give up. In many instances, each dose will have to be tackled in stages, cutting it down by half, a quarter, or even one-eighth before it can be entirely eliminated. Patients are asked to remain at each reduced level of intake for at least 1 week as withdrawal symptoms can take some time to develop, particularly with long-acting drugs, and some patients may have to remain at the same stage of withdrawal for several weeks before symptoms disappear or reduce to a tolerable level. A number of studies have provided empirical evidence for the superiority of gradual reduction of benzodiazepine intake over abrupt cessation (Rickels *et al.* 1984, 1990*a*; Cantopher *et al.* 1990; Schweizer *et al.* 1990). However, the extent to which benzodiazepine reduction should be determined by a decrease in withdrawal symptoms remains under debate. Onyett and Turpin (1988) argue that emphasis on minimization of withdrawal symptoms may encourage patients to remain at a certain dosage to avoid anxiety thus increasing rather than decreasing psychological dependency on the drug. Similarly, Sanchez-Craig *et al.* (1987) believe that there may be some advantage in exposing patients to withdrawal distress in order to provide a supervised learning opportunity.

Specific applications

Patients who experience prolonged and severe withdrawal reactions when their benzodiazepine medication is withdrawn report a multiplicity of physical and psychological symptoms (see Higgitt and Fonagy 1991). It may be useful to consider their resemblance to patients normally diagnosed as suffering from somatization disorder (APA 1987). Points in common among the two groups include: a preoccupation with fear of serious disease; a degree of physical pathology that is not commensurate with the degree of concern expressed about their symptoms, which can be hypothesized to be amplified by their excessive concern (Barsky and Wyshak 1990); a determination to seek professional help and advice, though some selectivity exists in their acceptance of opinions offered; a tendency to assume the worst possible explanation of any symptoms; and, finally, constant reassurance seeking and searching for information concerning their symptoms.

The clinical problem presented by patients with a somatization disorder (such as prolonged benzodiazepine dependence syndrome) will increase rather than decrease with the introduction of the new 'consumer-based' UK National Health Services. As Bass and Murphy (1990) point out, a large proportion of patients (perhaps as many as two-thirds) who consult physicians have no serious disease. The representation of ill health as a consumer need for diagnostic and treatment services that is implied by the White Paper leaves no room for an explanatory model of illness in terms of psychosocial factors. The encouragement of competition between service providers will draw patients who experience their distress in the idiom of bodily complaints (Lipowski 1988) to those doctors most sympathetic to their view. The patients will avoid those who wish to draw their attention to those painful aspects of their current life situation from which their physical difficulties temporarily distract them.

The proposed link of benzodiazepine dependence with hypochondriasis does not imply that the benzodiazepine withdrawal symptoms are in any sense imagined by patients. The usefulness of the comparison lies in the recent promising work on the cognitive–behavioural treatment approach in hypochondriasis (Warwick and Marks 1988), which may encourage similar attempts in benzodiazepine dependence. Here we describe in general terms the cognitive behavioural approach we have found to be of benefit (Higgitt *et al.* 1987; Higgitt and Fonagy 1991). Our views are concordant with those of other workers in the field (e.g. Tyrer *et al.* 1985; Sanchez-Craig *et al.* 1987; Hallström *et al.* 1988).

The cognitive–behavioural treatment approach

Patients with benzodiazepine dependence are encouraged to undertake a graded withdrawal of their benzodiazepines, titrated against their withdrawal symptoms. They are asked to take an active part in planning their withdrawal programme, along with their therapist(s). An educational input is offered along with a rationale of treatment. With the help of their therapists, they identify maladaptive thought patterns and learn to substitute more appropriate cognitions. A range of anxiety-management techniques are taught to the patients for use along with other coping strategies to deal with stress in the absence of medication.

This approach can be used in either a group or an individual setting. Which approach to use will, of course, depend upon number of referrals and availability of staff. As with other forms of drug dependency, the group approach has been found to be of benefit (Higgitt *et al.* 1987; Hamlin 1988; Hamlin and Hammersley 1989) and, provided that there are sufficient referrals of a similar type, offering a group may well be a more cost-effective approach. However, some patients will be equally well helped by one or two counselling sessions (Cormack *et al.* 1989) or by reading one of the currently available self-help guides (e.g. Curran and Golombok 1985; Trickett 1986), and attending a whole course of groups may be unnecessary. Since minimal intervention (Onyett and Turpin 1988; Fraser *et al.* 1990) seems as effective as more specialized psychologist help, we should reserve the latter for severe cases.

It is felt that the group members should be relatively homogeneous; those who are high-dose benzodiazepine abusers will require a different input (e.g. Busto *et al.* 1986; Seivewright 1990). If possible, there are benefits in having more than one therapist for the group. This allows for a multidisciplinary approach to be used, with a broadening of available therapeutic skills (see e.g. O'Leary 1989).

As noted above, the amount of therapeutic input required may well vary according to the severity of a particular case (presence of other psychopathology, etc.). Therapists should be prepared to be flexible; even if a fairly closely scheduled series of groups is planned, there should be the opportunity to add in extra input (Hayward *et al.* 1989) should particular problems arise (e.g. development of severe agoraphobia). Provision of hand-outs and audio tapes will be very useful to patients; it has been established that patients forget up to 30 per cent of information given to them verbally in a medical context.

Case-finding

Research data indicate that the proportion of long-term benzodiazepine users who are actually dependent on their medication varies. Due to the large amount of publicity that tranquillizer use and abuse have received over the past few years, those now requiring help in withdrawal may well have failed in previous withdrawal attempts and be reluctant again to undertake such a programme. Rather than seeking help themselves they may need to be sought out and persuaded to participate. It is likely that a large proportion of those who were just long-term users rather than dependent on their drugs will have already stopped their benzodiazepines. Each new article in the popular press (or other media attention) that addresses the issue of benzodiazepine dependence will, however, induce more patients to contact some health-care professional or self-help organization for advice. Within the context of primary care and hospital pharmacies the introduction of the microcomputer has made it easier to detect frequent prescriptions of any medication and hence can draw our attention to potential dependence. If it is hoped to treat these patients in a group setting, some limited advertising may need to be undertaken in order to attract sufficient referrals. A mail-shot to local general practitioners, mental health facilities, day centres, etc. may be all that is required.

Assessment

Prior to undertaking a withdrawal programme it is important that patients are fully assessed by a mental health professional with experience of the problems of those who are tranquillizer-dependent. Research data has accumulated to persuade us that one of the major prognostic factors in a withdrawal programme is the degree of pre-existing psychopathology (Schweizer *et al.* 1990); in particular, personality disorder is very important (Tyrer 1989). Thirty per cent of patients report significant symptoms 10 months to 3.5 years following withdrawal (Ashton 1987; Golombok *et al.* 1987; Holton and Tyrer 1990). Those whose problems persist in this manner will generally be found to have such poor prognostic factors.

Thus a full assessment, including the gathering of information on previous episodes of psychiatric illness and on current or past drug and alcohol use, is required. Using this information the patient can be given a realistic picture of likely outcome. If a patient is currently taking antidepressants they should be advised to remain on them until fully over the withdrawal period. The stress of benzodiazepine withdrawal may precipitate a depressive episode, especially in those with a previous history of depression. The assessment should also aim to establish the degree of social support available to patients during the stressful period of a withdrawal programme. The assessment may uncover reasons (such as agoraphobia) as to why a particular patient might not be able to take part in a group and require instead an individual approach. If very high-dose abuse of benzodiazepines is revealed an in-patient detoxification may be needed, at least initially. Particular attention should be given to the level (both current and in the past) of alcohol intake. There is a high risk that patients will substitute alcohol for their benzodiazepines as the latter are withdrawn unless they are warned of the risk and closely monitored. Some indication of motivation should also be evident following an initial interview and assessment.

Education prior to the start of a group or individual programme

A certain amount of propaganda work may be needed prior to engaging these patients in treatment, particularly if they have had previous unsuccessful attempts at withdrawal (e.g. Cantopher *et al.* 1990). Their belief in their ability to manage without the chemicals needs bolstering; they need empowering. In our cognitively framed model of benzodiazepine dependence, individuals are assumed to be capable of taking an active and responsible role in the change process required to tackle their addiction. The therapy offered to them is aimed at helping them to do this.

Specific components of the therapy

Rationale for the treatment approach

It can be suggested to the patient that the persistence of withdrawal symptoms may be understood in terms of an abnormality of thought processes, such as beliefs, expectancies, and attributions (all of which need explaining along with examples). These can be explained to occur along with, and in response to, psychological and bodily changes associated with loss of the drug's action, with withdrawal symptoms, and with anxiety, all of which are magnified by constant attention to normal bodily sensations. For example, the expectation that one is being offered an alcoholic drink has been shown to be more important in the amount of disinhibition produced than the actual amount of alcohol consumed (Goldman *et al.* 1987; Lang and Michaelec 1987; Marlatt 1987). This is a powerfully persuasive argument for the role of expectations in experience and behaviour. This theory can be shown to provide a wide range of approaches to tackling the problem.

Graded drug reduction

All patients will need to be persuaded to adhere to a graded drug withdrawal programme. This is generally more acceptable if the patient participates actively in any decision-making concerning the rate of drug reduction. The encouragement inherent in the decisions made being publicized in a group setting may well help patients to stick to and achieve their goals.

Self-monitoring—diaries, etc.

When first referred patients may have a very chaotic pattern of drug intake. Pills are taken in response to stress and perceived internal experiences. In order to break the link between these stresses and the taking of pills, a regular schedule of medication should be introduced. The patient should simultaneously be acquiring alternative effective coping strategies for use in management of stressful experiences. It is helpful for patients to keep a daily diary in which they record pill-taking and moments of particular stress. It can also be useful to keep a regular record of levels of withdrawal or other symptoms for discussion at therapy sessions. Such regular self-monitoring does not magnify symptomatology; in fact, it achieves the reverse.

Identifying and correcting false beliefs

The importance of the educational component of benzodiazepine withdrawal treatment cannot be overemphasized. There have been a number of publications that have stressed the severity of the withdrawal syndrome ('worse than withdrawing from heroin') and contained other misleading notions. It is of interest that those countries where media attention has been greater (UK) report more, and more severe, withdrawal problems than those countries where relatively little has been published on the topic (Germany) (Balter 1991). The catastrophic false beliefs of patients lead them to expect to find withdrawal almost impossible. Once identified, particular false beliefs can be corrected by the therapist or other group members—a process that can start in the context of the general educational approach. The forum of group discussion can reveal some of the underlying cognitions, but judicious probing from the therapist may be needed in addition. An example of an automatic thought that will tend to prolong drug intake, perhaps indefinitely, is 'Taking the pill is the only way I can cope.' We found that identifying and correcting such thoughts was a highly effective method of promoting attitudinal change (Higgitt *et al.* 1987).

The similarity of the symptoms of anxiety to those of benzodiazepine withdrawal should be highlighted. This opens up the possibility of a patient utilizing anxiety-management techniques as a coping mechanism. Patients should not be allowed to believe that, after a quarter of a century on tranquillizers, they will feel as they did as late adolescents. They would be expected still to have problems, but to find new ways of tackling them, other than by just taking a pill. However, the Alcoholics Anonymous type message indicating that patients should remain abstinent indefinitely may be overharsh. In a 5-year follow-up of 41 patients withdrawn from benzodiazepines, Holton and Tyrer (1990) found that 31 patients were re-exposed to benzodiazepines, some on several occasions. Yet at the time of follow-up, only 14 were taking the drugs. Thus, in the majority of cases short-term use was again possible, and perhaps a useful coping mechanism at the time.

Improving self-efficacy

As mentioned under education, patients' beliefs that they can cope without medication and that they are not bound to fail need bolstering (their self-efficacy needs to improve). This, of course, is closely linked to the identification and correction of false beliefs, education, and other components of the therapy.

Education within the group

Patients respond well to a clear exposition of physiological and psychological aspects of anxiety, common fears reported in the context of anxiety and panic, mechanisms of drug action, a simple account of withdrawal and the cause of symptoms, as well as some of the empirical findings on benzodiazepine withdrawal, etc. Patients in the context of anxiety-management groups have identified 'the explanation of anxiety' as the most helpful technique they were offered within the group (Cadbury *et al.* 1990). A relatively didactic approach to part of some sessions not only serves to correct some false beliefs but also provides patients with a language suitable for discussing their experiences. Reference to Rickels *et al.* (1990*a*) will provide the therapist with an up-to-date account of some withdrawal research. Patients should know that they can expect a widening of their range of emotional experiences as their drug intake is reduced. Many have commented on the loss of their previous blunting of emotions.

There are those who fear that too much information and education will only serve to increase reports of withdrawal symptoms and increase their severity. Green and Gossop (1988) have neatly demonstrated that the reverse is the case. They compared the intensity of the opiate withdrawal syndrome both with and without full information concerning the withdrawal programme and the withdrawal syndrome. Significantly fewer complaints were reported by the 'informed' group both during withdrawal and during the postmethadone phase of treatment. The provision of information has also been shown to reduce postoperative pain (e.g. Melamed 1977).

Alternative coping strategies

Teaching of a relaxation technique has been recommended by a number of workers (e.g. Higgitt *et al*. 1987; Onyett and Turpin 1988). This can be carried out in the group setting and the provision of suitable audio tapes helps to generalize this to the patient's home. Discussion of distraction techniques should be scheduled into the programme. It may well be that, when the subject is raised, patients will come forward with 'tricks' that have helped them, e.g. always carrying some reading material, reciting a particular poem, singing a song, telling themselves to 'stop'.

Patients may develop a range of problems during withdrawal for which a specially tailored input will be required. Some may develop panic attacks for the first time (or have a recurrence of them). In these cases attention to ventilatory control may be relevant (Clark *et al*. 1985).

In some cases relatives should be included in treatment programmes. Those undergoing withdrawal require support at home and relatives may be included as co-therapists should an exposure programme be needed in the case of those developing a severe phobia in the course of withdrawal or following it.

Follow-up

Some workers feel that, because of the high risk of emergence of depression, anxiety, or other symptomatology (e.g. Golombok *et al*. 1987; Rickels *et al*. 1990*b*), follow-up should be offered following the completion of a withdrawal programme. The high relapse rate (Golombok *et al*. 1987; Holton and Tyrer 1990) requires us to put some thought into relapse prevention; extra attention to stress management may be a useful approach here.

Outcome studies

The efficacy of psychological treatment in helping patients to withdraw from benzodiazepines has been examined in a number of outcome studies. In all of these investigations, gradual reduction of benzodiazepine intake has been accompanied by psychological intervention comprising both cognitive and behavioural approaches.

In an early study, Skinner (1984) examined the efficacy of a course of six weekly lessons in anxiety-management skills that focused on the provision of information about anxiety, instruction in relaxation training, techniques for cognitive control and for modifying inappropriate thought patterns, and advice on how to substitute anxiety-management skills for anxiolytic medication. The lessons were conducted with groups of approximately six patients in each, and follow-up sessions were held 3 months and 1 year after the course ended. Of the 35 anxious patients who participated, 29 were taking benzodiazepines and 1 was on Largactil when the course began. The average length of time on medication was 2 years 9 months. At the 1-year follow-up appointment, 24 of the patients were taking no medication, 5 were taking less than their original dose, and 6 were taking the same amount or more. In addition, 22 of the 35 patients reported that their main anxiety symptom was eliminated and 12 reported improvement. Although these results suggest that anxiety-management skills are effective in helping patients to reduce their medication, it is important to remember that some had been taking benzodiazepines for a short time only and may well have been able to reduce their pill consumption without the aid of the course. As no control group was used, it is not possible to conclude to what extent the high success rate was due to the psychological intervention *per se* or to other factors.

Cormack and Sinnott (1983) have also carried out a general-practice-based study. They compared 13 patients who had taken up the offer of group treatment to help them reduce their medication with 31 who had not. All of the patients had been taking benzodiazepines continuously for at least 1 year and had received a letter from their general practitioner asking them to cut down, followed by a letter from a psychologist inviting them to attend an interview. Group treatment involved training in anxiety management that combined physical relaxation with cognitive approaches such as self-monitoring and the substitution of positive for negative statements. Treatment lasted for 11–13 weeks according to the group, with follow-ups 5 and 10 weeks later. Five of the 11 patients who remained in the treatment group beyond the first session reported a significant reduction in pill consumption compared with 12 of the 31 patients who had not received psychological intervention, producing an overall success rate of approximately 40 per cent. No details were given, however, of the amount by which patients reduced their benzodiazepine intake. Although it was found that the letter or interview produced a similar success rate to psychological treatment, the authors failed to report whether those who joined the group differed in important ways from those who chose, or were chosen, not to. As the patients were not randomly allocated to the treatment group, it seems likely that those who had become dependent on benzodiazepines would have been more inclined to seek help than those who were able to cut down easily following the initial request from their general practitioner. Rather than showing that psychological treatment is no more effective than simple encouragement and advice, the findings suggest that minimal intervention may be sufficient to enable some long-term benzodiazepine users to reduce their pill consumption, while psychological treatment is more appropriate for those who experience difficulties.

In a randomized, controlled study of benzodiazepine reduction, Onyett and Turpin (1988) compared the effects of group psychological intervention with those of individual appointments with a general practitioner. Eighteen volunteer patients who had been on medication for 8 years on average were allocated on a partially randomized basis to one of the two treatment conditions. Group treatment involved relaxation training together with behavioural and cognitive techniques such as goal setting and challenging negative thoughts, while those who had individual contact with their general practitioner received praise and encouragement but no specific psychological advice. Following a 3-week baseline period, all patients had six sessions and a follow-up appointment 15 weeks later. At follow-up, the average dosage had been significantly reduced in both groups, with 77 per cent of patients taking a quarter or less of their original dose. However, those receiving psychological intervention were no more successful at benzodiazepine reduction than those with general practitioner contact only, and neither intervention significantly altered anxiety or depression. Although this finding is in line with that of Cormack and Sinnott (1983), thus providing further evidence to suggest that psychological intervention may have no advantage over normal intervention by a general practitioner, the authors concluded that their findings should be interpreted cautiously given the small sample size and because there was a pronounced drop in dosage over the baseline period across both conditions.

Similar findings have been reported, however, by Fraser *et al.* (1990) lending further support to the view that psychological treatment methods are no more effective in helping general practice patients to reduce their benzodiazepine intake than support from their general practitioner. Thirty patients who had been receiving repeat prescriptions for benzodiazepines for at least 1 year were randomly allocated to one of three groups: (1) 'no help'—patients were advised to terminate benzodiazepine use and no further appointments were given; (2) 'general practitioner help'—patients attended interviews in which the doctor inquired about withdrawal symptoms, gave support and encouragement, and instituted further dosage reduction; and (3) 'psychology help'—patients received group behavioural treatment with a psychologist including self-monitoring of anxiety, education about the problem and coping skills, and relaxation training. At 6-month follow-up, significantly fewer prescriptions had been requested by patients in the two groups receiving professional help than by patients who were given no help, but there was no difference in outcome according to whether they had been seen by the general practitioner or the psychologist.

Higgitt *et al.* (1987) describe the hospital out-patient treatment of chronic benzodiazepine users whose average length of time on medication was approaching 12 years and who had previously tried unsuccessfully to withdraw. Ten patients receiving group psychological treatment were compared with a matched control group of six patients who received telephone contact following the same schedule and content as the group meetings over a 28-week period. The focus of psychological treatment was on anxiety management. Information about the mechanisms of withdrawal was given and false beliefs about benzodiazepine dependence were challenged during the initial phases of the intervention. Relaxation techniques were taught and each patient was provided with a relaxation tape to use at home. In addition, various cognitive restructuring and problem-solving techniques were discussed with individual patients at different stages as the need arose, and the principles of systematic desensitization were explained and home-based, graded *in vivo* exposure was recommended to those with marked agoraphobic symptomatology. By the end of 7 months, eight patients who took part in group treatment and three who received telephone contact had achieved clinically and highly statistically significant reductions in their weekly drug intake; 25 per cent of the patients had completely withdrawn from medication and a further 66 per cent had reduced their benzodiazepine intake by more than half of their original dose. Anxiety, depression, and withdrawal symptoms were found to improve alongside the reduction in drug intake. Although the samples were too small to allow a meaningful statistical contrast between the treatment methods, visual examination of the data indicated that patients treated in a group setting fared better than those treated individually by telephone. The authors failed to include a control group who did not receive psychological treatment. However, the patients had all previously tried unsuccessfully to withdraw from medication, which suggests that the intervention was effective in helping them to reduce their benzodiazepine intake.

Tyrer *et al.* (1985) have also described a cognitive-behavioural approach to benzodiazepine reduction in patients who had previously failed to withdraw from lorazepam under medical supervision. Treatment concentrated on altering the patients' perceptions of, and attitudes towards, the symptoms of anxiety. Only three patients were included in the study, two of whom were randomly allocated to cognitive-behavioural treatment and one to relaxation therapy. After a 4-week baseline period, all three patients began to reduce their medication and saw a therapist at 2-weekly intervals over a 10-week period. The patient allocated to relaxation therapy was unable to reduce medication after week 6 and dropped out of the study. The two who received cognitive-behavioural therapy withdrew completely and remained abstinent 1 month later. Clearly, the superiority of the cognitive–behavioural approach over relaxation training cannot be concluded from a study of three patients. It is interesting to note, however, that the patients who received this treatment had failed to withdraw from their medication with a variety of other treatment approaches including behaviour therapy and day care at a psychiatric hospital.

A larger study of individual cognitive-behavioural out-patient treatment for benzodiazepine dependence has been conducted by Sanchez-Craig *et al.* (1987). Forty-two long-term users were assigned on a double-blind basis to either gradual tapering of their daily active dose or abrupt cessation of benzo-diazepine intake by substituting placebo tablets for active benzodiazepines. After a 2-week baseline period in which they took their benzodiazepines as usual, weekly 1-hour sessions of cognitive behavioural treatment were initiated for about 5 weeks for all patients. Therapy involved provision of information about withdrawal, identification of the circumstances of drug use, and instruction in behavioural and cognitive techniques for coping with these circumstances and with anxiety in general. By the end of treatment, 52 per cent of the patients in the drug group and 74 per cent of patients in the placebo group were abstinent or had reduced their medication by at least 50 per cent. At the 1-year follow-up, this was true for 39 and 47 per cent of patients in the drug and placebo groups, respectively. Although there were no overall differences in treatment outcome, those treated with placebo showed more prominent withdrawal symptoms but were significantly more successful in maintaining abstinence throughout the 1-year follow-up period.

Considering the studies together, it seems that psychological intervention in addition to gradual benzodiazepine reduction is effective in helping patients to withdraw from medication. Owing to the diverse nature of the samples studied and treatments offered, it is difficult to draw firm conclusions about which patients are most likely to benefit and which aspects of treatment are most useful. For some, simple encouragement and advice may be sufficient, while for others more intensive intervention using a variety of cognitive and behavioural techniques adapted to individual needs will be necessary for lasting reduction in pill consumption to take place. In general, it seems that psychological intervention does not have a great advantage over monitoring, encouragement, and support for patients in general practice, while out-patients who have experienced difficulties in previous attempts to reduce their medication appear to benefit from the psychological component of treatment. Particularly encouraging are the findings that patients who had been taking benzodiazepines for many years and who had failed at previous attempts to withdraw were able to reduce their medication with the aid of psychological therapy.

References

APA(American Psychiatric Association) (1987). *Diagnostic and statistical manual of mental disorders* (3rd edn, revised). APA, Washington, DC.

Ashton, H. (1987). Benzodiazepine withdrawal: outcome in 50 patients. *British Journal of Addiction*, **82**, 665–91.

Balter, M. (1991). Report to World Congress on Biological Psychiatry, Florence, Italy June 1991.

Barsky, A.J. and Wyshak, G. (1990). Hypochondriasis and somatosensory amplification. *British Journal of Psychiatry*, **157**, 404–9.

Bass, C. and Murphy, M. (1990). The chronic somatizer and the government White Paper. *Journal of the Royal Society of Medicine*, **83**, 203–5.

Busto, U., Sellers, E.M., Naranjo, C.A., Cappell, H.D., Sanchez-Craig, M., and Simpkins, J. (1986). Patterns of benzodiazepine use and dependence. *British Journal of Addiction*, **81**, 87–94.

Cadbury, S., Childs-Clark, A., and Sandhu, S. (1990). Group anxiety management: effectiveness, perceived helpfulness and follow-up. *British Journal of Clinical Psychology*, **29**, 245.

Cantopher, T., Olivieri, S., Cleave, N., and Edwards, J.G. (1990). Chronic benzo-diazepine dependence: a comparative study of abrupt withdrawal under propanolol cover versus gradual withdrawal. *British Journal of Psychiatry*, **156**, 406–11.

Clark, D., Salkovskis, P.M., and Chalbley, A.J. (1985). Respiratory control as a treatment for panic attacks. *Journal of Behavioural Therapy and Experimental Psychiatry*, **16**, 23–30.

Cormack, M.A. and Sinnott, A. (1983). Psychological alternatives to long-term benzodiazepine use. *Journal of the Royal College of General Practitioners*, **33**, 279–81.

Cormack, M.A., Owens, R.G., and Dewey, M.E. (1989). The effect of minimal intervention by general practitioners on long-term benzodiazepine use. *Journal of the Royal College of General Practitioners*, **39**, 408–11.

Curran, V. and Golombok, S. (1985). *Bottling it up*. Faber, London.

Fraser, D., Peterkin, G.S.D., Gamsu, C.V., and Baldwin, P.J. (1990). Benzodiazepine withdrawal: a pilot comparison of three methods, *British Journal of Clinical Psychology*, **29**, 231–3.

Goldman, M.S., Brown, S.A., and Christiansen, B.A. (1987). Expectancy theory: thinking about drinking. In *Psychological theories of drinking and alcoholism* (ed. H.T. Blane and K.S. Leonard). Guilford, New York.

Golombok, S., Higgitt, A., Fonagy, P., Dodds, S., Saper, J., and Lader, M. (1987). A follow up study of patients treated for benzodiazepine dependence, *British Journal of Medical Psychology*, **60**, 141–9.

Green, L. and Gossop, M. (1988). Effects of information on the opiate withdrawal syndome. *British Journal of Addiction*, **83**, 305–9.

Hallström, C., Crouch, G., Robson, M., and Shine, P. (1988). The treatment of tranquilliser dependence by propranolol. *Postgraduate Medical Journal*, **64** (suppl.2), 40–4.

Hamlin, M. (1988). An intergrated cognitive behavioural approach to withdrawal from tranquillisers. In *Developments in cognitive psychotherapy* (ed. W. Dryden and P. Trower), pp.153–76. Sage, London.

Hamlin, M. and Hammersley, D. (1989). Managing benzodiazepine withdrawal. In *Treating drug abusers* (ed. G. Bennett), pp.91–114. Routledge, London.

Hayward, P., Wardle, J., and Higgitt, A. (1989). Benzodiazepine research: current findings and practical consequences. *British Journal of Clinical Psychology*, **28**, 307–27.

Higgitt, A., Lader, M.H., and Fonagy, P. (1985). Clinical management of benzo-diazepine dependence, *British Medical Journal*, **291**, 688–90.

Higgitt, A., Golombok, S., Fonagy, P., and Lader, M.H. (1987). Group treatment of benzodiazepine dependence. *British Journal of Addiction*, **82**, 517–32.

Higgitt, A. and Fonagy, P. (1991). Withdrawal from benzodiazepines and the persistent benzodiazepine dependence syndrome. In *Recent advances in clinical psychiatry*, Vol. 7 (ed. K. Granville Grossman). Churchill Livingstone, London.

Holton, A. and Tyrer, P. (1990). Five year outcome in patients withdrawn from long term treatment with diazepam. *British Medical Journal*, **300**, 1241–2.

Lang, A. R. and Michaelec, E. M. (1987). Expectancy effects in reinforcement from alcohol. In *Why people drink: parameters of alcohol as a reinforcer*, (ed. W.M. Cox). Gardener, New York.

Lipowski, Z.T. (1988), Somatisation: the concept and its clinical application. *American Journal of Psychiatry*, **145**, 1358–68.

Marlatt, G.A. (1987). Alcohol the magic elixir: stress expectancy and the transformation of emotional states. In *Stress and addiction* (ed. E. Gottheil *et al.*). Bruner Mazel, New York.

Melamed, B.G. (1977). Psychological preparation for hospitalisation. In *Contribution to medical psychology* (ed. S. Radman). Pergamon Press, Oxford.

O'Leary, M. (1989). A novel approach to tackling the 'benzodiazepine problem in general practice. *Psychiatric Bulletin*, **13**, 180–1.

Onyett, S.R. and Turpin, G. (1988). Benzodiazepine withdrawal in primary care: a comparison of behavioural group training and individual sessions. *Behavioural Psychotherapy*, **16**, 297–312.

Rickels, K., Case, W.G., Winokur, A., and Swenson, C. (1984). Long-term benzodiazepine therapy: benefits and risks. *Psychopharmacology Bulletin*, **20**, 608–15.

Rickels, K., Case, W. G., and Greenblatt, D. J. (1990*a*). Long-term therapeutic use of benzodiazepines 1. Effects of abrupt discontinuation. *Archives of General Psychiatry*, **47**, 899–907.

Rickels, K., Case, W.G., Schweizer, E., Garcia-España, F., and Friedman, R. (1990*b*). Benzodiazepine dependence: management of discontinuation. *Psychopharmacology Bulletin*, **26**, 63–8.

Sanchez-Craig, M., Cappell, H., Busto, U., and Kay, G. (1987). Cognitive-behavioural treatment for benzodiazepine dependence: a comparison of gradual versus abrupt cessation of drug intake. *British Journal of Addiction*, **82**, 1317–27.

Schweizer, E., Rickels, K., Case, W.G., and Greenblatt, D.J. (1990). Long-term therapeutic use of benzodiazepines II. Effects of gradual taper. *Archives of General Psychiatry*, **47**, 908–15.

Seivewright, N. (1990). Treatment and outcome of drug dependence. *Current Opinion in Psychiatry*, **3**, 403–7.

Skinner, P.T. (1984). Skills not pills: learning to cope with anxiety symptoms. *Journal of the Royal College of General Practitioners*, **34**, 258–60.

Trickett, S. (1986). *Coming Off tranquillisers*. Thorson's, Northampton.

Tyrer, P. (1989). Risks of dependence on benzodiazepine drugs: the importance of patient selection, *British Medical Journal*, **298**, 102–5.

Tyrer, P., Murphy, S., Oates, G., and Kingdon, G. (1985). Psychological treatment for benzodiazepine dependence, *Lancet*, **i**, 1042–3.

Warwick, H.M.C. and Marks, I.M. (1988). Behavioural treatment of illness phobia and hypochondriasis: a pilot study of 17 cases. *British Journal of Psychiatry*, **152**, 239–41.

20 Pharmacological treatments for benzodiazepine dependence

Peter P. Roy-Byrne and James C. Ballenger

The greater part of the public and scientific controversy surrounding the long-term use of benzodiazepines has focused on the phenomenon of dependence. Even in the absence of abuse or significant cognitive/psychomotor impairment resulting from these medications, some clinicians continue to feel that the risk of dependence can outweigh their substantial anxiolytic efficacy. Although dependence hypothetically develops as the brain adapts to the constant presence of benzodiazepines and their potentiation of GABAergic neuronal inhibition, it can only be identified as the benzodiazepine is discontinued and there is sudden loss of GABAergic neuronal inhibition causing withdrawal symptoms (Haefely 1986). The exact neurochemical mechanisms underlying dependence are unknown, since adaptive changes in the brain during benzodiazepine treatment may occur at a molecular level, e.g. changes in receptor number or receptor coupling to effector mechanisms, or in neural systems that are affected subsequent to the primary action of the drug.

A frequent and troublesome clinical error is the tendency to equate dependence with addiction. Although individuals with any form of drug addiction are also 'dependent' on that drug, addicts by definition abuse their drug of choice and suffer, as a consequence, impairment in various life spheres. In addition to this tendency to take the drug for non-medically prescribed indications (usually to obtain euphoria), addiction is often associated with the development of tolerance and the resulting dose escalation (Rinaldi *et al.* 1988).

The contrast between dependence and addiction suggests that there are two kinds of chronic benzodiazepine users (Woods *et al.* 1988)—those who take benzodiazepines for medically prescribed and appropriate reasons, do not escalate dose, and achieve the benefits of improved social, occupational, and interpersonal function; and those who abuse benzodiazepines, usually as part of a pattern of abusing multiple substances, and have accompanying social, occupational, and interpersonal dysfunction. In this review, we will focus on the therapeutic user of benzodiazepines and the variety of pharmacological treatments that have been utilized to facilitate benzodiazepine discontinuation. Less emphasis will be placed on patients whose benzodiazepine dependence occurs as part of a pattern of multiple substance abuse.

The benzodiazepine discontinuation syndrome

When benzodiazepines are discontinued, the observed clinical response consists of several different phenomena (Roy-Byrne and Hommer 1988). A true physiological withdrawal syndrome can occur and consists of the brain's readjustment following the physiological adaptation that occurred during chronic benzodiazepine treatment (Nutt 1986). Reversal of the original neurochemical changes induced by the benzodiazepine result in a relative loss of GABAergic neuronal inhibition causing symptoms of anxiety, insomnia, restlessness, tremulousness, gastrointestinal upset, and increased muscle tension. Although these symptoms may be identical to the original anxiety syndrome for which the drug was prescribed, the presence of additional psychosensory symptoms (i.e. hyperacusis, photosensitivity, kinaesthetic illusions, and other perceptual distortions) is more specific for physiological withdrawal and rarely occurs as part of any but severe anxiety states (Roy-Byrne and Hommer 1988). This withdrawal syndrome may be complicated by the return of the original anxiety syndrome that was being treated. If the resulting symptoms of anxiety are more severe than they were prior to treatment, the syndrome is termed 'rebound' rather than just relapse (Fontaine et al. 1984). It is difficult, if not impossible, to distinguish relapse or rebound from withdrawal. Most commonly, the time course of onset and offset is used to distinguish them. Withdrawal occurs in a time-limited fashion corresponding to the pharmacokinetics of the benzodiazepine being tapered so that it begins to occur as the blood level of the drug drops precipitously and will wear off a number of days after the blood level reaches zero. Relapse, on the other hand, should emerge slowly and gradually as the drug is discontinued and persist well beyond discontinuation. Nonetheless, the true course of relapse may also depend on the intrinsic time course of action of the drug. Since benzodiazepines work 'fast' in contrast to the more slowly acting antidepressants, relapse appearing after these two medications may have a correspondingly different time course and profile. For these reasons, in practice, the two phenomena are inextricably intertwined and always contribute to some degree to clinical syndromes observed during discontinuation.

Clinicians frequently speak of the possibility of a longer-term withdrawal syndrome lasting many months, which may have many of the characteristics of rebound (i.e. anxiety worse than it ever was, even prior to treatment) (Higgitt et al. 1990). It is difficulty to distinguish this 'low-dose withdrawal syndrome' from the re-emergence of an anxiety syndrome whose hypothetical progression over time was masked by treatment and finally emerged following discontinuation, appearing worse than previously and perhaps of a different character. Even immediate and time-limited anxiety symptoms occurring at the point when withdrawal would be expected to be most prominent (i.e. panic attacks in panic disorder patients undergoing benzodiazepine discontinuation) are more likely to represent relapse. Despite these ambiguities, it is heuristically helpful to divide the benzodiazepine discontinuation syndrome into these overlapping yet theoretically distinct components of withdrawal and relapse/ rebound. There are, accordingly, two obvious therapeutic approaches to benzodiazepine discontinuation: withdrawal attenuation and relapse prevention. In this chapter we will focus on the first of these major approaches. However, it must be recognized that the two approaches are, in practice, difficult to distinguish, and so we will touch on the second approach in a more broad and non-specific way.

Withdrawal attenuation

General strategies

The major withdrawal attenuation strategy, often overlooked by clinicians, is to try and prevent the syndrome from occurring by the use of a careful, slow, and flexible tapered withdrawal. While recognizing that benzodiazepines should not be discontinued abruptly, clinicians often fail to taper them slowly enough. Although there is little comparative data on the relative effects of different withdrawal schedules, Pecknold (1990) reported no rebound and only 7 per cent mild withdrawal using a 2–4 month taper; this contrasts with the corresponding 35 and 35 per cent figures that he found using a 2–4 week taper schedule (Pecknold *et al*. 1988). Although there has been considerable discussion about the advantages of switching over to a longer-acting drug such as clonazepam prior to taper, Rickels *et al*. (1990) noted that long half-life drugs have no special advantage over short half-life drugs if tapered over 4 weeks. Clinicians continue to feel, however, that select cases may do better with such a switch-over strategy.

   Studies and case series have focused on three medications for the treatment of benzodiazepine withdrawal: beta-blockers, clonidine, and carbamazepine. Because none of these are now considered first-line treatments for most of the major anxiety disorders (Roy-Byrne and Wingerson, 1992), they would not be thought of as treatments targeted toward preventing relapse. However, while double-blind studies have failed to show antipanic efficacy for beta-blockers (Munjack *et al*. 1989) and carbamazepine (Uhde *et al*. 1988), some recent, albeit short-lived efficacy against panic attacks has been seen with clonidine (Hoehn-Saric *et al*. 1981; Liebowitz *et al*. 1981). Furthermore, beta-blockers are known to be an effective treatment for generalized symptoms of anxiety, and clonidine has some ability to attenuate non-panic anxiety symptoms in panic disorder patients (Uhde *et al*. 1989). Thus, the fact that these medications attenuate symptoms following benzodiazepine discontinuation does not prove that they are working entirely on the withdrawal as opposed to the relapse process. Nonetheless, since some time is usually required for anxiolytic efficacy to develop, beneficial effects following short periods of pre-treatment prior to benzodiazepine discontinuation make an effect on relapse less likely.

Propranolol

In a single case report, Abernethy *et al.* (1981) demonstrated that propranolol's major therapeutic effect on benzodiazepine withdrawal was reducing the increases in systolic and diastolic blood pressure and ventricular heart rate that occurred during discontinuation. In contrast, psychological symptoms of withdrawal-related dysphoria were unaffected. Thus, although beta-blockers may have more specific effects on the autonomic arousal that occurs during withdrawal, they are of little clinical benefit since patients usually do not 'feel' any better despite being less autonomically aroused. The efficacy of propranolol for benzodiazepine withdrawal symptoms was examined in a subsequent double-blind placebo-controlled trial (Tyrer *et al.* 1981). Although not statistically significant, a greater proportion of patients dropped out on placebo (55 per cent) than on propranolol (35 per cent). However, the propranolol group's final mean Hamilton Anxiety Scale score after discontinuation was slightly higher than that of the placebo group, offering little indication that this group was less symptomatic. Although the paper emphasized that the difference in the slopes of the regression lines formed by connecting Hamilton Anxiety Scale scores before and after discontinuation was significant at the $p < 0.05$ level, suggesting that the placebo group worsened more, the more rapid increase in anxiety during discontinuation was partially due to this group having significantly lower scores at baseline.

Hallström and colleagues (1988) attempted to contrast propranolol, placebo, and no-pill pre-treatment of benzodiazepine-dependent patients undergoing tapered discontinuation. Although they reported that symptom increase was greatest in the non-propranolol treatment groups, no statistics were provided. Moreover, with the rate of drop-out, only five patients took propranolol, 10 took placebo, and eight took 'no pill', making statistically significant differences unlikely to emerge.

A more recent study (Cantopher *et al.* 1990) contrasted abrupt benzodiazepine discontinuation under cover of propranolol with gradual discontinuation. Ten of 16 patients in the gradual discontinuation group successfully withdrew from their drugs, while only four of 15 in the abrupt propranolol discontinuation group did so. Unfortunately, this study confounds schedule of discontinuation with drug effect. Nonetheless, it shows that propranolol cannot compensate for the effects of abrupt discontinuation, unlike cognitive-behaviour therapy, which was shown in a recent study to do just that (Sanchez-Craig *et al.* 1986).

While better controlled studies have examined the efficacy of beta-blockers in the treatment of alcohol withdrawal, there are no other studies that have examined this issue in benzodiazepine withdrawal. Anecdotal reports favouring the use of beta-blockers continue to appear, although it is noteworthy that they are always tempered by statements suggesting that the usefulness of beta-blockers is somewhat limited. In sum, it can be said that the available studies provide little support for the routine use of beta-blockers as adjunctive treatment for benzodiazepine discontinuation, although it is possible that patients who complain of prominent symptoms of palpitations and tremor as part of their own benzodiazepine withdrawal syndrome might be helped by them. These findings suggest that the increases in central nervous system noradrenergic activity reported to be a consequence of benzodiazepine withdrawal are either less important contributors to the overall withdrawal syndrome or are not effectively antagonized by beta-blockers.

Clonidine

As with propranolol, there are few available reports or studies examining the efficacy of clonidine for benzodiazepine withdrawal. Prompted by earlier evidence of its efficacy against symptoms of opiate withdrawal, Ashton (1984) reported some limited benefit in four patients undergoing benzodiazepine withdrawal. A more detailed case report of a man who had previously failed medically supervised taper with the support of hospitalization was provided by Keshavan and Crammer (1985). Using a single-blind placebo-controlled design to control for pseudo-withdrawal (i.e. the negative placebo effect of perceived reduction in pills), physicians told the patient his lorazepam might be replaced by placebo (although it was not) and noted some mild increase in anxiety ('pseudowithdrawal'). Clonidine was then added at a dose of 0.6 mg per day with no other changes. After the patient was stabilized on this regime for 1 week, lorazepam was blindly tapered using placebo substitution over the next 2 weeks with no increase in symptoms. After another 2 weeks with no further symptoms, the clonidine was abruptly discontinued. Withdrawal symptoms immediately occurred and were abolished by re-institution of the clonidine at a slightly lower dose (0.4 mg).

In contrast to this case, three subsequent placebo-controlled cases were reported in which clonidine was ineffective in treating benzodiazepine withdrawal (Goodman et al. 1986). In this improved experimental design, patients received placebo clonidine for the first 1–2 weeks while they were maintained on their usual dose of benzodiazepine. The benzodiazepine was then abruptly discontinued and placebo substituted without the patient's knowledge. After withdrawal symptoms emerged, active clonidine was substituted for placebo clonidine. In contrast to the previously reported case, placebo control of the clonidine administration eliminated any possibility of a placebo effect on withdrawal. This is crucial, since one study has shown that patients whose benzodiazepines were abruptly discontinued with immediate blind placebo substitution had fewer symptoms compared to those who experienced abrupt discontinuation without placebo substitution

(Pecknold *et al.* 1982). This is consistent with other data showing that 58 per cent of patients achieve successful discontinuation with placebo (Rickels *et al.* 1990).

The most recently published report on clonidine studied a homogeneous population of panic disorder patients (Fyer *et al.* 1988). In this open study, patients were treated for 4–8 weeks with alprazolam, after which it was slowly tapered over the next 4 weeks. Investigators waited for withdrawal symptoms to appear before adding clonidine as tolerated in doses of 0.2 and 0.7 mg. All patients experienced severe rebound panic and anxiety. Lader *et al.* (unpublished observations) also report that their on-going placebo-controlled studies of clonidine have failed to note any degree of efficacy for benzodiazepine withdrawal in mixed patient populations. Because the two negative studies cited above administered clonidine *after* an abstinence syndrome appeared (in contrast to the initial positive report), it is still possible that pre-treatment with clonidine, prior to initiation of discontinuation, might be more effective.

Carbamazepine

Over the last 2 decades, four double-blind placebo-controlled studies and one large 2500-patient case series showed that carbamazepine was as effective as conventionally used medications such as barbital, tiapride, and chlomethiazole for ameliorating symptoms of alcohol withdrawal in mild cases of alcoholism (Ballenger and Post 1984). Some studies were actually done on an out-patient basis. A recent study of more seriously ill alcoholics (score of 20 or more on the Clinical Institute Withdrawal Assessment for Alcohol Scale) also showed that carbamazepine was as effective as oxazepam in treating symptoms of alcohol withdrawal (Malcolm *et al.* 1989).

In agreement with these results, unpublished clinical anecdotes from Scandinavia in the 1960s and 1970s claimed that carbamazepine was useful in attenuating benzodiazepine withdrawal. However, the first detailed, published account of carbamazepine's efficacy in attenuating benzodiazepine withdrawal did not appear until the last decade (Klein *et al.* 1986). These authors reported that three patients taking alprazolam for panic disorder who had failed multiple discontinuation trials, some with intensive clinical intervention, were able to discontinue alprazolam following carbamazepine treatment. A subsequent nine-patient case series (Ries *et al.* 1989) suggested that carbamazepine was specifically helpful in detoxifying patients with other diagnoses including substance abuse, more of whom were taking very high doses of benzodiazepines (i.e. 2 g of chlordiazepoxide, 13 mg of clonazepam). In both reports, doses of between 400 and 800 mg of carbamazepine were employed. In the second report, carbamazepine was only given to some patients the day prior to initiation of rapid taper (discontinuation over 1–3 days). Because the half-life of carbamazepine in the first 4 days, prior to enzyme induction, is over 24 h, large amounts or all of the daily dose was sometimes given at bedtime to capitalize on carbamazepine's sedative effects and to combat withdrawal-related insomnia.

Results of a recent placebo-controlled study by Schweizer *et al.* (1991) in a heterogeneous group of anxious patients show a trend in favour of a role for carbamazepine in attenuating withdrawal. Patients on carbamazepine showed a trend toward lower daily self-ratings of withdrawal intensity and were significantly less likely to resume benzodiazepines at 5-week follow-up. These effects seemed most evident in patients taking daily doses of at least 20 mg diazepam equivalents (patients more likely to have more intense withdrawal). In contrast to the modest results of this study, a larger collaborative study examining a homogeneous group of panic disorder patients found less impressive results (Ballenger 1991). In 103 patients withdrawing from alprazolam after a double-blind initiation of carbamazepine or placebo, there was no overall effect of carbamazepine on the rate of patients able to successfully discontinue according to schedule. This outcome primarily seemed to result from the rapid reduction in alprazolam serum levels caused by the addition of carbamazepine. However, the patients who remained in the study and on carbamazepine seemed to have a milder withdrawal syndrome than patients on placebo, suggesting some efficacy for carbamazepine.

One possible explanation for these contrasting results is that patients with panic disorder may respond less well because carbamazepine is not an effective treatment for panic attacks (Uhde *et al.* 1988), and hence will not prevent the re-emergence of panic symptoms. An alternative explanation is that panic disorder patients, who tend to be taking higher doses of benzodiazepines compared with other patients, could be more prone to develop tolerance, making them theoretically more vulnerable to withdrawal and more resistant to carbamazepine's effect. However, 45 per cent of the patients in the Schweizer *et al.* study (1991) had panic disorder, although the average daily benzodiazepine dose seemed a bit lower. In addition, these authors did not note any reduction in benzodiazepine levels during the first 1 to 2 weeks of carbamazepine prior to taper. Such a reduction, although present in only one of these studies, might suggest that rapid institution and taper over a single week as was done in the Ries *et al.* (1989) case series could alleviate this problem and improve carbamazepine's efficacy.

Recently, in an open report by Ries *et al.* (1991), carbamazepine was compared with the phenobarbital taper method previously used at three in-patient chemical dependency centres to detoxify patients from high-dose, chronically abused benzodiazepines. The carbamazepine method was routinely used for 1 year after many years of using the phenobarbital method. After the next year, the unit director and head nurse rated carbamazepine as superior to phenobarbital in attenuating withdrawal and also felt there were fewer sedative and cognitive impairing effects with carbamazepine. Again, this suggests that anticonvulsant treatment for benzodiazepine withdrawal may be particularly effective in patients with chemical dependency (drug abusers) as opposed to those taking benzodiazepines for therapeutically prescribed reasons (particularly patients with panic disorder). Nonetheless, mixed groups of anxious patients, as in the study by Schweizer *et al.* (1991), appeared to benefit to some degree.

Evidence that sodium valproate may also have some efficacy in attenuating benzodiazepine withdrawal is limited (Roy-Byrne *et al.* 1989; Alpelt and Emrich 1990). Roy-Byrne and colleagues (1989) reported a single case in which sodium valproate allowed successful discontinuation of alprazolam, 4 mg. daily, over an 8-day period. The patient had failed two prior taper attempts, one involving very slow (0.25 mg) reduction per week, and the other involving rapid substitution of clonazepam. Interpretation of efficacy was complicated by the patient's underlying bipolar disorder and the possibility that better control of this with sodium valproate facilitated withdrawal.

In contrast, in the series of four cases reported by Alpelt and Emrich (1990), valproate was always added several days *after* abstinence symptoms began. The late appearance of these symptoms and their somewhat atypical nature (psychosis in one case, vomiting and vertigo in another) make it hard to generalize from these cases. Nonetheless, because valproate may have antipanic efficacy and clearly does have a mood-stabilizing effect, it may be the anticonvulsant of choice for patients with mood and anxiety disorders. It is not clear how long anticonvulsants need be continued after discontinuation is complete, although several weeks is a reasonable guideline. Furthermore, there is no information on how quickly anticonvulsants should be tapered, if at all. A large study of epileptic patients taking either carbamazepine or sodium valproate failed to reveal evidence of withdrawal symptoms following abrupt discontinuation, although patients did not have underlying anxiety and increases in seizures (their underlying disorder) *were* reported (Duncan *et al.* 1988).

The mode of action of anticonvulsants with respect to this specific indication is unclear. Benzodiazepine discontinuation theoretically results in decreased GABAergic activity, which in turn produces increased neuronal excitability at multiple neurochemical sites. Both clonidine and beta-blockers, which have specific noradrenergic effects, only address the increases in noradrenergic activity that are part of the overall increased excitability. Thus they may have limited efficacy on overall symptomatic distress. In contrast, it is possible that the abovementioned anticonvulsants, by their effect on sodium channels, may have a direct effect on the more widespread increases in neuronal excitability that occur as a result of discontinuation. Valproate also has some GABAergic effects, partly based on slowing the enzymatic degradation of GABA but also probably due to more direct effects at the chloride channel (Roy-Byrne 1988). Finally, both carbamazepine and valproate are known to have the ability to block the development and/or expression of electrical kindling in animals (Post and Weiss 1988). If repeated episodes of alcohol and other drug withdrawal may sensitize or 'kindle' the brain over time making future episodes of symptomatic withdrawal more likely (Ballenger and Post 1984), this mode of action may contribute to the efficacy of anticonvulsants in the chemically dependent/drug abusing population.

Other strategies

Buspirone

The recent introduction of the novel anxiolytic buspirone has prompted interest in the possibility that it might be useful in facilitating successful withdrawal from benzodiazepines. The first study done by Schweizer and Rickels (1986) failed to show that buspirone had any efficacy in attenuating withdrawal. These authors used a one-to-one substitution of buspirone for the benzodiazepine withdrawn (no pre-treatment). Ashton and colleagues (1990) showed that, even when buspirone was given for 4 weeks *prior* to tapered discontinuation to chronic users of diazepam (mean 10 years), it failed to work and actually was *less* effective than placebo in attenuating symptoms during the withdrawal phases. These two reports contrast with that of Rickels *et al.* (1990), who showed that the institution of buspirone treatment for 4 weeks followed by a gradual 4-week discontinuation of the benzodiazepine allowed 11 of 13 patients (85 per cent) to remain off the benzodiazepine for at least 5 weeks. Contradictory results in these two sets of studies suggest that the type of patient might be more important than previously thought in determining discontinuation outcome and adjunctive treatment efficacy. The efficacy of buspirone in treating underlying symptoms of anxiety also makes it impossible to claim that has any direct effect on withdrawal *per se*. This is further reinforced by the failure to show efficacy with minimal or no pre-treatment.

Antidepressants

In contrast to numerous anecdotal reports suggesting that pre-treatment with antidepressants may facilitate benzodiazepine discontinuation (Ashton 1984), the one controlled study of this issue actually demonstrated that this strategy produced *worse* results (Woods *et al.*, 1992). In this study, patients were treated with imipramine for 8 weeks along with alprazolam or placebo for the initial 4 weeks. Following benzodiazepine taper during weeks 5 and 6 those individuals on the combined alprazolam–imipramine treatment dropped out at a much greater rate. Although this suggests that tricyclics have little efficacy in attenuating benzodiazepine withdrawal, a 2-week taper may be too rapid and 4 weeks of antidepressant pre-treatment may be too short for clinical efficacy to take effect.

In contrast, Rickels *et al.* (1990) showed that pre-treatment with imipramine was quite effective in facilitating a subsequent 4-week taper from long-acting benzodiazepines. For the final 3 weeks the adjunctive medications under double-blind conditions were replaced by placebo, and follow-up indicated that 11 of 14, or 79 per cent, of imipramine-treated patients were able to stay off for 5 weeks. This study treated a heterogeneous group of anxious patients in contrast to the homogeneous group of panic patients treated by Woods *et al.* (1992). The rate of successful discontinuation in the Rickels *et al.* (1990) study using carbamazepine pre-treatment was 12 of 13 (92 per cent). Of note, however, is that 26 of 45 placebo-treated patients (58 per cent) were also able to taper, indicating, as previously noted, that placebo may be quite effective in ameliorating withdrawal in some patients.

Our clinical experience (N. Ward, personal communication) indicates that discontinuation of benzodiazepines in some patients concomitantly taking monoamine oxidase inhibitors (MAOI) sometimes seems to produce symptom exacerbation. There is a theoretical possibility that potentiation by the MAOI of any noradrenergic increases due to discontinuation might override the relapse-preventing effect. Unfortunately, there is no study in the literature at this point looking at the efficacy of MAOI in facilitating benzodiazepine discontinuation, and, it should be emphasized, no case reports of adverse effects.

Conclusion

A number of conclusions can be reached from a review of this data. Beta-blockers appear to block the autonomic arousal associated with benzodiazepine discontinuation, but have no effect on psychological symptoms and, in general, are not effective in facilitating successful discontinuation. Clonidine appears to be ineffective in several placebo-controlled studies when given after discontinuation was initiated. Pre-treatment may work better since in the initial positive case report the patient was pre-treated with clonidine. Anecdotal reports suggest that carbamazepine may be effective on all aspects on benzodiazepine discontinuation, but subsequent placebo-controlled studies suggest perhaps greater utility in the addicted population and in mixed groups of anxious patients and less utility in more homogeneous groups of panic disorder patients.

Relapse prevention by the addition of anxiolytic agents prior to discontinuation is a common practice, but is not entirely supported by controlled studies. Negative results in some studies may be due to not administering the anxiolytic for long enough before discontinuation or discontinuing the benzodiazepines too rapidly. Nonetheless, Rickels *et al.*'s more recent study (1990) suggests that, even with 4-week substitution, there may be some efficacy of the azaspirone and tricyclic antidepressant compounds.

Finally, previous studies of discontinuation syndromes, while often addressing abuser/non-abuser typology, have not included other relevant typologies that will probably affect outcome. Variables that should be addressed in future research include: (1) addiction history, even if it is temporally remote and/or to socially accepted substance such as tobacco; (2) genetic loading for addictive disease (Ciraulo *et al.* 1989); (3) history of previous attempt to discontinue any psychotropic drug and the results of that attempt (Ballenger and Post 1984; Post and Weiss 1988); (4) at-risk personality traits (Tyrer *et al.* 1985; Rickels *et al.* 1988); and (5) severity and type of disorder.

References

Abernethy, D.R., Greenblatt, D.J., and Shader R.I. (1981). Treatment of diazepam withdrawal syndrome with propranolol. *Annals of Internal Medicine*, **94**, 354–5.

Alpelt, S. and Emrich, H.M. (1990). Sodium valproate in benzodiazepine withdrawal. *American Journal of Psychiatry*, **147**, 950–1.

Ashton, H. (1984). Benzodiazepine withdrawal: an unfinished story. *British Medical Journal*, **288**, 1135–40.

Ashton, C.H., Rawlings, M.D., and Tyrer, S.P. (1990). A double-blind placebo-controlled study of buspirone in diazepam withdrawal in chronic benzodiazepine users. *British Journal of Psychiatry*, **157**, 232–8.

Ballenger, J.C. (1991). Use of carbamazepine in alprozalam discontinuation. Payer presented at the 144th Annual Meeting of the American Psychiatric Association, May 11–16.

Ballenger, J.C. and Post, R.M. (1984). Carbamazepine in alcohol withdrawal syndromes and schizophrenic psychosis. *Psychopharmacology Bulletin.* **20**, 572–84.

Cantopher, T., Olivieri, S., Cleave, N., and Edward, J.G. (1990). Chronic benzodiazepine dependence: a comparative study of abrupt withdrawal under propranolol cover versus gradual withdrawal. *British Journal of Psychiatry*, **156**, 406–11.

Ciraulo, D.A., Barnhill, J.G., Ciraulo, A.M., Greenblatt, D.J., and Shader, R.J. (1989). Parental alcoholism as a risk factor in benzodiazepine abuse: a pilot study. *American Journal of Psychiatry*, **146**, 1333–5.

Duncan, J., Shorvon, S.D., and Trimble, M.R. (1988). Withdrawal symptoms from phenytoin, carbamazepine and sodium valproate. *Journal of Neurology, Neurosurgery and Psychiatry*, **51**, 924–48.

Fontaine, R., Chouinard, G., and Annable, L. (1984). Rebound anxiety in anxious patients after abrupt withdrawal of benzodiazepine treatment. *American Journal of Psychiatry*, **141**, 848–52.

Fyer, A.J., Liebowitz, M.R., Gorman, J.M., Campeas, R., Levin, A., Davies, S.O. *et al.* (1988). Effects of clonidine on alprazolam discontinuation in panic patients: a pilot study. *Journal of Clinical Psychopharmacology*, **8**, 270–5.

Goodman, W.K., Charney, D.S., and Price, L.H. (1986). Ineffectiveness of clonidine in the treatment of benzodiazepine withdrawal syndrome. *American Journal of Psychiatry*, **143**, 900–3.

Haefely, W. (1986). Biological basis for drug-induced tolerance, rebound and dependence: contribution of recent research on benzodiazepines. *Pharmacopsychiatry*, **19**, 353–61.

Hallström, C., Crock, G., Robson, M., and Shine, P. (1988). The treatment of tranquilizer dependence by propranolol. *Postgraduate Medical Journal*, **64**, (suppl. 2), 40–4.

Higgitt, A., Fonagy, P., Toone, B., and Shine, P. (1990). The prolonged benzodiazepine withdrawal syndrome: anxiety or hysteria? *Acta Psychiatrica Scandinavica*, **82**, 165–8.

Hoehn-Saric, R., Merchant, A.F., Keyser, M.L., and Smith, V.K. (1981). Effects of clonidine on anxiety disorders. *Archives of General Psychiatry*, **38**, 1278–82.

Keshavan, J.S. and Crammer, J.L. (1985). Clonidine in benzodiazepine withdrawal. *Lancet*, **i**, 1325–6.

Klein, E., Uhde, T.W., and Post, R.M. (1986). Preliminary evidence for the utility of carbamazepine in alprazolam withdrawal. *American Journal of Psychiatry*, **143**, 235–6.

Liebowitz, M.R., Fyer, A.J., McGrath, P., and Klein, D.F. (1981). Clonidine treatment of panic disorder. *Psychopharmacology Bulletin*, **17**, 122–3.

Malcolm, R., Ballenger, J.C., Sturgis, E.T., and Anton, R. (1989). Double-blind controlled trial comparing carbamazepine to oxapam treatment of alcohol withdrawal. *American Journal of Psychiatry*, **146**, 617–21.

Munjack, D.J., Crocker, B., Cabe, D., Brown, R., and Vsigh, R. (1989). Alprazolam, propranolol and placebo in the treatment of panic disorder and agoraphobia with panic attacks. *Journal of Clinical Psychopharmacology*, **9**, 22–6.

Nutt, D. (1986). Benzodiazepine dependence in the clinic: reason for anxiety trends. *Pharmacological Sciences*, **7**, 457–60.

Pecknold, J.C. (1990). Discontinuation Studies: Short-term and long-term. Presented at Panic and Anxiety: A decade of progress. Geneva, Switzerland, June 19–22.

Pecknold, J.C., McClure, D.J., Fleuri, D., and Chang, H. (1982). Benzodiazepine withdrawal effects. *Progress in Neuro-psychopharmacology and Biological Psychiatry*, **6**, 517–22.

Pecknold, J.C., Swinson, R.P., Kuch, K., and Lewis, C.P. (1988). Alprazolam in panic disorder and agoraphobia: discontinuation effects. *Archives of General Psychiatry*, **45**, 429–36.

Post, R.M. and Weiss, S.R.B. (1988). Sensitization and kindling: implications for the evolution of psychiatric symptomatology. In *Sensitization of the nervous system*, (ed. P.W. Kalivas and C.D. Barnes), Telford, New Jersey.

Rickels, K., Schweizer, E., Case, G.W., and Garcia-Espana, F. (1988). Benzodiazepine dependence, withdrawal, severity and clinical outcome: effects on personality. *Psychopharmacology Bulletin*, **24**, 415–20.

Rickels, K., Case, W.G., Schweizer, E., Garcia-España, F., and Fridman, R. (1990). Management of discontinuation. *Psychopharmacology Bulletin*, **26**, 63–8.

Ries, R., Roy-Byrne, P., Ward, N.G., Neppe, V., and Cullison, S. (1989). Carbamazepine treatment for benzodiazepine withdrawal. *American Journal of Psychiatry*, **146**, 536–7.

Ries, R.K., Cullison, S., Horn, R., and Ward, N. (1991). Benzodiazepine withdrawal: clinicians' ratings of carbamazepine treatment versus traditional taper methods. *Journal of Psychoactive Drugs*, **23**, 73–6.

Rinaldi, R.C., Steindler, E.M., Wilford, B.B., and Goodwin, D. (1988). Clarification and standardization of substance abuse terminology. *Journal of the American Medical Association*, **259**, 555–7.

Roy-Byrne, P.P. (1988). Anticonvulsants in anxiety and withdrawal syndromes: hypotheses for future research. In *Use of anticonvulsants in psychiatry* (ed. S.L.McElroy and H.G.Pope), pp.155–68. Oxford Health Care, Inc, Oxford.

Roy-Byrne, P. and Hommer, D. (1988). Benzodiazepine withdrawal: overview and implications for the treatment of anxiety. *American Journal of Medicine*, **84**, 1041–51.

Roy-Byrne, P. and Wingerson, D. (1992). Pharmacotherapy of the anxiety disorders. In *Annual review of psychiatry*, Vol. II (ed. A. Tasman), pp.260–84. American Psychiatric Press, Washington, DC.

Roy-Byrne, P., Ward, N.G., and Donnelly, P. (1989). Valproate in anxiety and withdrawal syndromes. *Journal of Clinical Psychiatry*, **50**, 44–8.

Sanchez-Craig, M., Kay, G., Busto, U., and Cappell, H. (1986). Cognitive–behavioral treatment for benzodiazepine dependence. *Lancet*, **i**, 388–9.

Schweizer, E. and Rickels, K. (1986). Failure of buspirone to manage benzodiazepine withdrawal. *American Journal of Psychiatry*, **143**, 1590–2.

Schweizer, E., Rickels, K., Case, W.G., and Greenblatt, D.J. (1991). Effects of carbamazepine treatment on withdrawal severity and outcome in patients on long-term benzodiazepine therapy. *Archives of General Psychiatry*, **48**, 448–52.

Tyrer, P., Rutherford, D., and Huggett, D. (1981). Benzodiazepine withdrawal symptoms and propranolol. *Lancet*, **i**, 520–2.

Tyrer, P., Murphy, S., Oates, G., and Kingdom, G. (1985). Psychological treatment for benzodiazepine dependence. *Lancet*, **i**, 1042–3.

Uhde, T.W., Stein, M.D., and Post, R.M. (1988). Lack of efficacy of carbamazepine in the treatment of panic disorder. *American Journal of Psychiatry*, **145**, 1104–9.

Uhde, T.W., Stein, M.D., Vittone, B.J., Siever, L.J., Boulenger, J.P., and Mellman, T.A. (1989). Behavioral and physiologic effects of short-term and long-term administration of clonidine in panic disorder. *Archives of General Psychiatry*, **46**, 170–7.

Woods, J.H., Katz, J.L., and Winger, G. (1988). Use and abuse of benzodiazepines. *Journal of the American Medical Association*, **260**, 3476–80.

Woods, S.W., Nagy, L.M., Koleszar, A.S., Krystal, J.H., Heninger, G.R., and Charney, D.S. (1992). Controlled trial of alprazolam supplementation during imipramine treament of panic disorder. *Journal of Clinical Psychopharmacology*, **12**, 32–42.

Self-help groups and benzodiazepine dependence

Mark Tattersall

Self-help groups probably cater for more unhappy benzodiazepine users than any other single type of caring agency. This chapter aims to describe what these groups do, and to present one (TRANX (UK) in more detail, with a study of its members, their experience of TRANX, and their outcome.

Self-help: what does it mean?

Self-help is a term that, despite wide usage, can be misleading. The *Oxford English dictionary* (1971, p. 2717) defines it as 'The action or faculty of providing for oneself without assistance from others'. The first use of the term is credited to Carlyle in 1831 in a work of fiction, although it is more commonly associated with Samuel Smiles, a Victorian surgeon who wrote the first self-help book, a best seller appropriately titled *Self help*, in 1859. Smiles was a champion of self-reliance, and believed that 'help from without is sometimes enfeebling in its effects, but help from within invariably invigorates' (Smiles 1986).

More recently and in the present context, self-help has come to mean something rather different, perhaps better described as mutual aid. Stephen Lock expanded on this in his definition of a self-help group as 'A voluntary organisation, usually of peers, who have come together for mutual help and support, in satisfying a common need, overcoming a common handicap or life disrupting problem, and bringing about desired social or personality change or both' (Lock 1986).

Self-help groups for benzodiazepine users: why they evolved and what they offer

Self-help health groups tend to be formed when there is a perceived failure of the professional care-givers to meet the needs of a particular group of patients, or where there are 'uncorrected failures in the larger system' (Gartner and Reissman 1977). If one can judge by the explosive development of self-help groups for benzodiazepine users in Britain from the first in 1982, to some 600 at the time of writing (MIND database, personal correspondence), such failures in provision have been perceived by a large number of those taking benzodiazepines, as well as by at least some health care workers in this field (Trickett 1983).

This may not be surprising in that the concept of benzodiazepine dependence had not achieved wide medical acceptance prior to the mid 1980s, and the kind of mutual support that many of those withdrawing from benzodiazepines seek does not fit easily into the prescriptive style of orthodox health care provision. The development of self-help groups to meet increasing demands for information, recognition, and support was then facilitated by the general rising tide in the self-help movement.

These groups were founded by ex-benzodiazepine users and concerned health care workers. Their work generally covers some or all of the following areas:

1. research into the effects of benzodiazepine use and withdrawal, increasing public awareness of these, and applying political pressure to curb inappropriate prescribing;

2. development and promotion of alternative therapeutic options to the prescription of minor tranquillizers;

3. support of individual users, helping them to withdraw from benzodiazepines and cope with stress without them.

The first two of these are, broadly speaking, political aims and involve disseminating information by means ranging from leaflets for the local general practitioner's waiting room to air time on national television and lobbying Members of Parliament.

The third of these aims is therapeutic and may be delivered by means of support groups, individual counselling, telephone counselling, newsletters, leaflets, and audio tapes. Self-help groups strive to educate their members, to demystify and demedicalize their problems, and to return the locus of control and responsibility to the individual in a supportive atmosphere of shared experience. Members are informed about and share their experience of withdrawal symptoms and together learn to cope with them. They are taught how to manage anxiety and stress without relying on drugs. A sense of belonging to a supportive subculture is encouraged, and may be further enhanced by the provision of emergency telephone support.

Despite the spirit of mutual aid, experience has shown that support groups for withdrawing benzodiazepine users work best if structured, and led by an identified member, and that self-help groups themselves benefit from the assistance of professional advisors (Wann *et al.* 1989). The National Self-Help Support Centre works to support all self-help groups, and can give practical advice on this and related issues. Their address is given in the appendix to this chapter.

The advantages and disadvantages of self-help groups

The advantages of self-help groups as compared to orthodox services include their ability to explore the unorthodox and find novel solutions that challenge conventional perspectives. They cater more to individuals, with the potential of being more flexible to their needs. They can provide specialized information, and a more personal type of support, based on shared experience, so that being a member of a self-help group fosters a sense of communality. This approach is one that empowers members as equals rather than reducing them to dependent consumers of a prescriptive health care system.

The disadvantages of self-help groups include their lack of accountability, and inconsistencies in the standard of training of their workers. As 95 per cent of the work tends to be done by 5 per cent of the members, the leaders may lose touch with the needs of the majority. Success by self-help groups in meeting some of the health care needs of their members might also have the adverse effect of allowing statutory services to avoid working to meet these needs.

Do self-help groups work for benzodiazepine users?

This key question can be broken down into the following principal components.

1. Do self-help groups add to our understanding of the effects of benzodiazepine use and withdrawal?

2. Do they increase public awareness of these effects?

3. Do they influence prescribing trends in a beneficial fashion by reducing inappropriate prescribing, without compromising appropriate use of benzodiazepines or other drugs, such as antidepressants?

4. Do they help their members withdraw from benzodiazepines?

5. Do they help their members develop adequate replacement coping skills?

6. Do they help their members to improve the quality of their lives?

7. Are they acceptable to those who need their help?

While there has been an increase in both medical and public knowledge of the effects of benzodiazepine use and withdrawal, and a parallel reduction in prescribing of benzodiazepines (Dunbar *et al.* 1989), a causal link with the concurrent growth of the self-help movement for this client group cannot be proven. Despite some preliminary research (Ettore 1986; TRANX 1988) and anecdotal evidence (Ashton 1984), there has been insufficient data available on which to base an answer to questions about the acceptability or benefit to members of joining such self-help groups. The study of TRANX (UK) presented in this chapter was designed with the aim of helping to answer these questions.

Self-help books for benzodiazepine users

Rather closer to the self-reliant model of self-help are the various self-help books for benzodiazepine users. These aim to help their readers understand the effects of benzodiazepine use and withdrawal and to advise users on how to give them up. The earlier books focus on exposing the nature and extent of the problems of benzodiazepine dependence, while the later ones give more guidance on how to withdraw from benzodiazepines and cope without them. A briefly annotated list of some of these books is included in the appendix to this chapter.

A study of TRANX (UK) Ltd

The first self-help group for benzodiazepine users in Britain was founded in 1982 by Joan Jerome, who had experienced withdrawal symptoms when she stopped taking benzodiazepines after 17 years. When she recovered she discussed the needs of those withdrawing from benzodiazepines with her local community health council. Although initially sceptical about the extent of the problem, they backed her plan to set up a self-help group after an encouraging response to an article she wrote for the local paper. She named the group TRANX (UK), standing for Tranquillizer Recovery And New eXistence.

By 1983 TRANX had obtained state funding from the Department of Health and Social Security, and continued to expand as the largest self-help group in the UK for benzodiazepine users, with 10 082 people having registered as members by the end of 1988 (TRANX 1988). Despite this, in June 1990 a funding crisis forced its closure.

TRANX's aims were to set up a network of self-help groups for people dependent on minor tranquillizers; to form a national advice, information, support, and referral service for people with the physical and psychological symptoms of tranquillizer withdrawal; and to create greater awareness in the community of the consequences of long-term tranquillizer use, which included applying political pressure to reduce the prescribing of benzo-diazepines.

TRANX was perhaps a victim of its own success. With the increasing numbers of local self-help groups throughout the country, the greater public and medical awareness of the risks of benzodiazepine use, and the downturn in benzodiazepine prescribing, many of its aims as a national organization were being achieved. Central government funding was then discontinued on the basis that local funding of local self-help groups might be more appropriate.

TRANX's services to members included telephone counselling and support; individual counselling; support groups (all of these provided or led by ex-benzodiazepine users trained by TRANX); a quarterly newsletter; information leaflets, including clear guidelines on how to withdraw from benzodiazepines; and an audio tape, on one side of which Joan Jerome described and discussed her own experience of benzodiazepine withdrawal, while the other side featured a guided relaxation session.

While based in London, TRANX supported members all over Britain by telephone and postal counselling and support. All potential members who contacted TRANX were sent an information package and invited to register as members at a cost of £10 per annum. This gave access to telephone counselling, and members were sent details of a slow detoxification regime to follow over many months, and of strategies to cope with withdrawal symptoms. The other services described above were available at further cost, and members' general practitioners were contacted where this was appropriate.

In 1988 this author, in collaboration with the editor of this book, commenced an evaluation of TRANX's therapeutic work, with the aim of understanding more about its members, what they thought of TRANX, and their outcome. We concentrated on members whose contact with TRANX was primarily by telephone or post as this provided the greatest contrast with what was on offer from statutory services.

Method

This was a prospective study of a sample biased to favour those using TRANX's remote (telephone and post) services by selecting only telephone self-referrals, and all 150 such enquirers consecutively contacting TRANX between 22nd March and 21st April 1988 were entered. They were initially interviewed at the time of self-referral by TRANX workers, trained for uniformity of data collection, and using a standard form for this purpose. Baseline data, as presented in Table 21.2 were elicited during this interview. At the same time the enquirers were asked for consent to a follow-up interview.

Follow-up data were collected independently of TRANX by the author after 9 months, using a semi-structured telephone interview lasting 15–20 min. The interviewer stated that he was a doctor working independently of TRANX, researching the experiences of people who take tranquillizers. Data was elicited on whether the enquirer had registered with TRANX, on their experience of both TRANX and other resources, and on their outcome.

As a variety of benzodiazepines were being used, doses were converted to an equivalent dose in milligrams of diazepam (mgDE) using a table (see Table 21.1) expanded from that used by Higgitt *et al.* (1985).

Table 21.1. Conversion table to give equivalent doses of diazepam

Benzodiazepine	Conversion factor equivalent dose of diazepam
Oxazepam and flurazepam	0.33
Temazepam and chlordiazepoxide	0.5
Clobazepam, nitrazepam, and diazepam	1.0
Clorazepate	2.0
Lorazepam	5.0
Alprazolam	10
Triazolam	20

Table 21.2. Members' characteristics at initial contact ($n=41$)

Sex ratio (female: male)	3:1
Age, mean (years)	47 (SD 12.6)
Married (no.)	33 (81%)
White British (no.)	39 (95%)
No. using as main benzodiazepine	
Diazepam	18 (44%)
Lorazepam	10 (24%)
Others	13 (32%)
More than one used	7 (17%)
No. using other psychotropic drugs	
Any prescribed	15 (37%)
Antidepressants	10 (24%)
Daily benzodiazepine dose	
mean (mgDE)	7.2 (SD 7.7)
Range (mgDE)	1–30
No. whose dose = 0 on the day of initial contact	9 (22%)
Mean dose (mgDE) excluding those whose dose = 0	9 (SD 7.6)
Previous dose (mgDE) (before attempts to withdraw)	
Mean	29 (SD 40.4)
Range	2–218
Duration of use, mean (years)	12 (SD 9.9)
No. who were previously in-patient for*	
Any psychiatric treatment	11 (27%)
Benzodiazepine withdrawal	4 (10%)

* Data elicited at follow-up

Results

It proved possible to follow up 117 of the 150 original enquirers (eight refused consent to follow-up when asked at initial contact, as did a further five at follow-up, and 20 were untraceable). Forty-one of these had registered with TRANX following their initial contact; these make up the sample for this study.

Members' characteristics

The members' characteristics at initial contact are presented in Table 21.2. The only significant difference between the 117 enquirers who were followed up and the 33 who were not was a younger mean age of the former (48 compared to 57 years, $p<0.001$, chi-squared test). The only significant difference between the 41 who became members and the 76 who did not was a higher female-to-male sex ratio of 8.5:1 among the non-members ($p<0.05$, chi-squared test).

Members' experience of TRANX and other resources

A breakdown of the use members reported having made of the various services available to them through TRANX, and whether they found these helpful is presented in Table 21.3. 'Helpfulness' was rated by members on a four-point scale of: unhelpful—slightly—moderately—very helpful. A breakdown of members' dissatisfactions with TRANX is presented in Table 21.4. This was rated by members on a four-point scale of: not a problem—slightly—moderately—very unhelpful.

When members were asked to rate the importance to them of TRANX counsellors being ex-benzodiazepine users (on a four-point scale of: unimportant—some benefit—important—very important), 35 (85 per cent) felt that this was either important (7 members), or very important (28 members).

Information collected at follow-up about other resources tried by members

Table 21.3. Use made by members of TRANX services, with their rating of the helpfulness of each ($n=41$)

TRANX service	Number (%) of members			
	Using this service		Rating it as helpful*	
Telephone counselling	31	(76%)	22	(71%)
Information leaflets	41	(100%)	27	(66%)
Newsletter	22	(54%)	14	(64%)
Case history/relaxation tape	17	(41%)	10	(59%)
Support group	7	(17%)	3	(43%)

* 'Helpful' means a rating of moderately or very helpful.

Table 21.4. Members' dissatisfactions with TRANX (*n*=41)

Dissatisfied with	Number (%) rating moderately–very dissatisfied	
Lack of a local TRANX service	18	(44)
Distance to attend support groups	17	(41)
TRANX's telephone lines being engaged	14	(34)
Cost of telephong TRANX	8	(20)
Lack of face-to-face contact	6	(15)
Counsellors not being professionals	5	(12)
Cost of registration fee	0	(0)

to assist them in withdrawing from benzodiazepines, and whether these were perceived as having been helpful, is summarized in Table 21.5.

Members' outcome

At the 9-months follow-up, 28 members (68 per cent) reported that they had stopped using benzodiazepines. This was reflected in a statistically very significant reduction in the mean benzodiazepine dose, from 7.2 to 2.2 mgDE ($p<0.000$, T test). 30 members (73 per cent) reported that the symptoms for which they had initially been prescribed benzodiazepines had improved. Members who rated symptoms as worse were either among those who had not reduced their dose at all (two of four) or among those who had withdrawn completely (seven of 28). Thirty-three members (80 per cent) reported that

Table 21.5. Other resources tried by members and whether they felt these helped them to withdraw from benzodiazepines (*n*=41)

Resource	Number (%) of members			
	using this resource		rating it as helpful*	
General practitioner	NA[†]		10	(24)[†]
Psychiatrist	23	(56)	10	(43)
Other orthodox counsellor (nurse, psychologist, social worker)	16	(39)	11	(69)
Alternative therapies (yoga, hypnotherapy, acupuncture)	34	(83)	16	(44)
Local support group	9	(22)	6	(67)

* 'Helpful' here means a rating of moderately or very helpful.
† All members had consulted their general practitioner, but could not always clarify whether this was with the aim of benzodiazepine withdrawal. The percentage 'helped by' their general practitioner was calculated from the assumption that all members had sought this help, and is likely to be an underestimate.

they were satisfied with their withdrawal in terms of subjective current quality of life. All but one of the eight members who were dissatisfied with their withdrawal were still taking benzodiazepines. A breakdown of this data is presented in Table 21.6 Of the 28 members who had stopped benzodiazepines at follow-up, two were taking antidepressants, and one a beta-blocker.

An indicator of overall outcome was derived by combining these measures. Seventeen members (41 per cent) had an excellent outcome: they had stopped all psychotropic medication, yet experienced an improvement in their symptoms, and were at least moderately satisfied with their withdrawal. A further 11 (27 per cent) had a moderate outcome: they had stopped taking benzodiazepines, but were still using other psychotropic drugs, and/or were finding that their symptoms had not improved, and/or were less than moderately satisfied with their withdrawal. The remaining 13 (32 per cent) had a poor outcome, defined as continued use of benzodiazepines.

In comparison, the 76 enquirers who did not become members of TRANX

Table 21.6. Outcome at follow-up as determined by three variables

	No. of members (%)	
Change in dose of benzodiazepine		
Stopped	28	(68)
Reduced dose by 3/4	4	(10)
Reduced dose by 1/2	3	(7)
Reduced dose by 1/4	2	(5)
Dose unchanged	4	(10)
Dose increased	0	(0)
Change in symptoms for which benzodiazepines were initially prescribed		
Much better	6	(15)
Better	24	(59)
Same	2	(5)
Worse	9	(22)
Much worse	0	(0)
Satisfaction with the withdrawal in terms of current quality of life		
Satisfied–very	18	(44)
Satisfied–moderate	9	(22)
Satisfied–slight	6	(15)
Dissatisfied	8	(20)

did less well despite a similar pattern of use of other resources: 21 per cent had an excellent outcome, 18 per cent a moderate outcome, and 61 per cent a poor outcome.

All nine of the members who claimed not to have taken benzodiazepines on the day of initial contact, for a period of time ranging from 1 to 65 weeks (median 2 weeks), were abstinent at follow-up.

The data collected at contact were analysed in the light of the outcome in an attempt to identify prognostic indicators. There was a trend towards 'being drug-free at the time of contact' being a positive prognostic indicator ($p=0.06$, chi-squared test) and 'use of lorazepam' being a negative prognostic indicator ($p=0.3$, chi-squared test), but no factor was found to operate at a significant level.

Discussion of results

Designing clinical studies of self-help groups involves a compromise between their philosophy and the need of the researcher for valid scientific data. In this study enquirers were not randomly allocated to either a treatment or a control group and, although the data was elicited in a standardized fashion, the follow-up interviewer was not blind to whether enquirers had become members of TRANX, and there was no independent confirmation of members' reporters of current and past benzodiazepine use. Caution should therefore be exercised in interpreting this study and in comparing it with studies of more orthodox treatments for benzodiazepine dependence.

The findings suggest that all the services offered by TRANX that we enquired about, other than the support groups, were both well used and perceived as helpful by the majority of members using them. Use of and attitudes towards the support groups may have been adversely influenced by the selection bias towards members living at some distance from TRANX's office, where the groups were held, and this is borne out by their most frequent dissatisfaction with TRANX being about this distance.

There seemed to be an acceptance of the self-help model among the members in that the large majority felt it was important that their counsellor was an ex-benzodiazepine user, and only a minority were dissatisfied by the lack of professional support offered them. However, as 65 per cent of active self-referrers decided not to register as members, this form of self-help may have a limited first-sight acceptability to benzodiazepine users in general. Whether this self-selection method results in the most productive matching of resources to clients remains unknown.

Comparing this study with other published studies of treatments for benzodiazepine dependence, the members' characteristics at initial contact are similar in terms of age, sex ratio, and the dose and duration of use of benzodiazepines (other studies report a range of mean age of 40–60 years, median 45 years; a sex ratio of 1:1–4:1 female: male, median 2:1; a mean daily benzodiazepine dose of 9–19 mgDE, median 13 mgDE; and a mean duration of use of 3–13 years, median 7.5 years). In addition, the high rate of psychiatric admission in this sample testifies to the severity of it's morbidity.

Outcome statistics too are comparable, with follow-up findings in other studies of some 60 per cent (range 25–92 per cent, median 60 per cent) withdrawn from benzodiazepines, and some 45 per cent (range 11–70 per cent, median 46 per cent), meeting the stricter overall criteria (where they are published, or can be derived) of being off all psychotropics, relatively asymptomatic, and satisfied with their current quality of life. This is true despite the fact that subjects of such studies generally receive considerable professional treatment from specialist units (Tyrer *et al.* 1981, 1983; Hopkins *et al.* 1982; Teare Skinner 1984; Busto *et al.* 1986; Rickels *et al.* 1986; Ashton 1987; Golombok *et al.* 1987; Higgitt *et al.* 1987; Hallström *et al.* 1988; Cantopher *et al.* 1990).

Although the sample size was small, this study did indicate that joining TRANX was likely to be of benefit to those trying to withdraw from benzodiazepines. This is in line with the viewpoint of Cantopher *et al.* (1990) that, with gradual withdrawal and sympathetic, but not necessarily professional support, most of those who wish to stop taking benzodiazepines achieve this. As TRANX members often used other resources as well this may have been an additive effect, although the non-members had a poorer outcome despite a similar use of these other resources.

Conclusion

Self-help groups differ, but in general have much to offer both the community and the individual that is not available elsewhere, and they may well be effective in helping benzodiazepine users to withdraw from their drug use. That they are not a panacea is also clear, but then, neither is orthodox health care. In order to fully utilize this additional resource, orthodox therapists need to find ways to work in tandem with, and facilitate the development of self-help organizations, so that those in need may experience the benefits of both approaches.

Acknowledgements

With regard to the study of TRANX, the author would like to thank Joan Jerome and all the staff at TRANX (UK) Ltd who helped with the initial data collection, the Charing Cross and Westminster Medical School Computing department for assistance in analysing the data, and the North West Thames Regional Health Authority for financial assistance.

Appendix

How to contact self-help groups for benzodiazepine users

MIND, National Association For Mental Health, 22 Harley Street, London W1N 2ED, UK. Telephone: 071–637 0741; Fax: 071–323 0061.

Information about groups throughout Britain is available from MIND head office.

Information about self-help groups anywhere in the USA is available from the Illinois Self-Help Centre. Telephone (312) 328–0470.

Agencies and publications for those starting up and running self-help groups

The National Self-Help Support Centre, National Council for Voluntary Organisations, 26 Bedford Square, London WC1B 3HU, UK. Telephone: 071–636 4066.

Capper, S., Unell, J., and Weyman, A. (1989). *Starting and running a voluntary group*. Bedford Square Press, London.

Holloway, C. and Otto, S. (1988). *Getting organised: a handbook for non-statutory organisations*. Bedford Square Press, London.

Wilson, J. (1986). *Self-help groups: getting started; keeping going*. Longman, Harlow.

Chronological bibliography of self-help books for benzodiazepine users

Haddon, C. (1984). *Women and tranquillizers*. Sheldon Press, London.

Celia Haddon is a journalist, and her book is primarily an exposé of the benzodiazepine problem, with particular reference to women, and includes a brief and simple plan for withdrawing from benzodiazepines.

Melville, J. (1984). *The tranquillizer trap and how to get out of it*. Fontana· Books, London.

Joy Melville is also a journalist. Her book includes a history of the benzodiazepine problem, and of the early stages of the development of self-help groups for benzodiazepine users.

Coleman, V. (1985). *Life without tranquillizers*. Corgi Books, London.

Dr Vernon Coleman is a former general practitioner. His book discusses how to cope with stress, but does not focus on how to withdraw from benzodiazepines.

Curran, V. and Golombok, S. (1985). *Bottling it up*. Faber & Faber, London.

Drs Valerie Curran and Susan Golombok are psychologists. Their book explores the social and political issues surrounding the prescribing of benzo-diazepines. They describe the different treatment options available, both orthodox and unorthodox, and include a clear and comprehensive self-help withdrawal programme.

Tyrer, P. (1986). *How to stop taking tranquillizers*. Sheldon Press, London.

Dr Peter Tyrer is a consultant psychiatrist. In addition to discussing the background to the development and recognition of the benzodiazepine problem, he gives detailed advice about how to withdraw from benzodiazepines.

Neild, L. (1990). *Escape from tranquillisers and sleeping pills*. Ebury Press, London.

Larry Neild is lay worker with a self-help group for benzodiazepine users. His book includes a comprehensive self-help withdrawal programme.

Trickett, S. (1991). *Coming off tranquillizers and sleeping pills* (2nd edn). Thorsons, Wellingborough.

Shirley Trickett is a nurse who founded one of the first benzodiazepine self-help groups. Her book presents a self-help withdrawal programme that includes a spiritual dimension.

References

Ashton, H. (1984). Benzodiazepine withdrawal: an unfinished story. *British Medical Journal*, **288**, 1135–40.
Ashton, H. (1987). Benzodiazepine Withdrawal: outcome in 50 patients. *British Journal of Addiction*, **82**, 665–71.
Busto, U., Sellers, E.M., Naranjo, C.A., Cappell, H., Sanchez-Craig, M., and Sykora, K. (1986). Withdrawal reactions after long-term use of benzodiazepines. *New England Journal of Medicine*, **315**, 854–9.
Cantopher, T., Olivieri, S., Clesve, N., and Guy Edwards, J. (1990). Chronic benzodiazepine dependence. A comparative study of abrupt withdrawal under propranolol cover versus gradual withdrawal. *British Journal of Psychiatry*, **156**, 406–11.
Dunbar, G.C., Perera, M.H., and Jenner, F.A. (1989). Patterns of benzodiazepine use in Great Britain as measured by a population survey. *British Journal of Psychiatry*, **155**, 836–41.
Ettorre, E.M. (1986). Self-help groups as an alternative to benzodiazepine use. In *Tranquillisers* (ed. J. Gabe and P. Williams), pp.180–93. Tavistock Publications, London.

Gartner, A. and Reissman, F. (1977). *Self-help in the human services*. Jossey-Bass, San Francisco.

Golombok, S., Higgitt, A., Fonagy, P., Dodds, S., Sapper, J., and Lader, M. (1987). A follow up study of patients treated for benzodiazepine dependence. *British Journal of Medical Psychology*, **60**, 141–9.

Hallström, C., Crouch, G., and Robson, M. (1988). The treatment of tranquillizer dependence by propranolol. *Postgraduate Medical Journal*, **64** (suppl. 2), 40–4.

Higgitt, A., Lader, M.H., and Fonagy, P. (1985). Clinical management of benzodiazepine dependence. *British Medical Journal*, **291**, 688–90.

Higgitt, A., Golombok, S., Fonagy, P., and Lader, M. (1987). Group treatment of benzodiazepine dependence. *British Journal of Addiction*, **82**, 517–32.

Hopkins, D., Sethi, K., and Mucklow, J. (1982). Benzodiazepine withdrawal in General Practice. *Journal of the Royal College of General Practitioners*, **32**, 758–62.

Lock, S. (1986). Self help groups: the fourth estate in medicine? *British Medical Journal*, **293**, 1596–600.

Oxford English Dictionary, (1971). *Oxford English Dictionary* (compact edn). Oxford University Press, Oxford.

Rickels, K., Case, G.W., Schweizer, E.E., Swenson, C., and Fridman, R.B. (1986). Low-dose dependence in chronic benzodiazepine users: a preliminary report on 119 patients. *Psychopharmacology Bulletin*, **22**, 407–15.

Smiles, S. (1986). *Self help* (ed. G. Bull and K. Joseph) (revised edn). Penguin, Harmondsworth.

Teare Skinner, P. (1984). Skills not pills: learning to cope with anxiety symptoms. *Journal of the Royal College of General Practitioners*, **34**, 258–60.

TRANX (UK) Ltd (1988). *Annual report* 1988. TRANX, London.

Trickett, S. (1983). Withdrawal from benzodiazepines. *Journal of the Royal College of General Practitioners*, **33**, 608.

Tyrer, P., Rutherford, D., and Huggett, T. (1981). Benzodiazepine withdrawal symptoms and propranolol. *Lancet*, **i**, 520–2.

Tyrer, P., Owen, R., and Dawling, S. (1983). Gradual withdrawal of diazepam after long term therapy. *Lancet*, **i**, 1402–6.

Wann, M., Warren, J., and Walls, J. (1989). Women and tranquillisers group. *The Bulletin of the National Self-Help Support Centre*, **12**, 3–6.

22 Benzodiazepines and the pharmaceutical industry

Frank Wells

In considering the role of the pharmaceutical industry in relation to the benzodiazepines, it is essential that the regulatory and legal aspects of their use are linked with the clinical aspects. In the course of this chapter, therefore—in establishing this relationship—the indications and contraindications for their use set out in detail by others may well be repeated, but the reasons for this will hopefully be apparent. In a book of this nature, there is bound to be some overlap among the topics covered by the various contributors.

The need to recognize dependence as a potential problem was not immediately obvious when the benzodiazepines were first introduced. They were invaluable as a therapeutic tool in weaning patients off barbiturates, but relatively few doctors at the time, even those who were specialists in the fields recognized that their dependence potential was likely to assume considerable proportions (Wells 1973). It was therefore not surprising that it was some years before anyone actually confirmed that benzodiazepines were themselves associated with dependence. However, it made sense then, and it certainly makes sense now, that no medicine should be prescribed in perpetuity for any condition that ought to be self-limiting, curable, or, at the very least, controllable for long periods without the need for medication.

It does seem inappropriate, therefore, that pressure groups blame the pharmaceutical industry for irresponsible promotion, when the evidence shows that the irresponsible ones were those doctors who prescribed long-term benzodiazepines without ensuring that their patients were positively continuing to benefit from them. Undoubtedly, some patients will benefit from the short-term use of benzodiazepines, though some of them, quite legitimately, will require a further course, a few of them repeatedly, but only for short-term treatment.

There is no doubt that the virtual demise of barbiturates as therapeutic products followed better understanding by doctors of the ways in which they behaved—and misbehaved—together with the development of safer alternatives by the pharmaceutical industry. The CURB campaign to reduce their use was highly successful in this regard. Better understanding by doctors of the ways in which benzodiazepines behave should also have led to better prescribing—but in many instances this did not happen. However, the usefulness of benzodiazepines as hypnotics or tranquillizers *is* much greater than that of barbiturates, given the very considerable difference in risk/benefit ratio between the two—in favour of benzodiazepines.

Prescribing patterns for benzodiazepines

The benzodiazepines first became available in the UK in the early 1960s, when the hypnotic/tranquillizer market was virtually dominated by the barbiturates. Nearly 28 million general practitioner National Health Service (NHS) prescriptions were dispensed in 1960 classified either as hypnotics or tranquillizers; 15 million of these were for barbiturates. The pattern had changed by 1974, when 40 million NHS general practitioner prescriptions were dispensed; by then 24.6 million were for benzodiazepines, and only 8 million were for barbiturates.

Data from the UK Department of Health for the period 1974–89 show that the total number of benzodiazepine prescriptions rose from 24.6 million in 1974 to a peak of 31 million in 1979 and then fell back to 21.4 million in 1989.

Despite the introduction of the restricted list of medicines prescribable on the NHS in 1985 (the 'limited list'), whereby only a restricted number of benzodiazepines were allowed to be prescribed—and then only by approved

Table 22.1. Prescriptions of benzodiazepines in Great Britain, 1989

Drug group	No. of prescriptions ($\times 10^6$)[†]
Tempazepam	7.1
Nitrazepam	4.2
Diazepam	4.1
Triazolam	2.1
Lorazepam	1.7
Chlordiazepoxide	0.8
Oxazepam	0.5
Lormetazepam	0.2
Loprazolam	0.2
Clonazepam	0.1
Clobazam	0.1
Total	22.1

* Source: Department of Health (1990).
† These estimates are based on a sample of prescriptions of approximately 1 in 200 in England and Wales and 1 in 100 in Scotland that were dispensed by community pharmacists.

name—the annual number of prescriptions levelled off in 1990 at just over 21 million, which is about the same absolute level as for barbiturates 20 years earlier. This raises the query as to whether there might always be a finite group of patients within the population of the UK who will always expect to receive anxiolytic medication, knowing that it is relatively freely available, and it would be interesting to research this further.

It is possible to separate the indications for which various benzodiazepines are licensed into hypnotics and tranquillizers. If the prescribed numbers of each are compared, some interesting facts are unearthed. Two quite different patterns are seen. Hypnotic prescribing rose throughout the 1970s from less than 5 million general practitioner prescriptions in 1970 to 14 million in 1989. By contrast, the benzodiazepine tranquillizer general practitioner prescriptions were estimated at 10 million in 1970, peaked at 18 million in 1978, and came down again to about 7 million in 1989. This obviously shows a significant shift in the balance of usage, and it is products such as temazepam with a short plasma half-life that are now preferred as hypnotics. The number of prescriptions for each individual benzodiazepine dispensed by community pharmacists during 1989 is shown in Table 22.1. The total number is 9 per cent smaller than in 1988 (*Hansard* 1990).

The above paragraphs give some indication of the previous and the current positions regarding numbers of prescriptions; the pattern of prescription dispensing over the years 1973 to 1989 is demonstrated in Fig. 22.1. It is not possible, however, with the current available facilities, to estimate with any

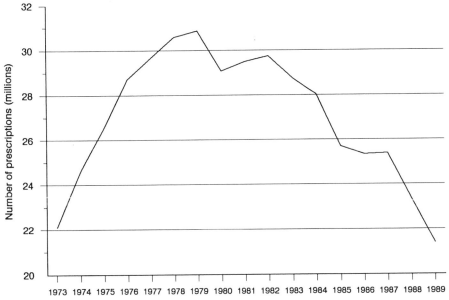

Fig. 22.1. Benzodiazepines. Prescription items dispensed by pharmacists in Great Britain. (Source: Department of Health Pharmaceutical Division.)

real degree of accuracy how many of these prescriptions were for long-term users of benzodiazepines, and how many were for medium-term, short-term, occasional, or one-off users. It is also not possible to give any indication of the likelihood or incidence of withdrawal symptoms if benzodiazepines are suddenly stopped. The best estimate we have is that three out of four benzodiazepine tranquillizer prescriptions are repeat prescriptions and that five out of six benzodiazepine hypnotic prescriptions are repeats. Together with other data that probably means, again as a best estimate, that about 3 million consumers in the UK take benzodiazepines on a short-term basis (arbitrarily set at up to 6 months in the year) and between 500 000 and 1 million take them on a long-term basis.

These are inevitably very rough calculations and even these may need to be modified further: perhaps up to 10 per cent of benzodiazepine prescriptions are for use other than as a tranquillizer or hypnotic; and some—possibly many—long-term benzodiazepine users are taking them on an intermittent or 'as required' basis. By no criteria are such patients either physically or psychologically dependent on benzodiazepines. So, although the Department of Health states that in mid-1986 there were perhaps half a million people in the UK dependent on benzodiazepines, it is impossible to estimate accurately the true number of benzodiazepine-dependent patients in this country, in terms of those who are at significant risk of developing unpleasant withdrawal symptoms if their prescription is stopped. Of course, this is not to argue that there is any justification for having any patients dependent on this class of medicine, but it is important to point out that the number of patients stated to have been dependent may have been inaccurately estimated.

When should benzodiazepine be prescribed?

Because the numbers of patients estimated to be dependent on benzo-diazepines may be too high, this might account for the frequency and vehemence of the comments made about the 'dangerous nature' of this particular class of medicines. Nevertheless, used in the way in which the manufacturers advise, for which they are licensed, and which is now rec-ommended by the British Medical Association and the Royal College of General Practitioners, they are useful and effective without being unduly hazardous. Furthermore (just as with alcohol) dependence does not always occur even with regular use, though the qualification that they should *not* be used for more than 4 months without a break is vitally important. Ill-advised benzodiazepine prescribing has and probably does still occur, and it can lead to a minority of consumers experiencing distress and be responsible for the majority of cases of genuine dependence.

Much has been written about the 'state of the art' of anxiolytic prescribing, and some commentators have queried whether patients in general would have been better off without the benzodiazepines at all. My personal view on this was, as a prescriber, and is, as an observer in the field, emphatically negative. People tend to forget that the products that they replaced, the barbiturates, were far more hazardous, in that they had a much greater dependence potential and were lethal in quite a small overdose, which the benzodiazepines are not. Doctors are, therefore, acting quite in accordance with responsible medical opinion when they prescribe benzodiazepines for the short-term treatment of acute anxiety. That is the current position and is reflected in the relevant recommendations issued by the Committee on Safety of Medicines (CSM) in January 1988, referred to in the next section. Adequate warnings on the use of benzodiazepines for other than short-term use for anxiety (or for hypnosis) have been provided by the pharmaceutical companies with product licences for benzodiazepines and have been available for many years; they were merely consolidated by the CSM when they issued their recommendations.

The CSM recommendations

It must therefore be acknowledged that, for a considerable period of time, there has been recognition by the pharmaceutical industry of and increasing concern over the problem of benzodiazepine dependence (Owen and Tyrer 1983; Pétursson and Lader 1984; Murphy and Tyrer 1987). It was only to be expected, therefore, that the CSM would eventually publish recommendations for limiting the prescribing of benzodiazepines, and the CSM issued such rec-ommendations in January 1988, commenting at the time that the occurrence of dependency was becoming increasingly worrying.

Although the industry had itself taken action on the hazard of dependence potential some years previously, it found itself caught up in the aftermath of the CSM recommendations. What became a concern to pharmaceutical companies producing benzodiazepines, and which to some extent remains a concern, was that the increase in dependence was not strongly supported by evidence of morbidity in other respects, and that the CSM comments were based partially on emotive evidence. Although such comments have the status of advice rather than of a mandatory requirement, the practical effects of this advice for prescribers can be far-reaching.

The CSM itself, in its (1988) recommendation, stated that, although there had been concern for many years, this concern was not in fact supported by any good case studies providing hard data. It was, presumably, the efforts of vociferous pressure groups, whose activities achieved prominent media coverage, the steady build-up of this pressure to take some action, and the claims of some experts in the field that their clinical experience had begun to point to there being a sizeable problem of benzodiazepine dependence that led the CSM to take this action. The message of these pressure groups can be summarized as alleging that large numbers of patients suffer from addiction and withdrawal symptoms due to their long-term use of prescribed benzodiazepines.

The 'limited list' and the UK Misuse of Drugs Act

Ever since the so-called 'limited list' was introduced by the UK government in 1984, certain benzodiazepines have not been available on NHS prescription. The symbol ̶N̶H̶S̶ has been placed against such preparations where they appear in the *British national formulary* (BNF). Although some benzodiazepines cannot be prescribed under the NHS at all, others, though not prescribable by brand name, may be prescribed by their approved or non-proprietary name and, indeed, the brand in question may nevertheless be dispensed if no generic preparation is marketed.

The Misuse of Drugs Act also applies to 33 benzodiazepines, which include all those available on prescription in the UK. However, most of these benzodiazepines are included in Schedule 4 of the Act, which means that none of the drug prescription restrictions affecting drugs in schedules 1.2, and 3 are required, nor are they subject to the safe custody regulations that apply to drugs in Schedules 1 and 2. Nevertheless, their inclusion in the Act at all implies—or, it could be said, confirms—that they are recognized as drugs of abuse.

Advice from the BNF

That being so, it is appropriate to quote the advice to prescribers given in the BNF on drugs likely to cause dependence or abuse (British Medical Association and Royal Pharmaceutical Society of Great Britain 1989). The prescriber has three main responsibilities:

1. To avoid creating dependence by introducing drugs to patients without sufficient reason. In this context, the proper use of drugs is well understood. The dangers of other controlled drugs are less clear because recognition of dependence is not easy and its effects, and those of withdrawal, are less obvious. Perhaps the most notable result of uninhibited prescribing is that a very large number of patients in the country take tablets that do them neither much good nor much harm, but they are committed to them indefinitely because they cannot readily be stopped.

2. To see that the patient does not gradually increase the dose of a drug, given for good medical reasons, to the point where dependence becomes more likely. This tendency is seen especially with hypnotics and anxiolytics. The prescriber should keep a close eye on the amount prescribed to prevent patients from accumulating stocks that would enable them to arrange their own dosage or even that of their families and friends. A minimal amount should be prescribed in the first instance, or when seeing a new patient for the first time.

3. To avoid being used as an unwitting source of supply for addicts. Methods include visiting more than one doctor, fabricating stories, and forging

prescriptions. A doctor should therefore be wary of prescribing for strangers and may be able to get information about suspected opioid addicts from the UK Home Office.

Additional advice is given in the BNF under the general section on hypnotics and anxiolytics, and in the specific subsections under the individual headings, 'Hypnotics' and 'anxiolytics'. The advice cannot be faulted, as it is entirely compatible with the details given in the specific data sheets of individual benzodiazepines.

Data sheets for branded preparations

It is important to take careful note of what a data sheet, provided by an innovative company for a branded preparation, actually says. Paradoxically, such information is no longer available for any benzodiazepines prescribed under the UK NHS, following the introduction of the 'limited list' referred to above. Nevertheless, most branded versions of the various benzodiazepines currently available in the UK remain on the market, and therefore *their* data sheets remain in print and are published in the *Data sheet compendium* (ABPI (1993–94). It must be remembered that data sheets are supplied in order to comply with the requirements of the Medicines Act 1968, and are prepared by the individual companies concerned who are required to follow the Medicines (Data Sheet) Regulations 1972. Each data sheet is required to be compatible with the conditions of the product licence granted for each individual product—so each one has the status of effectively being statutorily approved. That is important and gives the data sheet a legal status not shared by entries in the *British national formulary*—or, indeed, by any other publication regarding the use of medicines.

A typical data sheet produced by a pharmaceutical company for a benzodiazepine used as a hypnotic states very clearly that it can be administered effectively for *short-term moderate* or *severe* insomnia and *occasional* use in patients with recurring insomnia, and that its long-term chronic use is *not recommended*. The data sheet also emphasizes that the patient should be reassessed at the end of *no longer than* 4 weeks of *treatment*. Important additional statements include reminders to prescribers that depression may be intensified, that extreme caution should be used in patients who are prone to substance abuse, and that, in cases of loss or bereavement, psychological adjustment may be inhibited—a fairly clear contraindication.

The data sheet for a typical benzodiazepine used as an anxiolytic makes equally clear statements about its justified though limited indications, including short-term (2–4 weeks) symptomatic treatment of anxiety that is severe, disabling, or subjecting the patient to unacceptable distress. The dose should be the *lowest* that can control symptoms, and treatment should not be continued at the full dose *beyond* 4 weeks. In both the hypnotic and the anxiolytic data sheets extensive lists of contraindications and precautions are given.

The BNF confirms that benzodiazepine anxiolytics can indeed be effective in alleviating genuine anxiety states, and that, as hypnotics, appropriate benzodiazepines can be used occasionally for transient insomnia, and intermittently for short-term or chronic insomnia. Hypnotics should *not* (says the BNF) be prescribed indiscriminately and routine prescribing is undesirable.

The prescribing figures over the past 18 years, referred to earlier, demonstrate the popularity of the benzodiazepines. But there has been a tendency to prescribe these particular medicines to almost anyone with stress-related symptoms, unhappiness, or minor physical disease, although these are not given as indications in the data sheet of the product concerned, and their use is unjustified in many such situations. They should not be used to treat depression, phobia, or obsessional state, or chronic psychosis, but again pharmaceutical companies do not give these as indications in the data sheets.

Pharmacological alternatives to benzodiazepines

Other medicines have product licences that confirm their use as anxiolytics: these include buspirone, meprobamate, and certain beta-blockers. Buspirone is indicated for the treatment of anxiety, but it is still relatively new though its dependence potential appears to be low. It is metabolized differently from the benzodiazepines, and it consequently has no effect in preventing benzodiazepine withdrawal symptoms, where these might occur.

Meprobamate is much less effective than the benzodiazepines, and more hazardous in overdosage, with a recognized potential for inducing dependence. It has never been as popular as the benzodiazepines, and its use is dwindling: in 1989 only 26 000 prescriptions were issued, compared with the peak of over 90 000 in 1975.

Certain beta-blockers are also licensed as anxiolytics since, although they do not affect psychological symptoms such as worry, tension, and fear, they do reduce autonomic symptoms including palpitations, sweating, and tremor. If the predominantly somatic symptoms are controlled, this may prevent the onset of worry and fear. However, patients with predominantly psychological symptoms will not obtain any benefit from beta-blockers at all, and they should not be used inappropriately for unlicensed indications.

The role of the pharmaceutical industry in education about benzodiazepines

Pharmaceutical companies are well aware of the comments and queries that arise regarding the benzodiazepines. Indeed the innovative companies with licensed products in this group possess a wealth of information, which is probably unsurpassed and which can readily be called upon. It tends to be forgotten that, for at least the past 10 years, these companies have been advising doctors of the dependence potential of benzodiazepines, and that they are fully in agreement with the parliamentarians who wish to remind doctors of this potential. Ministers are frequently called upon to answer parliamentary questions on this subject, and their answers reflect the current views of the industry. The then Minister for Health, for example (*Hansard* 1989*b*) commented that whatever form of treatment is appropriate for particular patients, including the prescription of benzodiazepines, is a matter for the clinical judgement of their doctors, and that ministers would not wish to seek to promote particular forms of treatment.

The same minister, in a second parliamentary answer (*Hansard* 1989*a*) to a query as to why people dependent on benzodiazepines are classed by the Department of Health as drug misusers, emphasized his concern, and that of his department, over the prevention and treatment of drug dependence irrespective of whether the condition arises from illicit or prescribed drug use. Equally, he commented, the funds that the department has made available are for the development of services both for those dependent on prescribed drugs and those experiencing problems with illicit drug use.

The attitude of the pharmaceutical industry towards the sum total of medicines currently recommended in the UK as anxiolytics is that their prescribing requires considerable skill to ensure that they are both maximally effective and minimally hazardous. The benzodiazepines remain exceedingly useful medicines when used in accordance with the advice given in the data sheets for those benzodiazepines prescribed privately by brand name or with the advice given in the BNF for those prescribed generically and under the NHS.

As has already been stated, there is some irony in the fact that data sheets for products prescribed by the approved name generically are not required and that one effect of the 'limited list' has in theory been to deny doctors important prescribing information about this group of medicines! However, much information does abound, and it is very important that doctors read and understand it. The intermittent or short-term use of benzodiazepine *tranquillizers* is therefore therapeutic in appropriate cases, but this should never be allowed to slide into long-term continuous use. Pharmaceutical companies are staunch supporters of the well publicized advice from the CSM on this aspect of prescribing policy.

Benzodiazepines are also licensed as *hypnotics* and their occasional and intermittent use is entirely justified for those patients who genuinely suffer as a result of insomnia; again their continued use is undesirable. Although it is less than it was during the 1970s and early 1980s, there is still considerable psychological dependence on them in the general community, although this may eventually be self-limiting. The problem is undoubtedly exaggerated by the media, and the hazards *are* less than those of barbiturate dependence; in my own past experience, the treatment of benzodiazepine dependence did not present such a challenge as the treatment of barbiturate dependence.

Turning to the promotion of benzodiazepines, it must be accepted that this might have been considered inappropriate since approximately 10 years ago. That, though, is with the benefit of hindsight. The situation now is quite different, and a worldwide trawl of promotional and patient-orientated literature produced by the pharmaceutical industry on benzodiazepines, which was prepared for an exhibit at the United Nations International Conference on Drug Abuse and Illicit Trafficking held in Vienna in 1987, revealed that no overt promotion of benzodiazepines to the medical profession has occurred for a number of years; it also revealed that patient information leaflets advising on the use of benzodiazepines, and including warnings about possible dependence, were produced as long as 10 years ago. Also during 1987, the Association of the British Pharmaceutical Industry (ABPI) produced a poster for doctors to put up in their surgeries and waiting rooms that reminded patients that for the treatment of their anxiety it was frequently not necessary to have any prescribed medicine at all, and that it was at the discretion of their doctors whether drug therapy was considered desirable or necessary.

This valuable activity of the industry is not fully appreciated and it should be recognized that the pharmaceutical industry strives very hard to achieve a responsible attitude towards the medicines it produces, particularly in this field. It would after all be quite counterproductive if it were promoting, or even associated with, the irresponsible use of its own products.

Pharmaceutical industry initiatives to assist in benzodiazepine withdrawal

Several pharmaceutical company initiatives are worthy of comment. One particular company producing a specific benzodiazepine recently decided to market in the UK an original pack—called a 'Planpak'—containing reducing doses of temazepam. This is specifically designed to help wean those patients who had become dependent off this particular product, and to encourage a return to normal sleep without the need for a hypnotic at all. That is a good example of highly responsible marketing. Two recently published papers confirm the efficacy of planned withdrawal of benzodiazepine hypnotics in general practice using this 'Planpak' (Drake 1991a,b). The success of this withdrawal is measured in terms of 71 per cent of the original chronic users taking no hypnotic at all after a follow-up period of several months (Drake 1991b). The same company has also collaborated with another manufacturer in a reformulation programme designed to prevent abuse, by making capsules whose active ingredients cannot be extracted before ingestion. The liquid-filled softgel capsules they have produced are known as Temazepam Gelthix (Launchbury et al. 1991).

Another company—the original manufacturer of diazepam—has produced a benzodiazepine management programme. This is a set of leaflets for various groups of patients written in user-friendly terms, together with guidance notes for doctors on the management of patients for whom the benzodiazepines are both indicated and contraindicated. The leaflets for patients were prepared in liaison with TRANX, the consumer organization representing the interests of patients with problems associated with the use of benzodiazepines. This demonstrates a very positive attitude towards tackling responsible prescribing by a company, which, circumstantially, has little continuing interest in this market, following the introduction of the 'limited list' referred to previously.

Pharmaceutical companies readily acknowledge that patients who have inadvertently become dependent need a great deal of help to enable them to withdraw their benzodiazepines with the minimum of distress. Several doctors, too, have documented their own preferred methods of benzodiazepine withdrawal. For example, a Buckinghamshire general practitioner recently described a method which he had used since 1981 involving diazepam elixir (Clark 1989). This presentation enables whatever benzodiazepine is involved to be switched to diazepam, which, in liquid format, can be gradually reduced in smaller increments than can otherwise be achieved. That method has nevertheless been challenged by pharmacists (Elcock 1989) on the grounds of contamination and the possibility of the growth of micro-organisms. Nevertheless, the concept of assisting patients to minimize withdrawal symptoms and, psychologically as well as physically, to encourage and enable them to improve their own treatment seems sound. Clearly, this outweighs the theoretical pharmaceutical objections.

Further pharmaceutical professional advice, again supported by the industry, came from the Council of the Royal Pharmaceutical Society of Great Britain (RPSGB), which in 1989 issued a statement advising pharmacists who receive medium or long-term prescriptions for benzodiazepines to counsel the patient, but without impairing the patient's confidence in his or her own doctor. This coincided with a report from the Association of Community Health Councils for England and Wales (1989, p.22) which, while acknowledging the value of benzodiazepines when prescribed properly, commented on their frequently inappropriate prescribing, suggested policies for reducing prescribing levels, and emphasized the support needed for those who had become dependent.

Once again, these sentiments were publicly endorsed by the pharmaceutical industry when the report was published, though it was pointed out that prescribing—and consumption—in accordance with the existing recommendations on indications, dose, and duration of use would have considerably reduced the incidence of the problem in the first place.

Not surprisingly, the statement from the RSPGB (1989) produced a vigorous response from doctors who felt it would be quite impossible to counsel patients against taking benzodiazepines without impairing the patients' confidence in their doctors. An example of such a response came from two psychiatrists at New Cross Hospital in Wolverhampton (Farid and

Butto 1989) who emphasized that the difficulty they faced was not that of long-term prescribing of benzodiazepines, but rather that of too quick a reduction of the prescribed dose with little or no other forms of help being offered. Reference to the above mentioned benzodiazepine management programme, and the use of patient-orientated leaflets to back up their own advice might have been useful.

Legal liability in benzodiazepine dependence

Mention must be made of the UK Consumer Protection Act 1987, which came into force on 1 March 1988. The act introduces strict liability in the UK for the first time, and the supplier of a product can be sued under the act if the product is defective in any way, the supplier being defined as the proven originator of the product in the form in which it was supplied to the consumer. No cases have yet arisen under this act as far as anxiolytics are concerned, but a number of cases are still being considered under the previous law—because the product was supplied before the new law came into effect.

It is the dependence potential of the benzodiazepines that has currently brought about their involvement in product liability cases. This dependence was initially unrecognized, because of the undoubtedly greater safety of the benzodiazepines as compared to the barbiturates. Many general practitioners appear to have prescribed and maintained patients on benzodiazepines over periods of several years, often issuing repeat prescriptions without seeing the patient. These court cases are currently making legal history, and it will be interesting to see whether the date of issue of the CSM warning on the prescribing of benzodiazepines has any bearing on the court cases.

Conclusion

In concluding this chapter, the positive roles of the pharmaceutical industry and of individual companies in making medicines appropriately available and in giving accurate information about them to those who need to know must be remembered. When used in accordance with the licensed indications, benzodiazepines continue to provide useful therapy. Research continues both inside and outside the pharmaceutical industry to find better medicines, but the continued widespread prescribing of benzodiazepines, which, for the majority of patients who take them, present no problems, must be seen as some indication of their success. Nevertheless, even though the problems associated with dependence may be somewhat exaggerated, the industry has no complacency whatsoever about such problems and supports every objective intended to ensure that benzodiazepine use in the future is appropriate.

Acknowledgement

The views expressed in this chapter are strictly personal and do not represent ABPI policy.

References

ABPI (Association of the British Pharmaceutical Industry) (1991–92). *ABPI data sheet compendium* 1991–92. Datapharm Publications, London.

Association of Community Health Councils for England and Wales (1989). *Benzodiazepines: a suitable case for treatment*. Her Majesty's Stationery Office, London.

British Medical Association and Royal Pharmaceutical Society of Great Britain (1989). Prescribing drugs likely to cause dependence or abuse. In *British national formulary*, no. 18, p. 8. Pharmaceutical Press, London.

Clark, W.I.C. (1989). Benzodiazepine withdrawal. *Lancet*, **ii**, 986–7.

CSM (Committee on Safety of Medicines) (1988). Prescribing of benzodiazepines. *Current Problems*, January 1988.

Drake, J. (1991*a*). Temazepam 'Planpak': a multicentre practice trial in planned benzodiazepine hypnotic withdrawal. *Current Medical Research and Opinion*, **12**(6), 390–3.

Drake, J. (1991*b*). Temazepam 'Planpak': a fixed-dose reduction regimen for withdrawing benzodiazepine hypnotics: results of a general practice survey. *Current Medical Research and Opinion*, **12**(6), 394–400.

Elcock, P. (1989). Benzodiazepine withdrawal. *Lancet*, **ii**, 1402.

Farid, B.T. and Bulto, M. (1989). Benzodiazepine prescribing. *Lancet*, **ii**, 917.

Hansard (1989*a*). *Hansard*, Column 169, 19 December 1989.

Hansard (1989*b*). *Hansard*, Column 381, 21, December 1989.

Hansard (1990). *Hansard*, Column 75, 4 December 1990.

Launchbury, A.P., Morton, F.S.S., and Lacy, J.E. (1991). The development of Temazepam Gelthix. *Manufacturing Chemist*, December, 38–40.

Murphy, S.M. and Tyrer, P. (1987). The essence of benzodiazepine dependence. *British Journal of Psychiatry*, **151**, 719–23.

Owen, R.T. and Tyrer, P. (1983). Benzodiazepine dependence: a review of the evidence. *Drugs*, **25**, 385–98.

Pétursson, H. and Lader, M. (1984). *Dependence on tranquillizers*. Oxford University Press, London.

RPSGB (Royal Pharmaceutical Society of Great Britain) Council Statement (1989). Benzodiazepines. *Pharmaceutical Journal*, **243**, 200.

Wells, F.O. (1973). Prescribing barbiturates: drug substitution in general practice. *Journal of the Royal College of General Practitioners*, **25**, 164–7.

23 Women and tranquillizer use: a case study in the social politics of health and health care

Jonathan Gabe

One of the most consistent findings in the epidemiological literature on benzodiazepines has been the marked gender difference in their receipt and usage. Throughout the industrialized world women have been found to be being prescribed and to be using minor tranquillizers and hypnotics twice as often as men. Pharmacy prescription audits (Cooperstock and Sims 1971; Isacson *et al.* 1988), regional studies of physician prescribing (Parish 1971; Skegg *et al.* 1977), prescription audits in specific general practices (Catalan *et al.* 1988; Rodrigo *et al.* 1988), and sample surveys of psychotropic drug use in the community (Murray *et al.* 1981; Mellinger *et al.* 1984; Ashton and Golding 1989) have demonstrated this gender difference in the general rate of benzodiazepine prescribing and use/prolonged use. It is not surprising, therefore, that women have been identified as twice as likely to be dependent on these drugs as men (Ettorre 1985).

The purpose of this chapter is to try and explain the gendered nature of benzodiazepine use by drawing on the limited amount of sociological work that has been undertaken on women's use of these drugs and relating this to the growing sociological and feminist literature on women's health. It is intended to focus on the social and material factors implicated in women's use of benzodiazepines, the impact of a changing cultural context on their drug usage, the part played by doctors, and the social and political consequences for women of their taking these drugs.

Social and material factors

Much of the work on inequalities in women's health has been conceived of and conceptualized in terms of role analysis. It has been argued by some that marriage is detrimental to women's physical and mental health because of the nurturant role that they are expected to occupy in undertaking the essential household tasks and caring for all the other household members without the opportunity to rest and relax (Gove 1984). Others have suggested, however, that the parental role provides health benefits by counteracting the monotony and isolation of the housework role (Nathanson 1975). The effects of paid employment have similarly been interpreted in contradictory ways with some arguing that it is beneficial for women's health because it provides an extra source of self-esteem and social contacts (Nathanson 1980; Verbrugge 1983), while others have suggested that it is responsible for role strain and overload because women have to do it in conjunction with their domestic and parental responsibilities (Cleary and Mechanic 1983).

This 'role-based' analysis has in turn been criticized for failing to analyse the effects of these roles within the structural context of women's lives (Arber 1990). It has been suggested that the material circumstances (income, class position, housing tenure) in which women's roles are enacted also need to be considered if inequalities in women's health are to be understood. Research following this line of argument has established that the health status (limited long-standing illness) of married women varies according to class position and employment status, with those in full-time, non-manual jobs experiencing the least illness, and those currently unemployed or housewives who previously had manual jobs being the most disadvantaged in terms of their health (Arber 1991). Being divorced, separated, or widowed; living in local authority housing; and not having dependent children also appear to be disadvantageous for health status (Arber 1991). Thus groups of women who are disadvantaged in terms of family roles, employment status, and material circumstances appear to experience particularly poor health status.

The literature on inequalities in women's health thus suggests that there is likely to be some relationship between women's roles and position in the social structure and their use of tranquillizers, even if the nature of this relationship is not necessarily clear-cut. Evidence of such a link has been provided by research on the social origins of tranquillizer use. This has highlighted the part played by parental and marital roles and social position in determining women's use of these drugs. Survey research by Cafferata *et al.* (1983) and Kaufert and Gilbert (1986) in North America suggests that women's parental role in caring for young children helps reduce the likelihood of tranquillizer use, in line with Nathanson's (1975) argument about parenting counteracting the monotony and isolation of housework. Cafferata *et al.* (1983), like Linn and Davis (1971) and Mellinger *et al.* (1978) before them, have also found that a changed marital status, through separation or divorce, increases the chances of using these drugs, and have attributed this to the stress of such a life event and the loss of potential social support that follows. On the other hand, Isacson and Haglund (1988) have concluded, on the basis of Swedish pharmacy data, that married women are as likely as the divorced to be in receipt of hypnotics and tranquillizers and that the major difference is between married women and single women aged 35–44 who use such drugs to a greater extent. They explained this finding in terms of the stresses and strains of single parenthood or the unhappiness caused by regretting not having a partner/husband or children as the menopause approaches.

The position of women in the social structure has been implicated in tranquillizer use by Isacson and Haglund (1986) and by Riska and Klaukka (1984) who found that women in blue collar jobs were more likely to be using these drugs than their white collar counterparts, and by Kaufert and Gilbert (1986) who reported that concern with money, housing, and work problems increased the likelihood of tranquillizer use amongst women in mid-life.

Ethnographic research on the continuing or long-term use of benzo-diazepines by women has also highlighted the role of social and material factors. For example, Cooperstock and Lennard (1979) focused on how these drugs were used by the Canadian women in their study ($n=38$) to enable them to maintain themselves in the traditional female roles of wife, mother, and houseworker. Frequently, they indicated that they resented being restricted to this caring and nurturing role but said that they saw no alternative.

As one of the women in their sample put it:

> I take it to protect the family from my irritability because the kids are kids. I don't think it's fair for me to start yelling at them because their normal activity is bothering me . . . So I take Valium to keep me calm . . . Peace and calm. That's what my husband wants because frankly the kids get on his nerves, too. But he will not take anything . . . He blows his top . . . He can blow but I can't. And this I have resented over the years, but I've accepted it. I'm biding my time. One of these days I'm going to leave the whole kit and kaboodle and walk out on him. Then maybe I won't need any more Valium.'

Others described their drug use as enabling them to cope with some unresolved conflict, often concerning their relationship with a spouse or child, while a few talked about taking tranquillizers as a learned habitual mode of reacting to stressful life events.

Another ethnographic study, undertaken in the UK by Gabe and Thorogood (1986), was used to develop a more structural analysis of long-term tran-quillizer use among working-class white women. They interviewed 45 such women and found that access to resources like paid work and children and partners explained why some of them were more likely than others to take tranquillizers on a long-term basis. As regards paid work they noted that long-term users were not only less likely to have a full-time job than other working-class women, but that those who were so employed were more likely to express mixed feelings about their situation. It would thus seem that, while the absence of paid work may deprive long-term users of a resource that might make their lives easier, thereby reducing their need for tranquillizers, those users with access to this resource did not experience it in a sufficiently positive way to enable them to change the nature of their drug use.

Gabe and Thorogood also found that women who were long-term users were more likely to be divorced and not to have children living at home. Moreover, if these benzodiazepine users were living with partners and/or their children they were less likely than other women to find these kin supportive. It would thus appear that long-term users either lack access to potentially supportive social resources or find that those that are available are unsupportive and a poor substitute for tranquillizers. In such circumstances the existing pattern of drug use is likely to be maintained.

In sum, the evidence from studies of both the social origins of and the continuing use of tranquillizers suggest that women take these drugs in part at least because of their roles at home and/or as paid workers and because of their position in the social structure. These social and material factors combine in a complex way to make such women's lives sufficiently stressful that they turn to tranquillizers, often on a long-term basis, to help them get by.

The cultural context

In order to understand fully the preponderance of women taking benzo-diazepines it is also necessary to understand the shifting cultural context in which these drugs have been used. In particular, we need to consider the extent to which the gendered pattern of tranquillizer use has been influenced by changes in the degree of discomfort felt to be tolerable for women in an industrialized society and changes in beliefs about using prescribed drugs like benzodiazepines to alleviate such discomfort.

According to a number of commentators, the period of the 1960s and early 1970s was a time when it was culturally more acceptable for women to recognize emotional problems in themselves and turn to the doctor for help than it was for men (Philips and Segal 1969; Cooperstock 1971). Women had been encouraged in this belief by the mass media, which had proclaimed the value of medical solutions to problems in their everyday lives in articles with headlines such as 'Happiness by prescription', and 'Peace of mind pills' (Smith 1985). It was in this era of 'pharmacological enthusiasm' (Pellegrino 1976) that women expressed generally positive views about using tranquillizers (Linn and Davis 1971), and prescriptions for these drugs grew dramatically (Williams 1980).

Since the mid-1970s, however, women's views about managing distress with the help of prescribed drugs seem to have changed. There has been a shift in attitudes away from a belief in the right to happiness and an unwillingness to tolerate 'normal' discomfort and malaise towards a more puritanical view of life, based on abstinence, stoicism, and self-reliance (Hall 1983). This is illustrated by the research of Scambler et al. (1981) on symptom episodes and medical consultations among women in Britain. They noted that the women in their study were often likely to report 'suffering in silence' when experiencing 'nerves, depression, and irritability' instead of seeking a consultation with the doctor. Interestingly, a similar finding was reported over 50 years ago by Spring Rice (1939) in her survey of working-class wives, illustrating the extent to which the current emphasis on self-reliance and stoicism reflects the dominant values of a previous era.

The return to a more puritanical view of health maintenance and illness prevention has gone hand in hand with the development of an attitude to drugs that can be described as 'pharmacological Calvinism' (Klerman 1971). Simply stated this means 'if it makes you feel good it is wrong' (Blackwell 1977). The popularity of this antidrug culture amongst women (Gabe and Lipshitz-Phillips 1982) has also been fuelled by the media, who have over the last decade been continuously voicing concern about tranquillizer dependence (Gabe and Bury 1988). This coverage has often been sensationalist in tone, presenting tranquillizer users as 'innocent victims' of therapeutic drugs that they took in good faith, as the following headlines from British national and local newspapers and a woman's magazine illustrate:

'The tranquilliser trap' (*Mail on Sunday*, 1982)
'Tranquillisers—the shocking truth' (*Woman's Own*, 1984)
'Ativan—the devil drug' (*The Star*, 1988)
'Forgotten victims of the pill-popping generation' (*Western Morning Post*, Plymouth, 1988)

Frequently, alongside these headlines are pictures or silhouettes of women, often surrounded by bottles of pills, in order to make it clear to readers who are the 'victims' of these drugs.

The image of the female tranquillizer user is in turn reinforced by the newspaper and magazine copy. This compares and contrasts her with heroin users who are, by implication, seen as culpable for their addiction, and emphasizes her role as a wife and mother, suggesting that any innocent woman could become 'addicted' (Gabe *et al.* 1991). Indeed the impression is given that every woman taking tranquillizers is dependent on them, even though studies of such women have shown this not to be the case (Helman 1981; Gabe and Thorogood 1986).

It seems likely that this 'trial by media' (Cohen 1983) may have encouraged the more ambivalent feelings about using these drugs found amongst female long-term users in the 1980s, and reinforced the negative attitudes of those who have taken them intermittently or have never done so (Gabe and Lipshitz-Phillips 1982; Gabe and Thorogood 1986). This shift in attitudes towards tranquillizers, together with the stress on self-reliance and stoicism, may in turn help explain the 16 per cent reduction in the use of these drugs between 1979 and 1985 (Taylor 1987). Even so there are still estimated to be 1.2 million long-term tranquillizer users in Britain alone (Balter *et al.* 1984; Taylor 1987) and they are still twice as likely to be female as male (Ettorre 1985).

The role of the medical profession

In addition to the shifting cultural climate, the gendered nature of tranquillizer use can also be explained in terms of the stereotyped imagery employed by the medical profession when deciding who should be prescribed these drugs.

In recent years feminists have paid particular attention to the images of women held by the male-dominated medical profession and the extent to which these influence the outcome of the consultation in terms of diagnosis and prescription. Two basic ideas are said to underpin contemporary medicine's view of women (Doyal 1979). First, it is suggested that women's health is judged against the male standard, with women being defined as 'abnormal' and defective. Second, this abnormality is said to stem from women's 'natural' reproductive role which determines their personality structure and psychological well-being. These ideas are said to encourage (male) doctors to perceive the illnesses of their women patients as psychogenic in origin, stemming from their greater emotionality and hazardous menstrual and reproductive cycles (Clarke 1983).

Feminists and sociologists frequently attribute these fundamentally sexist ideas about the nature of women and their place in society to medical education. It is argued that women are often treated as sexual objects of ridicule by (male) lecturers in medical schools (Campbell 1974), medical textbooks are said to reflect stereotypes regarding women's social roles and behaviour as patients (Scully and Bart 1973; Clark *et al.* 1991), and advertisements in medical journals are criticized for attributing women's physical complaints to emotional problems (Prather and Fidell 1975). The result, it is suggested, is the perpetuation of masculine ideologies about the care and cure involved in medicine, even in the face of the growing number of women now entering the profession (Clarke 1983).

If doctors see emotional distress as more 'normal' for women than men, they may be more likely to define female patients as neurotic and in need of tranquillizers than are their male counterparts. Is there any evidence that this is the case? Early research by Cooperstock (1971) and Linn (1971) in North America did provide some support for this proposition. Cooperstock reported that over three-quarters of the general practitioners ($n=68$) interviewed said that they wrote more mood-modifying drug prescriptions for their female than for their male patients and explained this discrepancy in terms of factors such as biological vulnerability and self-indulgence as well as male reluctance to seek help. For example,

It's constitutional. The female's nervous system is more sensitive. They're affected by problems and emotional upsets more. That's the way the Lord made them.

Females have more time to indulge in neurosis than men. They're bored, often, and frustrated. As they get older, there's the menopause, which we men don't indulge in.

Similarly, Linn (1971) found that, when he asked 124 general practitioners and specialists in internal medicine through a postal questionnaire whether they agreed with certain general statements about the legitimate use of tranquillizers, they expressed a wide range of opinions. However, there was one exception. The great majority (87 per cent) agreed that the daily use of this drug for nervousness by a middle-aged housewife was legitimate.

Research conducted in the early 1970s thus suggests that doctor stereotyping may have played a part in determining the gender imbalance in tranquillizer use. However, a more recent ethnographic study of 14 general practitioners in Britain conducted by Gabe and Lipshitz-Phillips (1984) has produced equivocal results. On the one hand, the doctors they interviewed acknowledged that they prescribed more benzodiazepines to women than to men and explained this excess not only in terms of the stresses that women experience because of their social position (e.g. having two jobs, one inside and one outside the home), but also as a result of their greater emotionality and difficulties relating to reproduction. On the other hand, nearly all the doctors maintained that they did not respond to their patients in terms of preconceived ideas about gender differences in illness and psychological make-up. Instead they pointed out that more women than men experiencing anxiety symptoms came to the surgery: consequently, they prescribed more benzodiazepines to women. Moreover, most of the doctors in the study maintained that they were not influenced by drug companies, either by their literature or by visits from their representatives. Indeed almost half the sample said they had a policy of not seeing representatives of drug companies at all. Of course, doctors frequently deny being influenced by such promotional pressure (Melrose 1982), in part perhaps to project themselves as independent, judicious prescribers. However, as the doctors in this study expressed views about benzodiazepine prescribing that were consistent with their comments about the pharmaceutical industry, it was concluded that they were not trying to project themselves in this way.

Nonetheless, many doctors do read advertising in medical journals to provide them with information about new drugs (Linn and Davis 1972; Krupka and Vener 1985) and are likely to have been influenced by the pharmaceutical industry's attempts to target particular populations as tranquillizer users. It is therefore important to consider briefly research which has been undertaken on the content of advertisements for these drugs and the ways in which they work with readers.

Researchers who have analysed these advertisements have produced a series of findings that are relevant to our concerns here. To start with, it has frequently been reported that women have outnumbered men in the pictorial imagery used in psychotropic drug advertisements (Mant and Darroch 1975; Prather and Fidell 1975; Stimson 1975) and that such advertisements have been more frequently rerun if they portrayed women (King 1980). Moreover, the pictures and captions used in these psychotropic drug advertisements generally seem to have been constructed in terms of gender stereotypes, with women being portrayed as helpless and passive, as harrassed housewives, or as causing difficulties for others (e.g. a retired husband), while men have been presented as suffering from the stresses of paid work or physical illness (Mant and Darroch 1975; Prather and Fidell 1975; Stimson 1975; King 1980). It has also been found that advertisements featuring women are more likely to have involved non-rational appeals suggesting humour, sex appeal, and curiosity, whereas those featuring men have more frequently contained rational appeals, with information about the product, its clinical use, and the reputation of the company (Smith and Griffin 1977).

According to Chapman (1979) these advertisements have worked with doctors because they present a problem—vague symptoms of emotional distress—which is commonly encountered, and suggest a solution—the writing of a prescription—which it is easy for them to perform. In this way the advertisements suggest the possibility of 'at a glance diagnosis' (Stimson 1975) and reassure doctors that they can be of help. Furthermore, advertisements portraying women in stereotyped roles are said to work with male medical readers because they appeal to and reinforce the cultural ideals about the role of women held by these readers (Chapman 1979).

In sum it would seem that the pharmaceutical industry has targeted women as tranquillizer users and their advertisements have been successful in convincing a sizeable number of doctors, at least in the 1960s and 1970s, that women need tranquillizers in order to manage their everyday lives. Recently, however, it seems that pharmaceutical companies have changed their advertising strategy and relied less on sexual stereotyping and more on impersonal images such bottles of tablets, test tubes, flowers, and light shining through an open door to promote tranquillizer prescribing (Prather 1991). Moreover, there are far fewer advertisements for these drugs than there were previously (Krupka and Vener 1985; Smith 1985). Yet, by targeting women as a key group of potential tranquillizer users in past decades, the pharmaceutical industry has arguably helped to create the problem of tranquillizer dependence currently faced by a significant number of women in the industrialized world.

Social and political consequences

In addition to considering the social, material, and cultural factors and medical images that might explain the gender imbalance in tranquillizer use, attention also needs to be given to the social and political consequences for women of taking these drugs and, in particular, the extent to which their use represents a form of social control.

Those concerned with this issue have drawn on that body of literature that suggests that the institution of medicine, through the medical profession, is centrally involved in maintaining social order and stability. Two mechanisms are generally identified in this literature: the medicalization of everyday life and the reinforcement of existing hierarchical social relations.

Doctors, it is said, medicalize everyday life by defining patients' problems that have a social origin in terms of a medical model and an individualized aetiology, thereby reifying the person and their illness and focusing solely on their symptoms (Zola 1972; Ehrenreich and Ehrenreich 1978; Waitzkin 1979). In so doing they encourage patients to be dependent on them and their medicines, discredit lay advice and help, and generally make little attempt to help patients handle their own lives or to become aware of the links between social structure and ill health (Illich 1972; Ehrenreich 1978; Waitzkin 1979).

In addition, doctors are said to legitimize and reinforce existing hierarchical social relations by their attitudes and behaviour towards patients. A frequently quoted example of such behaviour is the doctor indicating to a female patient that her symptoms are merely a reflection of her sex's inherently unstable physiology and personality or of her unwillingness to direct herself to her natural maternal role (Barrett and Roberts 1978; Doyal 1979; Oakley 1981). Both mechanisms, it is held, minimize the likelihood of people attempting by collective action to change the way in which their society is organized.

In applying the concept of social control to tranquillizer use most writers have focused on the first of these mechanisms—the medicalization of everyday life. They argue that benzodiazepines are generally prescribed for socially induced symptoms, that in prescribing them doctors are encouraging patients to deny the social concomitants of distress, and that in this way they help to minimize the pressure for social change (Waldron 1977; Koumjian 1981).

While this social control model is useful in that it has brought into relief the influence of structural factors on tranquillizer use by women, we need to ask to what extent such a model is supported empirically.

One study that has explored this issue in relation to women was conducted by Gabe and Lipshitz-Phillips (1984). They interviewed 87 'middle-aged' women patients, of whom two-thirds were long-term users of benzodiazepines, and 14 general practitioners from two practices in London, England.

When they analysed their data they found little support for tranquillizers' involvement in the medicalization of the women's everyday lives in that there was little to indicate that the prescribing and use of these drugs necessarily involved the individualization of social problems. For example, the majority of doctors operated with a multicausal rather than a monocausal model when explaining their women patients' symptoms and seemed unlikely to impose individualized explanations on a patient if they felt that interpersonal factors were relevant to her predicament. The women, on the other hand, were rather more likely both to perceive a single cause for their symptoms and to suggest physical and psychosomatic factors as their cause. This was, however, less the case with long-term users than with other women patients.

Turning to the second mechanism of social control, the legitimation of existing gender relations, the evidence here was more equivocal. There were grounds for suggesting that not only the doctors (as mentioned earlier) but also the patients operated with negative stereotypes such as perceiving women as psychologically and physiologically more fragile than men and as limited by their reproductive function. They employed these stereotypes to explain why women received and used benzodiazepines more than men. The proponents of social control would contend that, to a considerable extent, it is the pattern of differential prescribing that reinforces such negative stereotypes.

At the same time there was much in Gabe and Lipshitz-Phillips' data that would appear to contradict the social control thesis. Thus, as we have already noted, nearly all the doctors maintained that they did not respond to their patients in terms of preconceived ideas about gender differences in illness or psychological make-up. It could therefore be argued that it was the women patients who were acting in terms of negative gender stereotypes independently of their doctors.

Furthermore, even if the women patients showed signs of operating in terms of these negative stereotypes, there was no evidence to suggest that their experience of the consultation reproduced or enhanced such stereotypes. Although a number of long-term users made a link between gender inequalities and benzodiazepine use in general, they seldom made such a link as far as they themselves were concerned.

In sum it would seem that the contention that tranquillizers represent a form of social control received only limited empirical support from Gabe and Lipshitz-Phillips' study. While there was little to suggest that the prescribing of these drugs medicalized the women's everyday lives there was some, albeit equivocal, support for the proposition that it legitimized gender relations. This suggests that, while the concept of social control has made a valuable contribution to understanding social action and the impact of structural factors on the doctor–patient relationship, its application to tranquillizers has been too mechanistic and has resulted in overgeneralizations. While the prescribing of these drugs may result in the social control of women, this is not necessarily the case and should not be assumed in advance.

Conclusion

In this chapter I have tried to account for the gender imbalance in benzo-diazepine use by looking at the role of social and material factors, changing attitudes towards the suffering of discomfort and its amelioration through the use of prescribed drugs, and the extent to which the male-dominated medical profession operates with negative gender stereotypes. Having reviewed the available literature it has been suggested that all these factors have played at least some part in the use of benzodiazepines by women over the last 30 years.

In addition, attention has been given to the social and political consequences for women of their disproportionate use of these drugs and the extent to which this has resulted in their social control. The empirical evidence on this point is more equivocal and suggests that, while some women may be socially controlled by doctors prescribing them tranquillizers, this is not always the case. Nor should women be conceived of as simply passive victims of this process as has often been the case in the past. Not all doctors think and act in terms of negative gender stereotypes and not all women passively accept all their doctors tell them, regardless of other influences on their consciousness. Indeed, to cast women as simply passive victims of this process is, as Reisman (1983) has argued, to perpetuate the very kinds of assumptions about women that feminists have been trying to challenge. Researchers therefore need to be aware of this danger as they try to unravel the complex reasons for and consequences of women's overrepresentation among tranquillizer users.

References

Arber, S. (1990). Opening the 'black box': inequalities in women's health. In *New directions in the sociology of health* (ed. P. Abbott and G. Payne), pp.37–56. Falmer Press, London.

Arber, S. (1991). Class, paid employment and family roles: making sense of structural disadvantage, gender and health status. *Social Science and Medicine*, **32**, 425–36.

Ashton, H. and Golding, J. (1989). Tranquillisers: prevalence and possible consequences. Data from a large United Kingdom survey. *British Journal of Addiction*, **84**, 541–6.

Balter, M., Manheimer, G.D., and Uhlenhuth, E.H. (1984). A cross-national comparison of anti-anxiety/sedative drug use. *Current Medical Research and Opinion*, **8** (suppl. 4), 5–20.

Barrett, M. and Roberts, H. (1978). Doctors and their patients: the social control of women in general practice. In *Women sexuality and social control*, (ed. C. Smart and B. Smart), pp.41–52. Routledge and Kegan Paul, London.

Blackwell, B. (1977). Medical, social and ethical issues in minor tranquilliser use. Paper presented at the *World Congress in Mental Health*, Vancouver.

Cafferata, G.L., Kasper, J., and Bernstein, A. (1983). Family roles, structure and stressors in relation to sex differences in obtaining psychotropic drugs. *Journal of Health and Social Behaviour*, **24**, 132–43.

Campbell, M.A. (1974). *Why would a girl go into medicine?* The Feminist Press, New York.

Catalan, J., Gath, D., Bond, A., Edmonds, G., Martin, P., and Ennis, J. (1988). General practice patients on long-term psychotropic drugs. A controlled investigation. *British Journal of Psychiatry*, **152**, 399–405.

Chapman, S. (1979). Advertising and psychotropic drugs: the place of myth in ideological reproduction. *Social Science and Medicine*, **13A**, 751–64.

Clark, J.A., Potter, D., and McKinlay, J.B. (1991). Bringing social structure back into clinical decision making. *Social Science and Medicine*, **32**, 853–66.

Clarke, J. (1983). Sexism, feminism and medicalism: a decade review of literature on gender and illness. *Sociology of Health and Illness*, **5**, 62–82.

Cleary, P. and Mechanic, D. (1983). Sex differences in psychological distress among married people. *Journal of Health and Social Behaviour*, **24**, 111–21.

Cohen, S. (1983). Current attitudes about benzodiazepines: trial by media. *Journal of Psychoactive Drugs*, **15**, 109–13.

Cooperstock, R. (1971). Sex differences in the use of mood-modifying drugs: an explanatory model. *Journal of Health and Social Behaviour*, **12**, 238–44.

Cooperstock, R. and Lennard, H.L. (1979). Some social meanings of tranquilizer use. *Sociology of Health and Illness*, **1**, 331–47.

Cooperstock, R. and Sims, M. (1971). Mood-modifying drugs prescribed in a Canadian city: hidden problems. *American Journal of Public Health*, **61**, 1007–16.

Doyal, L. (1979). *The political economy of health*. Pluto Press, London.

Ehrenreich, B. and Ehrenreich, J. (1978). Medicine and social control. In *The cultural crisis of modern medicine* (ed. J. Ehrenreich), pp.39–79. Monthly Review Press, New York.

Ehrenreich, J. (1978). Introduction. In *The cultural crisis of modern medicine* (ed. J. Ehrenreich), pp.1–35. Monthly Review Press, New York.

Ettorre, E. (1985). Psychotropics, passivity and the pharmaceutical industry. In *Big deal: the politics of the illicit drugs business.* (ed. A. Henman, R. Lewis, and T. Maylon), pp.108–17. Pluto Press, London.

Gabe, J. and Bury, M. (1988). Tranquillisers as a social problem. *Sociological Review*, **36**, 320–52.

Gabe, J. and Lipshitz-Phillips, S. (1982). Evil necessity? The meaning of benzo-diazepine use for women patients from one general practice. *Sociology of Health and Illness*, **4**, 201–9.

Gabe, J. and Lipshitz-Phillips, S. (1984). Tranquillisers as social control? *Sociological Review*, **32**, 524–46.

Gabe, J. and Thorogood, N. (1986). Prescribed drugs and the management of everyday life: the experiences of black and white working class women. *Sociological Review*, **34**, 737–72.

Gabe, J., Gustafsson, U., and Bury, M. (1991). Mediating illness: newspaper coverage of tranquilliser dependence. *Sociology of Health and Illness*, **13**, 332–53.

Gove, W.R. (1984). Gender differences in mental and physical illness: the effects of fixed roles and nurturant roles. *Social Science and Medicine*, **19**, 77–91.

Hall, S. (1983). The great moving right show. In *The politics of Thatcherism* (ed. S. Hall and M. Jacques), pp.19–39. Lawrence and Wishart, London.

Helman, C. (1981). Tonic, fuel and food: social and symbolic aspects of the long-term use of psychotropic drugs. *Social Science and Medicine*, **15B**, 521–33.

Illich, I. (1972). *Medical nemesis*. Calder and Boyars, London.

Isacson, D. and Haglund, B. (1988). Psychotropic drug use in a Swedish community—the importance of demographic and socioeconomic factors. *Social Science and Medicine*, **26**, 477–83.

Isacson, D., Carsjo, K., Haglund, B., and Smedby, B. (1988). Psychotropic drug use in a Swedish community—patterns of use during two years. *Social Science and Medicine*, **27**, 263–7.

Kaufert, P. and Gilbert, p. (1986). The context of the menopause: psychotropic drug use and menopausal status. *Social Science and Medicine*, **23**, 747–55.

King, E. (1980). Sex bias in psychoactive drug advertisements. *Psychiatry*, **43**, 129–37.

Klerman, G.L. (1971). Drugs and social values. *International Journal of Addictions*, **5**, 313–19.

Koumjian, K. (1981). The use of Valium as a form of social control. *Social Science and Medicine*, **15E**, 245–9.

Krupka, L.R. and Vener, M.A. (1985). Prescription drug advertising: trends and implications. *Social Science and Medicine*, **20**, 191–7.

Linn, L.S. (1971). Physician characteristics and attitudes toward legitimate use of psychotherapeutic drugs. *Journal of Health and Social Behaviour*, **12**, 132–40.

Linn, L.S. and Davis, M.S. (1971). The use of psychotherapeutic drugs by middle-aged women. *Journal of Health and Social Behaviour*, **12**, 331–40.

Linn, L.S. and Davis, M.S. (1972). Physicians' orientation towards the legitimacy of drug use and their preferred source of new drug information. *Social Science and Medicine*, **6**, 199–203.

Mant, A. and Darroch, D.B. (1975). Media images and medical images. *Social Science and Medicine*, **9**, 613–18.

Mellinger, G.D., Balter, M.B., Manheimer, M.A., Cisin, I.H., and Parry, H.J. (1978). Psychic distress, life crisis, and use of psychotherapeutic medications. *Archives of General Psychiatry*, **35**, 1045–52.

Mellinger, G.D., Balter, M.B., and Uhlenhuth, E.H. (1984). Prevalence and correlates of long term regular use of anxiolytics. *Journal of the American Medical Association*, **251**, 375–9.

Melrose, D. (1982). *Bitter pills. Medicines and the third world poor*. Oxfam, Oxford.

Murray, J., Dunn, G., Williams, P., and Tarnopolosky, A. (1981). Factors affecting the consumption of psychotropic drugs. *Psychological Medicine*, **11**, 551–60.

Nathanson, C. 1975. Illness and the feminine role: a theoretical review. *Social Science and Medicine*, **9**, 57–62.

Nathanson, C. (1980). Social roles and health status among women: the significance of employment. *Social Science and Medicine*, **14A**, 463–71.

Oakley, A. (1981). Normal motherhood: an exercise in self control? In *Controlling women: the normal and the deviant* (ed. B. Hutter and G. Williams), pp.79–107. Croom Helm, London.

Parish, P. (1971). The prescribing of psychotropic drugs in general practice. *Journal of the Royal College of General Practitioners*, **21**, (suppl. 4), 1–77.

Pellegrino, E.D. (1976). Prescribing and drug ingestion: symbols and substances. *Drug Intelligence and Clinical Pharmacy*, **10**, 624–30.

Philips, D. and Segal, B. (1969). Sexual status and psychiatric symptoms. *American Sociological Review*, **34**, 58–72.

Prather, J. (1991). Decoding advertisements: the role of communication studies in explaining the popularity of minor tranquillisers. In *Understanding tranquilliser use. The role of the social sciences* (ed. J. Gabe), pp.112–35. Tavistock/Routledge, London.

Prather, J. and Fidell, L. (1975). Sex differences in the content and style of medical advertisements. *Social Science and Medicine*, **9**, 23–6.

Reisman, C.K. (1983). Women and medicalization: a new perspective. *Social Policy*, Summer, 3–18.

Riska, E. and Klaukka, T. (1984). Use of psychotropic drugs in Finland. *Social Science and Medicine*, **19**, 983–9.

Rodrigo, E.K., King, M.B., and Williams, P. (1988). Health of long term benzo-diazepine users. *British Medical Journal*, **296**, 603–6.

Scambler, A., Scambler, G., and Craig, D. (1981). Kinship and friendship networks and women's demand for primary care. *Journal of the Royal College of General Practitioners*, **26**, 746–50.

Scully, D. and Bart, P. (1973). A funny thing happened on the way to the orifice: women in gynecology textbooks. *American Journal of Sociology*, **78**, 1045–50.

Skegg, D.G., Doll, R., and Perry, J. (1977). Use of medicines in general practice. *British Medical Journal*, **i**, 1561–3.

Smith, M.C. (1985). *Small comfort: a history of the minor tranquillisers*. Praeger, New York.

Smith, M.C. and Griffin, L. (1977). Rationality of appeals used in the promotion of psychotropic drugs. A comparison of male and female models. *Social Science and Medicine*, **11**, 409–14.

Spring Rice, M. (1939). *Working class wives: their health and conditions*. Penguin. [Republished by Virago, London, 1981.]

Stimson, G.V. (1975). The message of psychotropic drug ads. *Journal of Communication*, **25**, 153–60.

Taylor, D. (1987). Current usage of benzodiazepines in Britain. In *Benzodiazepines in current clinical practice* (ed. H. Freeman and Y. Rue), pp.13–17. Royal Society of Medicine Services, London.

Verbrugge, L.M. (1983). Marital status and health. *Journal of Marriage and the Family*, **41**, 267–85.

Waitzkin, H. (1979). Medicine, superstructure and micropolitics. *Social Science and Medicine*, **13A**, 601–9.

Waldron, I. (1977). Increased prescribing of Valium, Librium and other drugs—an example of economic and social factors in the practice of medicine. *International Journal of Health Services*, **7**, 37–62.

Williams, P. (1980). The use of prescribed psychotropic medicines. *Public Health Reviews*, **9**, 215–47.

Zola, I. (1972). Medicine as an institution of social control. *Sociological Review*, **20**, 487–503.

Index

prescription of benzodiazepines
hospitals' role 205
prescription in UK 4, 205–10
regular drugs 204
social consequences, women's health 357–9
social and material factors 350–3
social phobia 268
social worker help, and parsimonious use of
benzodiazepines 216–17
sodium valproate, effect on benzodiazepine
withdrawal 317
somatization disorder, similarity to
benzodiazepine withdrawal 297–8
stress
anxiety-management skills 303–7
posttraumatic stress reaction 35
stress-management clinics 264
see also anxiety; group therapy
substance use disorders
and alcoholism 193–5
benzodiazepine supplements 131–2
defined 162–7
DSM-III-R criteria 168–9
epidemiology 162–85
data 169–70
prevalence 173–5
surveys 191–3
multiple drug abuse 131–2, 191
see also abuse of benzodiazepines
suicide risk 35

temazepam
elderly patients 247
intravenous abuse 134–5
pharmacology and dependence
potential 232–3
'Planpak' 346
prescribing pattern (1989) 338
relative strength 217, 328
softgel capsules 134, 346
tolerance
development 97–103
to anticonvulsant effects 98–9
to anxiolytic effects 101–2
to sedative effects 97–101
investigations 84–6
see also dependence; withdrawal
toxicity, elderly patients 16
tranquillizers, *see* anxiolytics
TRANX (UK) Ltd, (self-help group) 326–33
treatment
alternative therapy, *see* benzodiazepines,
alternatives
biological risks 34–5
continuing psychiatric illness 7
efficacy 7–8
elderly patients, compliance 241–2

psychological counselling 10, 16, 35
psychological risks 35–40
mental health 35–6
subjective sedation 36
psychological therapy
as alternatives to benzodiazepine 282–95
for benzodiazepine dependence 296–309
relapse rate 7
sedation
objective effects in patients 38–9
objective effects in volunteers 36–8
social risks 40–2
vs prevention of dependence 216
triazolam
elderly patients 247
intravenous abuse 134–5
pharmacology and dependence
potential 222–4
prescribing pattern (1989) 338
relative strength 217, 328
tribulin, and GABA function 73

United Nations Convention on
Psychotropic Substances (1971) 195–6
urine, detection of benzodiazepines 121
usage rates 13, 58–9
clinical syndromes 58–9
sex differences in benzodiazepine use
rates 59, 350

WHO
'defined daily doses' 187
review process 196
withdrawal
assessment (CIWA-B) scale 61
attenuation 312–18
dangers and benefits 263
effect of propranolol 313–14
outcome studies 303–7
patients wishing 218
pharmaceutical industry initiatives
to assist in benzodiazepine
withdrawal 346–8
re-exposure 302
similarity to somatization disorder 297–8
withdrawal syndromes 58–70
and anxiety 145–8
biological markers 154
criteria 61
development 97–103
early estimates 51–5
elderly patients 243–6
high-dose dependence 67–8
link with hypochondriasis 298
neurotransmitter changes 154–5
new symptoms 150